THE GENESIS OF CANCER

THE GENESIS OF CANCER
A Study in the History of Ideas

L. J. RATHER

THE JOHNS HOPKINS UNIVERSITY PRESS
Baltimore and London

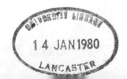

Manufactured in the United States of America

The Johns Hopkins University Press, Baltimore, Maryland 21218
The Johns Hopkins Press Ltd., London

Library of Congress Catalog Card Number 78-2785
ISBN 0-8018-2103-7

Library of Congress Cataloging in Publication data
will be found on the last printed page of this book.

To Patricia, Leland, and Noël

Wer nicht von dreitausend Jahren
Sich weiss Rechenschaft zu geben,
Bleib im Dunkeln unerfahren,
Mag von Tag zu Tage leben.

Goethe

CONTENTS

PREFACE   xiii

INTRODUCTION   3

1 TUMORS AND THE DEVELOPMENT OF HUMORAL
   THEORY, FIFTH CENTURY B.C. TO 1800   8
   PALEOPATHOLOGY OF ANIMAL TUMORS   8
   TUMOR THEORY   9
      Classical Greece   9
      Renaissance Europe   13
   MOVEMENT OF THE BLOOD   19
   IATROCHEMICAL HUMORALISM   26
   LYMPH   30
      Discovery of Lymphatic Circulation   30
      Cancer "Seeds"   32
      Solidistic Lymphatic Theory   35
      *Dominance of Lymphatic Humoralism in Eighteenth-Century
      Cancer Theory*   39
      Hunter's "Coagulating Lymph"   41

2 TUMORS AND TISSUE THEORY, FIFTH CENTURY B.C.
   TO 1838   46
   ANATOMICAL SCIENCE   46
      Sources   46
      Similar and Dissimilar Parts; The Ultimate Fiber   47
   TISSUE THEORY   52
      "Cellular Tissue"   52
      Bichat   52
   TISSUES AND TUMORS   58
      Tissu Cellulaire   58
      The French School   59
      The Third Version of Humoralism   64
      Formative Molecules   67
      Andral   69
   ENGLISH AND SCOTCH INVESTIGATORS   70
      Hodgkin's Generative Membranes   72
      Carswell   74
      Hodgkin's Amplification   76
   GERM-LAYER THEORY   77

ix

3 CELL THEORY AND THE GENESIS OF CELLS IN TUMORS, 1838-52 82

USE OF THE MICROSCOPE 82
   Globules and Cells 83
   Mueller 83
SCHWANN'S PAPERS OF 1838 AND THEIR RECEPTION BY MUELLER 84
REVISION OF MUELLER'S THEORY 88
   Mueller's "Cells" 88
   Mueller's Cancer "Seeds"; Return to the Blastema Theory 90
TISSUES REDEFINED IN THE LIGHT OF SCHWANN'S CELL THEORY 92
CELL THEORY; GENESIS OF CELLS IN TUMORS 95
   Vogel 95
   Rokitansky 99
   Virchow 100
DEBATES OVER THE SPECIFICITY OF CANCER CELLS 104
   Mechanism of Metastasis 104
   Origin and Nature of Cancroids 112

4 CELL THEORY AND THE GENESIS OF CELLS IN TUMORS, 1852-1900 118

BLASTEMA THEORY 118
   Cytogenetic Uncertainty 118
   Embryology 119
   Remak's Argument 120
   Remak and Cell Potency 122
   German Rejection of the Blastema Theory 122
FOERSTER AND THE NEW CELLULAR PATHOLOGY 124
   Origins of Epithelial Tumors 127
VIRCHOW AND THE NEW CELLULAR PATHOLOGY 128
   Neoplasms and Connective Tissue 128
   Objections to Remak's Derivation of Epithelial Cells 130
   Virchow's Treatise on Tumors 135
MICHEL'S CRITICISM OF VIRCHOW'S CONNECTIVE TISSUE THEORY 137
DECLINE OF VIRCHOW'S CONNECTIVE TISSUE THEORY 138
   Thiersch's Epithelial Theory 139
   Billroth's Conversion 141
   Neoplasia and Inflammation Distinguished 142
   French Conservatism 143
   The Debate in Germany 145
LIMITS OF CELL SPECIFICITY 148
   Waldeyer's First Paper 149
   Histogenetic Inference: Tibial Adamantinoma 154
   Waldeyer's Second Paper 162
   Inflammation and Neoplasia: New Developments 167
   Cohnheim's Cell Rests 169

Virchow: Neoplasia and Metaplasia 174
Bard: Specificity of Cellular Elements 176
MOLECULAR BIOLOGY FORESHADOWED 178

NOTES 181
BIBLIOGRAPHY 231
Books and Articles Cited 231
Bibliographic Supplement 247
ABBREVIATIONS 249
INDEX 251

PREFACE

Here the phrase "tumor genesis" refers chiefly to the material and formal genesis of tumors; their etiology, or causal genesis, is not an issue. The questions are, from what component of the body, whether fluid or solid, are tumors derived, and what are the factors determinative of their gross and microscopic structure? While avoiding, as far as possible, the prejudiced assessment of older theories in the light of newer theories or findings, I have attempted to show that a thread of logical continuity runs through the long history of Western medical thought on the genesis of tumors. A rather skeptical view of the inferential character of histogenetic classifications of tumors appears in the fourth chapter. But the reader should understand that I do not mean to depreciate either the validity of the findings on which such classifications have been based or the validity of correlations that have been established between the structure and the clinical behavior of tumors.

All translations, unless otherwise indicated, are my own. I thank the staff of the Lane Medical Library at Stanford University for their always ready assistance, and Patricia L. Rather for aiding me in bibliographical searches and for preparing the typescript. My greatest debt is to John B. Frerichs, M.D., who scrutinized every line of the text and notes while the manuscript was in preparation. The work was supported in part by NIH Grant LM 02058, and I am grateful to the administrators and librarians of the National Library of Medicine for their unfailing cooperation. I am grateful also to the personnel of The Johns Hopkins University Press —to my editor, David Farnham, in particular—for their various contributions to the final product.

THE GENESIS OF CANCER

INTRODUCTION

Before the end of the nineteenth century widespread agreement on the origin and nature of benign and malignant tumors had been reached among investigators working within the tradition of Western university medical science. So-called true tumors, it was agreed, constituted a separate class from inflammatory tumors of both specific and nonspecific character, and from retention cysts, parasitic cysts, and other localized masses with which they had been grouped in common for well over two thousand years. It was agreed that a true tumor was composed essentially of tumor cells, which derived from normal cells at the primary site of origin of the tumor in question and thereafter continued to multiply in the host organism, for the most part by mitotic division. Tumor cells, even the "rebellious" cells of cancers (the term dates from the 1840s), were thought to resemble, more or less, the normal cells from which they developed. Likewise, the tissue or organoid patterns displayed by tumor cells were thought to resemble the tissues or organs composed by the cells thought to be their normal precursors. It was further agreed that the essential constituents of tumors, the tumor cells, were in all instances nourished by the host organism's blood, and that in all but the simplest tumors a variable proportion of their bulk consisted of a supporting and nourishing stroma of blood vessels and connective tissue that was contributed, gratuitously it seemed, by the host toward the sustenance of a growth that was at best useless, and at worst lethal. Certain tumors, termed malignant, were characterized by infiltrative or destructive local spread and by their ability to generate secondary deposits, called metastases, in distant organs and tissues. It was agreed that the tumor cells were the responsible agents in both instances, in one case by pushing aggressively into and multiplying within the adjacent tissues, and in the other by moving, chiefly via the blood and lymph streams, to distant sites and there colonizing the organs and tissues.

Malignant tumors were of two kinds, carcinomas and sarcomas. Carcinomas consisted of cells more or less epithelial in character and were thought to be derived from true epithelial cells only, i.e., not from the flattened cells that line the blood and lymph vessels or the similar cells that line the body cavities: these were designated "endothelial" and "mesothelial," respectively. Sarcomas consisted of and arose from nonepithelial cells, i.e., from connective tissue cells in the broadest sense. It was generally agreed that even in the aberrant and atypical course of neo-

3

plastic cell proliferation the barrier between epithelial and nonepithelial cells—the origin of which was traced to the separation of the three germ layers early in embryonic life—remained in place. Benign tumors were also of two kinds, one deriving from and consisting of epithelial cells, and the other deriving from and consisting of connective tissue cells. Thus a *lipoma* arose from and consisted of fat cells; a *myoma* of muscle cells; a *chondroma* of cartilage cells; and so on. In the 1880s this notion acquired aphorismic form: *omnis cellula e cellula ejusdem naturae*, all cells arise from cells of the same kind. This made tracing a tumor to its cell and tissue of origin seem relatively simple.

Today there is still general agreement on all these points. Two hundred years ago the situation was otherwise. Tumors, cysts, inflammatory masses, and the like were thought to consist of fluid or semifluid substances ultimately derived from the blood, in particular from its so-called plastic, coagulable, or coagulating "lymph." François Bichat's revitalization of the tissue doctrine, which revolutionized pathological anatomy and the study of tumors, did not take place until the opening years of the nineteenth century. Pathological anatomy remained at the gross level until the 1830s, when a new dimension was explored with the recently improved microscope. At the end of that decade came Theodor Schwann's cell theory and Johannes Mueller's pioneering application of both microscope and cell theory to the study of tumors. In the eighteenth century the relation between embryology and pathology was distant, if it existed at all; in the nineteenth century the development of theories of tumor genesis and embryogenesis went hand in hand, with the same investigators, for example, Wilhelm His and Wilhelm Waldeyer, often contributing significantly to both fields of study. Germ-layer theory, resting for the most part on naked-eye observations interpreted in light of tissue theory, made its appearance early in the nineteenth century with the work of Christian Pander; at mid-century Robert Remak carried it to the microscopic level and, in conjunction with a revised Schwannian cell theory, first applied it to the study of tumor histocytogenesis. At the end of the eighteenth century bacteriology did not exist as a science; at the end of the nineteenth, the systematic study of bacteria as agents of disease, combined with the new, "biological" concept of inflammation, had added a teleological element to the distinction already made between true and inflammatory tumors. Chemistry, a science still in its Stahlian phase in the last quarter of the eighteenth century, was so far advanced one hundred years later that in 1884 Carl Wilhelm Naegeli was able to sketch the recognizable lineaments of the molecular biology of our day.

Developments in the sciences bearing on the genesis of tumors took place so rapidly in the first half of the nineteenth century that terminology was unable to keep pace. Under penalty of failing to understand the real course of events, the historian must continually be on the lookout for instances in which the same term designates different things at different times and, contrariwise, instances in which different terms designate what is more or less the same thing. Bichat, for example, thought that all tumors arose from ubiquitous *tissu cellulaire*, by which he meant tissue composed of fine plates and fibers as described by Albrecht von Haller in the mid-eighteenth century. Bichat's cellular tissue had, of course, no more to do with the mid-nineteenth-century notion—which is also our own—of a cell than did von Haller's *tela cellulosa*. Contrary to Bichat, some histologists at the beginning of the nineteenth century held that the fibers and plates were really postmortem artifacts; that the so-called tissue was actually an amorphous semifluid or gellike substance. In 1839, Schwann claimed that the real units constitutive of the tissues, namely, the cells, arose *de novo* from an amorphous semifluid substance called the blastema, or cytoblastema. Johannes Mueller's theory of tumor histogenesis and cytogenesis, as well as all subsequent theories put forth in the 1840s and early 1850s, were based on this notion. Robert Remak and Rudolf Virchow, to name only these two, then reached the conclusion that every cell arose from a preexisting cell in the adult organism as well as in the embryo, the ultimate source being the fertilized eggcell. Virchow's aphorism to this effect, *omnis cellula a cellula*, was formulated in 1855. Virchow held that all, or almost all, tumors arose from *connective tissue* (*Bindegewebe*, the new name for the *cellular tissue* of the earlier histologists). But, largely as a result of his own studies, he had come to believe that the ubiquitous connective tissue was composed of cells throughout and that some of these cells remained at a stage of "indifference" (*Indifferenz*). He thought these indifferent cells capable of multiplying by division and undergoing transformation into the constitutive cells of inflammatory tumors, tubercles, cancers, and tumors generally. It is not difficult to see that Virchow's connective tissue is the cellular equivalent of Bichat's *tissu cellulaire*. But the relation of Schwann's cytoblastema to the alternative version of the *tissu cellulaire*, i.e., that it was an amorphous gel, is easily overlooked. So, too, are the facts that Bichat's *tissu cellulaire*, Schwann's cytoblastema and Virchow's connective tissue were successively substituted for each other as the primary source of origin of all tumors; that John Hunter's coagulating lymph, with roots in earlier physiopathological thought, is represented in Schwann's cytoblastema; and that the conceptual precursor of Schwann's cell is neither the eighteenth-century cell nor that of Robert Hooke and Francis Bacon, but rather the fiber of eighteenth- and early-nineteenth-century anatomists, who held to the venerable belief in the ultimately fibrous constitution of plant and animal substance. Schwann's cell, like Johann Christian Reil's fiber before it, was supposed to arise *de novo* from an amorphous blastema, the formation of fibers in coagulating blood furnishing a paradigm.

Scientists at the beginning of the nineteenth century were of course not free to delineate their observations and interpretations on a *tabula rasa*. Perhaps Goethe went too far in his aphorism to the effect that everything clever has already been thought, our task being merely to think it over once again (*Alles Gescheite ist schon gedacht worden, man muss es nur versuchen, es noch einmal zu denken*). To one who reads widely in the record of intellectual history, however, Karl Mannheim's related dictum seems incontestable: "Strictly speaking, it is incorrect to say that the single individual thinks. Rather it is more correct to insist that he participates in thinking further what other men have thought before him." Behind the early-nineteenth-century scientists lay centuries of scientific tradition. For six hundred years anatomy, physiology (including physiological chemistry in its various forms, from the humoralism of Galen through spagyrical chemistry, the later iatrochemistry, and Stahlian phlogistic chemistry), and pathology had been studied and taught in the medical schools of European universities. Like scientists of all times, those of the early nineteenth century were on the one hand convinced of the fundamental soundness of their shared views, and on the other of the need for change as new observations and ideas made their appearance. To understand why students of tumor genesis in the early nineteenth century worked as they did with the new materials at their disposal, we must take account of eighteenth-century science. Behind eighteenth-century science lay five centuries of university scientific tradition, and behind the universities was an unbroken intellectual tradition reaching back to classical Greece.[1]

All of this bears on the history of the idea of tumor genesis presented here. In the first chapter, changing ideas of the genesis of tumors during the past two thousand years of the Western medical tradition are reviewed. In the second an account is given of the development of knowledge of the fine structure of animal bodies over an equally long period, which culminated in the rise of tissue theory at the end of the eighteenth century and its application to the problem of tumor genesis in the first third of the nineteenth. The third chapter is devoted to the study of the structure and genesis of tumors in the light of Schwannian cell theory in Germany in the 1840s; the fourth to the overthrow of Virchow's concept of the connective-tissue genesis of epithelial cancer some twenty years later. (Incidentally, the reader will find that cancer of the female breast, which is the prototypical cancer, plays a central role in the story from beginning to end.) The fourth chapter does not carry the story past the 1880s. By presenting a particular case in point, an attempt is made to show that both the character of the evidence and the methodological presuppositions underlying inferences drawn from that evidence as to the histogenesis and cytogenesis of tumors underwent little significant change during the subsequent seventy to eighty years. Only in very recent times have techniques been introduced that may perhaps shed new light on the genesis of tumors and, in so doing, upset some of our long-cherished preconceptions. Should this occur, it will have to be dealt with by a future historian of the problem.

1

TUMORS AND THE DEVELOPMENT
OF HUMORAL THEORY,
FIFTH CENTURY B.C. TO 1800

PALEOPATHOLOGY OF ANIMAL TUMORS

Tumors involving bone have been found in the petrified remnants of reptiles and mammals of remote geological times.[1] Although positive proof is lacking, it seems likely on general grounds that tumors of the soft tissues also occurred in these animals. The same may be said of the protohominids, but here, too, the evidence is scanty. The case is otherwise when we turn from the immense time scale of geology to the short span of recorded history. In mummified human remains from Egypt and other cultures, paleopathologists have found tumors involving both soft tissues and bone.[2] Paleopathology, the study of the primary evidence of disease in times past, is pursued in the light of current pathological theory and with the aid of contemporary investigative techniques. The present book, however, will be concerned only with interpretations of disease, or, more properly, of anatomical lesions, made in the past by investigators who used the techniques then available and the theory then current. Specifically, we shall be concerned with the historical development of Western medical concepts of the material constitution and mode of origin of tumors thought to be derived from other components of the human body. But it would be misleading to conclude that paleopathology is a relatively "hard" science, treating of diseases per se, whereas the present study is concerned with no more than what has been "thought about" tumors. However flattering to modern ears, this would be to overlook the inescapable fact that the investigator is always at the mercy of current theory, whatever the object under investigation. If paleopathology itself were old enough as a discipline it could be studied from the historical standpoint and the time-bound aspect of its ideas revealed. This is not to deny that there is a difference between studying a fossil bone tumor by means of a roentgenogram and perusing an ancient manuscript on bone tumors, but merely to insist that in both instances the modern investigator can only come up with a time-bound interpretation.

TUMOR THEORY

Classical Greece

The older writings on tumors must be approached with due caution. For example in Jacob Wolff's monumental study of the literature on cancerous diseases, one reads that Atossa, the wife of Darius the Great, was cured of cancer of the breast by a captive Greek physician, Democedes.[3] Awareness of the difficulty sometimes encountered today in distinguishing benign tumors of the breast from malignant or cancerous tumors—and both from a number of inflammatory and dysplastic lesions—justifies circumspection. Did Atossa have a cancer of the breast by today's diagnostic standards or a lesion called a cancer at the time? Or did she have neither? The third alternative actually fits the historical record best. Herodotus, the source of the tale, calls the lesion in question a *phyma* (growth or swelling) on the breast, rather than a cancer (*karkinos, karkinōma*). Furthermore, the readiness—vouched for by Herodotus—with which Democedes promised a cure to Atossa and the ease with which he seems to have effected it suggest that the lesion was not a cancer by our standards, or by his own. The exceedingly poor prognosis of breast cancer was, as we shall see, well known to the physicians of ancient Greece.[4]

In the Hippocratic writings the terms *phyma, oidēma, karkinos,* and *karkinōma* are used to designate several kinds of growth or swelling, some of which are fairly clearly cancerous in the current sense. Others are, equally clearly, inflammatory rather than cancerous lesions. The verb "to cancerize" (*karkinoō*) is used in a discussion of ulcers involving the female genitals; the writer stated that some of these ulcers, in consequence of faulty treatment, became *cancerized* (*karkinōthenai ta helkea*).[5] In the case of a woman of Abdera who had a *karkinōma* of the breast, we are told that although the physician successfully checked a bloody discharge from the nipple, the patient died. By today's standards the lesion may well have been a breast carcinoma. This diagnosis seems less likely in another instance where the Hippocratic writer uses the term *karkinōma*: a *karkinōma* of the throat is said to have been cured by cauterization.[6] Noncancerous tumors are usually referred to as *phymata* (growths) or *oidēmata* (soft swellings), and suppurating growths (said to be rare in adults but common in children) receive the designation *phymata empya;* possibly these were tuberculous lymph nodes. Many of the lesions termed *karkinos* by the Hippocratic writer seem to have been cancers, judging from the descriptions and the clinical course. Mentioned in the treatise on diseases of women are hard growths (*phymata sklēra*) in the breasts that do not suppurate but increasingly harden (*aiei sklērotera*) and develop into occult cancers (*karkinoi kryptoi*). Pain extends from the breast region to the neck and shoulder blades and the body becomes wasted; treatment at this stage is without avail, and death ensues.[7] Occult and deeply seated (*hypobrychthoi*) cancers are said to occur in mature adults; in older persons both occult and superficial cancers (*karkinoi hoi kryptoi kai hoi akropathoi*) are met with.[8] Noncongenital cancer (*karkinos mē symphytos*) is said not to occur before the age of puberty.[9] One of the best-known remarks on the subject of cancer in the Hippocratic corpus is the aphorism (XI, 38) to the effect that occult cancers are best left untreated: the patient will live longer that way.[10]

The use by physicians of the classical world of such terms as *karkinos* and *karkinōma* (as well as the Latin term *cancer*, which was used in a medical context by Cato the Elder around 200 B.C. and by Celsus two centuries later[11]) should not mislead us into supposing that cancerous lesions were at that time distinguished from benign tumors and inflammatory growths as these are now understood. In ancient medical theory lesions of all three classes were accounted for on the basis of a humoral theory of disease, in accordance with which they represented local aggregates of more or less abnormal *chymoi*, or "humors." A line of demarcation between inflammatory and neoplastic tumors was not drawn until the second half of the nineteenth century; more than sixty years after the first studies of tumors conducted in the light of tissue theory, and more than twenty-five after the similar application of Schwannian cell theory. In the Western medical tradition, which extends back through an unbroken line of Greek, Arab, and Latin transmitters to the fifth or sixth century B.C., all theories of the genesis—we cannot yet say, the *histo*genesis—of tumors fall into one category before the nineteenth century and another thereafter. The turning point came with the work of François Bichat (1771-1802), after which it became necessary for theorists to account for the genesis of tumor *tissues*. With the emergence of cell theory a few decades after Bichat's death, it became necessary to account for the genesis of tumor cells. The emergence of cell theory occurred simultaneously with a shift of attention from the gross to the microscopic level: Johannes Mueller's application of Schwann's cell theory to the study of tumors in 1838 was at the same time the first full-scale study of the microscopic structure of tumors. The earlier category of theories regarding tumor genesis (it could be labeled simply humoral were it not that the first theories of tumor histogenesis and cytogenesis were also humoral, albeit in a different sense) deserves our attention, not only because of its enormous historical staying power but also because of its influence on nineteenth-century tumor theory.

It has been noted above that the line of demarcation between inflammatory and neoplastic tumors was first drawn in relatively recent times.

The four so-called cardinal signs of inflammation — redness, heat, swelling, and pain (the *rubor, calor, tumor,* and *dolor* of Celsus, to which Galen did *not* add disturbance of function or *functio laesa* as a fifth)[12] — properly apply to only one of the forms of inflammation (termed *exquisite* by later writers) recognized by ancient physicians, and to that form only when it occurred on or near a body surface. The third cardinal sign, *tumor,* signified nothing more than a swelling or mass, but it is easy to see how it came to be used as a synecdoche for *inflammation* (Gr. *phlegmonē, phlogōsis*): not all forms of inflammation recognized by ancient physicians were painful, and redness and heat lose much of their value as signs when inflammation is deeply seated or internal. *Tumor* is used throughout for *inflammatio* in the writings of the fifth-century Latin physician Caelius Aurelianus; his book on acute and chronic diseases is a translation of the work of the second-century Greek physician Soranus of Ephesus.[13] And in the writings of Galen, too, the term *tumor* (*onkos*) most often refers to inflammation: his paradigmatic essay *On Praeternatural Tumors* (*Peri tōn para physin onkōn, De tumoribus praeter naturam*) is only marginally concerned with neoplasms as we know them today.

At a very early stage in the development of ancient Greek medicine and natural science the four universal elements (*stoicheia*), designated fire, air, water, and earth, were brought into relationship with four potencies or qualities (*dynameis*), hot, cold, moist, and dry. The *dynamis* "cold" seems first to have been assigned to air, and "moist" to water, with earth receiving "dry," and fire, of course, "hot." Aristotle, however, not only assigned two qualities or potencies, one primary and the other secondary, to each of the four elements, but also interchanged the qualities of water and air in a manner that at first seems arbitrary: water is said to be primarily cold and secondarily moist, air primarily moist and secondarily hot, fire hot and dry, and earth dry and cold.[14] With respect to the microcosmos, the *dynameis* were parceled out to the four humors of the body by the Hippocratic writers. Hot, cold, moist, and dry were assigned to blood, phlegm, yellow bile, and black bile (melancholy) with varying degrees of precision. *On the Nature of the Human Being* states that phlegm is the coldest of the humors, blood is moist and hot (akin to the season of spring), black bile is evidently cold, and the quality of yellow bile is not given. In some manner, the historical details of which are by no means clear, blood came to be associated with hot and moist (air, spring), phlegm with cold and moist (water, winter), yellow bile with hot and dry (fire, summer), and black bile with cold and dry (earth, autumn). Further correspondences, which do not concern us, were worked out later.[15] As modified by Galen, the scheme became canonical for medicine and remained so down to the seventeenth century. Galen's doctrine of the temperaments, as Erich Schoener has pointed out, rests less on the four humors than on the four *dynameis* ("qualities" or "potencies").[16] According to Galen a perfect state of health implies the right mixture (*eukrasis*) of the hot, moist, cold, and dry, while the more usual state involves an imperfect mixture (*dyskrasis*) or imbalance of these factors. There are eight dyscrasias: four simple, where hot, moist, cold, or dry predominates; and four combined, where hot and moist, dry and hot, cold and moist, or moist and dry predominate.[17]

For the physiologists in this tradition the ultimate material source of the humors was ingested food. The term *pepsis* ("ripening," "maturation") was applied to the transformation brought about by cooking, whereby the harsh and bitter qualities of foodstuffs were mitigated by heat. The meaning of *pepsis* was later broadened to include the series of changes, resulting in the formation of the humors, successively undergone by foodstuffs in the stomach, blood vessels, and local parts under the influence of innate body heat (*calor innatus, emphyton thermon*). The Latin term equivalent to *pepsis* is *coctio* or *concoctio* ("coction," "cooking"), although *digestio* ("digestion") is used as an equivalent term. Galen, in his commentary on the Hippocratic treatise *On Diet in Acute Disease,* discussed the rationale of the various meanings of *pepsis* and broadened the scope of the term still further by applying it to the ripening of excrementitious or noxious humors prior to their discharge from the body. Food underwent its first digestion or coction (*prōtē pepsis*) in the stomach and intestines. The resulting chyle was then drawn off via the portal vein to the liver, where yellow bile (choler) was separated out. The earthy, cold components of the nutriment were assembled in the spleen as black bile (melancholy). In the Galenic system of physiology only three of the four chief humors had physiological functions—phlegm apparently was no more than a waste product—and of these the blood was by far the most important. But it should be understood that for Galen and his followers down through the seventeenth century, the fluid substance contained in the veins and arteries, although called blood, was in fact a mixture of all the humors and some of their breakdown products as well. It carried, for example, the earthy humor, black bile, to distant parts of the body, there to strengthen the constituent fibers; it also carried the concocted breakdown products to be separated off as sweat and urine.[18]

Galen's most thorough study of the pathophysiology of inflammation (and thereby also of neoplasia) is found in the second part of his essay *On Therapeutic Method.* In that essay moist inflammation—which includes not only exquisite inflammation, or *phlegmonē* in the specific sense, but also inflammation in the generic sense—is presented as the manifestation of a flux or flow (*rheuma, fluxus*) of humors, single or admixed, to any part of the body. In addition to the large number of inflammatory lesions subsumed under the heading of "moist inflammation," Galen recognized a single species (*eidos*) of dry inflammation, manifested by an increased flow of heat to the involved part. This local fever (*pyretos*) was the sole form of inflammation in which no flux of humors took place; hence the only form in which *tumor* was lacking. (Galen might well have termed it a dynamic inflammation since only a single *dynamis*, the hot (*to thermon*), was involved.) Bearing in mind that Galen's category of moist inflammation includes our category of true tumors or neoplasia, we can see that it embraces almost the entire spectrum of visible lesions; just as today the combined categories of inflammation and neoplasia include everything other than congenital malformations and the so-called degenerative lesions.

Exquisite inflammation or *phlegmonē*, the species of inflammation that had, as Galen tells us, given its name to the genus, was due to the flux of blood to a part. Its exciting causes might be local, e.g., wounds, contusions, fractures, dislocations, even overexercise. Or it might be due to the relief of a general plethora of blood in the veins by the discharge of blood into some local part that was, as Galen put it, "most apt to receive" the excess. Of the other species of moist inflammation the more important are *herpēs* (yellow bile predominating in the flux of humors), *erysipelas* (predominance of a very hot form of bile), *anthrax* (a flux of hot, thick blood), and *oidēma* (a flux of phlegm, giving rise to a soft, painless tumor seen most often in the legs). A flux of black bile mixed with blood gave rise, according to Galen, to a kind of inflammation called scirrhus, one form of which was related to, or capable of converting into, cancer. A flux of black bile unmixed with blood gave rise to cancers (*karkinous*) forthwith.[19] Cancers (*karkinōmata*), says Galen, arise in many parts of the body but most often in the female breast; there they can be treated by excision and cauterization.[20] Hidden cancers, those in the depths of the body, are best left untreated, he says in his commentary on the Hippocratic aphorisms, for only in the case of superficial cancers is it possible, "so to speak, to cut out and extirpate the roots" (*ut sic loquar, radicibus exscindere et exstirpare*). The roots of a cancer should not be confused with adjacent veins filled with "melancholic blood."[21] Cancer of the breast is so-called because of the fancied resemblance to a crab (*karkinos*) given by the lateral prolongations of the tumor and the adjacent distended veins.[22]

Renaissance Europe

As already mentioned, Galen's essay *On Praeternatural Tumors* (*Peri tōn para physin onkōn; De tumoribus praeter naturam*) is a treatise on inflammation, in the broad sense of that term, rather than on tumors as now understood.[23] The various forms of *phlegmonē*, including cancer, are briefly presented, but only insofar as the surface of the body is concerned. It was pointed out in 1907 by Paul Richter that Galen's essay can best be regarded as the first treatise on dermatology, i.e., on diseases of the skin, mucous membranes, and superficial glands. Richter's article contains a brief account of medical writings, (in Greek, Arabic, and Latin, successively) through which this categorization of lesions, under various headings, was transmitted to the university physicians of sixteenth-century Europe.[24] A few remarks here on representative sixteenth-century medical texts will suffice for our purpose, which is no more than to indicate that the ancient system of pathophysiology remained almost intact. In the *Universa medicina* of Jean Fernel, first published in 1554, the category of *tumores praeter naturam* is expanded to include all lesions of the external parts of the body—whether or not there is associated "tumor" or swelling —all caused alike by fluxes of the humors, *serum* and *flatus.* According to Fernel, a *tumor* is larger than a *tuberculum,* and this in turn is larger than a *pustula.* Under the heading of *tumor,* Fernel lists phlegmon, bubo, phyma, erysipelas, oedema, hydrocephalus, hydrocele, scirrhus, ganglion, bronchocele, struma, and cancer. Under the heading of *tuberculum* are carbuncle and furuncle. *Pustulae* include herpes, scabies, psora, lepra, and callus, among others.[25] Fernel uses the term *phlegmon* rather than *inflammation.*[26] A phlegmon is a hot, preternatural tumor (*tumor callidus praeter naturam*) due to a flux, in which blood is present not only in veins and arteries but also in the empty spaces between the fibers composing muscles, membranes, and so on (*spacia vacua quae inter fibras sunt*). "Pure" blood gives rise to exquisite phlegmon. Admixtures of other humors give rise, variously, to *phlegmonē erysipelatōdes, phlegmonē oedematōdes, phlegmonē scirrhōdes,* and so on. A cancer is a hard, rounded, livid, or blackish *tumor praeter naturam,* surrounded by turgid veins. It is seen in the ear, eyes, uterus, anus and, most often, in the breast. The humors involved are "fervid blood" and black bile (*atra bilis*). Such lesions begin obscurely, often painlessly, but continue to increase in size. Eventually the overlying skin is "consumed"; an ulcerating cancer results. *Sarcoma* according to Fernel, is a tubercle or tumor that does *not* arise from an afflux of humors; it is due to a local disturbance of the nutritional process. Examples are *epulis* (in the gums) and *polyps.*[27]

Gabriele Falloppio, who will be mentioned later in connection with his admirably systematic survey of the "similar" and "dissimilar" parts (roughly equivalent to our *tissues* and *organs*) of the body, was the author of an equally admirable study of *tumores praeter naturam.*[28] As would be expected, there is no bond of any kind between Falloppio's histology —if we may here anticipate terms that were not introduced until the nineteenth century—and his oncology. The lesions discussed in the two parts of his treatise *De tumoribus praeter naturam* are inflammation, carbuncle, erysipelas, gangrene, scirrhus, cancer, elephantiasis, leprosy, aneurysm, struma, ranula, hernia, hemorrhoids, clavus, and swellings of superficial glands, i.e., of the lymph nodes.[29] Of these only the lesions designated scirrhus and cancer require comment. A scirrhus, says Falloppio, is so-called because of its hardness (only tumors of bone are harder than scirrhi); its other characteristic feature is indolence. One sign that a scirrhus is changing into cancer is the onset of pain. In his discussion of the etiology of scirrhus, Falloppio makes use of the Aristotelian categorization of four causes, material, efficient, formal, and final. Only the first two are dealt with, presumably because preternatural tumors, as Aristotle pointed out in the beginning, have no formal or final rationale insofar as a living organism is concerned. Falloppio writes:

> The efficient causes of scirrhous tumors are all causes of other tumors, external or internal: external, such as contusions, burns, the application of hot medicaments, and even extreme cooling. For we have two kinds of scirrhus: one that begins *per se* and the other derived from the transmutation of another tumor, from erysipelas for example, in which a scirrhus arises due to the application of coolants. A beginning, pure scirrhus always has extreme cooling as its cause. Such are the external causes. The internal efficient causes, however, are laxity of a receiving part and a propensity for receiving by reason of site or weakness; further, the arising in a part of heat, which attracts; further, a flow of thick viscous humors, with their causes, as by a vigorous expulsion of the humors of a scirrhus due to extreme heat and agitated motion of the members.[30]

After some additional remarks on the efficient causes of scirrhous tumors, including dietary errors or deficiency and suppression of menses and other forms of natural purgation, Falloppio continues:

> The material causes are the humors themselves, in regard to which the Greeks differ from the moderns. For the moderns say that black bile (*atram bilem*) or melancholy juice (*succum melancholicum*) is itself divided into the natural and the non-natural (*in naturalem et non naturalem*). Hence, since there are different species of black bile, so also are they followed by different kinds of scirrhous tumors. But the chief kinds of black bile are two: one termed hypostative, settling or sedimental, the other superabounding, excremential and non-natural. The first, a settling out of the blood and a melancholy juice or sediment of the blood, Galen terms natural; it is sent from the liver to the spleen, and it sinks down from the blood just as the coarse sediment does from wine while the must is concocted into wine; it is the natural melancholy, one part of which, according to them, is carried with the blood for the nourishment of the body and the cool parts, while the other part is sent off to the spleen, from which it is afterwards required by the stomach to make and arouse the appetite, and this savor, they say, is midway between sweet and bitter, and they call it semisweet or bridging (*ponticum*), and the same people say that from such a humor the exquisite,

true and pure scirrhus is generated. Secondly, they say that from non-natural melancholy arise scirrhous tumors differing in four ways, in accordance with what they say are the four species of non-natural melancholy. The first species exists when the sediment (*faex*) of the blood is burnt, from which comes the illegitimate scirrhus (*scirrhus non legitimus*); the second species exists when the burnt melancholy (*melancholia exusta*) comes from humors other than melancholy; the third species exists when the humors are rendered thick by cooling or in consequence of excessive drying, perhaps from medicaments, which species coincides with the first species of natural melancholy; the fourth non-natural species of melancholy exists when melancholy is admixed with blood, bile or phlegm (*pituita*). From all these they derive diverse species of scirrhus corresponding to the diversity of the species of melancholy just enumerated.[31]

For the understanding of the above it is essential to know that the "burning" or "overheating" (*exustio,* sometimes *adustio*) of yellow bile, blood, or phlegm was thought to yield melancholy. Falloppio goes on to show how the views of the "moderns" differ from those of Galen; but we need not concern ourselves here with the details of these differences or with his discussion of the prognosis and treatment of scirrhous tumors.

On broaching the topic of cancer Falloppio, citing Galen, Aetius of Amida, Paul of Aegina, and Avicenna, gives three reasons why cancers are so named. We are already familiar with the first; the second is that cancers seize on the surrounding parts with the tenacity of a crab seizing on its prey; the third is that cancers are extremely hard, rough tumors, resembling a crab in this respect as well.[32] It is understood that these characteristics are found in certain kinds of cancer only, the genus as a whole receiving its name from the most distinctive of its species. As in the case of scirrhus, the material cause of cancer is black bile, variously concocted and mixed with other humors:

> The material cause of a cancerous tumor (*cancerosi tumoris*) is an atrabiliary juice (*atrabiliaris succus*) which is either a melancholy humor and mild sediment (*faex mitis*), whereby the cancer itself is mild (*mitis*), or it is a true and adust atrabiliary matter (*atrabiliaris materia vera et adusta*) which, since it is malignant, gives rise also to malignant cancers; or it is black bile mixed with phlegm, a benign matter from which comes a mild cancer; or it is black bile admixed with blood, thus giving rise to inflammatory cancer (*cancer phlegmonōdes*); or it is mixed with [yellow] bile, and becomes erysipeloid. And all these matters may be with or without putrefaction. If the matter putrefies it produces an ulcerated cancer. . . .[33]

Falloppio explains why these black humors produce a mild cancer (*cancer mitis*) on one occasion and a malignant (*cancer malignus*) on another, but not why they give rise to a cancer rather than a scirrhus. However, it is true that in Falloppio's discussion of the efficient causes of cancer no external causes are listed, as they are in the case of scirrhus:

The efficient cause of cancer, however is a flux of atrabiliary humor, for only in the spleen and the liver can this tumor arise from congestion (*per congestionem*), because it is there that this humor is generated. But if any other place suffers from cancer, it suffers due to a flux. The flux, indeed, may be due to the strength of the transmitting parts, or to the quantity of matter [transmitted], or to its goading pungency; the cause of the attraction, indeed, weakness, pain or heat of the part; but the cause of the flux is a faulty mixture of the humors (*cacochymia*) due to bad food, as from lentils, turnips, the flesh of cows, asses and oxen, radishes, snails, salty and all bitter foods, and also from suppression of evacuations in any way customary, or from the suppression of varices that were wont to break open; also a cause of *cacochymia*, according to Galen, *lib. 2 ad Glauc., cap.* 10, is hot, dry air.[34]

Apparently the efficient causes of cancer are mainly intrinsic, whereas scirrhus often results from an external injury. It is likely that many of Falloppio's scirrhous tumors would be classified as indurated chronic inflammatory lesions or as scars by a modern histopathologist. But, in most instances, the lesions that Falloppio termed cancers would seem to have been genuine tumors, although we cannot know whether all were malignant.

Falloppio's sliding scale of distinction between benign and malignant tumors is worthy of further examination. The many varieties of black bile give rise to a corresponding variety of cancers, of which some are more benign, others more malignant (*alii benigniores sunt, alii maligniores*). Whether ulcerated or not, cancerous tumors can be subdivided into benign and malignant forms (*in benignos et malignos*). Falloppio continues:

In benign tumors the symptoms are not severe, and such tumors, unless they are irritated, do not greatly trouble men, for pain is not present or, if it is, is slight. Sometimes ulcerated [cancers] are benign, and so benign that they may persist for many years in the absence of much harm, sometimes they even persist for twelve years or more. Nevertheless, all such are malignant, but some more, some less.

Now the signs of benign cancer are, first, black or bluish [overlying] skin, by reason of the peccant humor (*humoris peccantis*), which is atrabiliary juice; second, no heat is apparent to the tactile sense, whether of the physician or patient. Indeed, some coolness is felt on occasion; it comes from the melancholy matter or the phlegm, which are cold. Third, the surrounding veins stand out, somewhat blackish and swollen. It is to be noted also—and this I ask you to observe, for it is mine—that, although such veins are regarded by everyone as a sign, they are nevertheless not a sure sign, since out of a hundred cancers four will not have them, and if they are found they are most obvious chiefly when the tumors are in the breasts....[35]

Some of the tumors classified by Falloppio as benign cancers would probably, to judge from their prolonged course, fall under the modern category of benign tumors. Falloppio's statement that all such tumors are more or less malignant simply means that all are more or less harmful to the patient. Lacking a term equivalent to our *tumor* he makes use of the term *cancer* in a generic sense. Falloppio's listing of the signs of malignant cancer makes this plain enough:

> The signs of malignant cancer (*maligni cancri*), however, are: first, a huge, hard tumor, for large tumors are never mild. The second sign is that to the sight the tumor seems single, but to the touch it seems otherwise, for to the sight the skin appears transparent and soft, but to the touch all is hard, and this points to ulceration and corruption of the part. The third sign is irregularity of the tumor, for when the tumor is rounded, small, regular, smooth and symptomless it is benign, whereas irregularity is a sure sign of malignancy even if pain is absent. If [the tumor] stubbornly adheres with widely extended roots this is a fourth sign, for cancer is of two kinds, to wit, separable by pulling and not separable by pulling, or adherent: cancers separable by pulling are those which, when gathered up in the hand and moved about, are not felt to adhere to the adjacent parts: of the adherent tumors almost none can be cured, while of those separable by pulling some are removed. Adherent [tumors], however, are sometimes attached to the muscles and bones, and hence in these a cure is not to be expected. The fifth sign is [the presence of] dilated, swollen veins resembling the legs of a crab, and this I single out from many signs, because from it a malignant cancer is called a "touch me not" (*noli me tangere*), since if its cure be undertaken the man nevertheless dies from this same cancer, hence the task of [curing] a malignant [tumor] ought not be undertaken, if you do not wish to receive the name of a bad physician. The sixth sign is a rather ashen color, with something added of black, and also a somewhat lustrous surface. The seventh sign is lancinating pain: for the patients say that they feel as it were a sharp sword or nail passing through the tumor; this is due to an acrid, malignant exhalation derived from the melancholy matter, which begins to putrefy. Such prickings also indicate cancer in the deeper parts. The eighth sign is some heat, sharp and piercing, perceptible to the touch of the physician or patient; this is a sign of extreme malignancy. For when inflammation or erysipelas is combined with a cancerous tumor it becomes extremely malignant and harmful.[36]

Obviously, Falloppio's view of the genesis of tumors, groundless as it may seem to a modern oncologist, did not blur his view of their symptomatology and semiology, for his list contains many items that have continued to retain their validity. Although he lays stress on the contrasting views of the Greeks and the "moderns" (*recentiores*), the differences, seen retrospectively, are slight, and there is no real breach in Galenical theory to be discerned. Briefly stated, the theory postulates that preternatural tumors result from the flow of humors to a part, where they accumulate and undergo a variety of alterations. Cancerous tumors, and their close relatives the scirrhous tumors, always contain an atrabiliary component, but one variable in type and origin. The tumor itself is an unformed fluid mass, unlike the similar and dissimilar parts (discussed in the following chapter), which are formed structures. Finally, the fluid make-up—that is, the chemical constitution—of a cancerous or scirrhous tumor determines its subsequent clinical behavior.

MOVEMENT OF THE BLOOD

This well-developed body of theory and observations was at the service of university physicians in Europe at the opening of the seventeenth century. Behind it was the hardly challenged Galenical theory of blood circulation with all that it implied regarding the movement of humors from place to place, together with accessory bits of Galenical theory such as that allowing for the expulsion, by a physiological faculty (*dynamis*), of corrupt or superfluous humors from the central and more important organs of the body to the periphery. This body of theory faced an immense challenge with the publication in 1628 of William Harvey's *De motu cordis*, in which modern circulatory theory made its first appearance —and not only theory, but practice as well, for the treatment of many "tumorous," i.e., inflammatory, lesions involved bloodletting, which had an elaborate rationale based on the Galenical theory of the movement of blood.[37] (There were in fact two rationales, one Greek and one Arab, for bloodletting, but since both Greeks and Arabs subscribed to Galen's theory, their differences do not concern us here.)

In order to understand the transformation of pathophysiological theory brought about by Harvey's innovation it is necessary to turn back to the Greeks. The Hippocratic treatise *On aliments* (*peri trophēs*) states that the liver is the root of the veins (*phlebōn*, vessels) as the heart is that of the arteries (*artēriōn*, "air-passages"). The veins distribute blood *to* the parts; the arteries, *pneuma* ("breath," "spirit") and heat—*pneuma* being considered a tenuous but material substance inhaled from the surrounding air.[38] Aristotle, on the contrary, held that the heart was the single source of both arteries and veins, as well as the organ in which blood was endowed with heat and life. Whereas the Hippocratic writer has a double system of vessels, rooted in different organs, for distributing nutriment on the one hand and pneuma on the other, Aristotle specifies that the blood is *one* thing, and that the blood vessels are two in number because animals have anterior and posterior parts.[39] In the period immediately following Aristotle's, however, the idea—attributed on somewhat uncertain grounds to Praxagoras of Kos—arose that arteries carried only *pneuma* and the veins only blood. This idea was taken up by the medical school of Alexandria, and it was Herophilus of that school who named the thick-walled vessel (the pulmonary artery) connecting the right ventricle to the lung the *phleps artēriōdes*, or "arterial vein," and the thin-walled vessel between the left ventricle and the lung (the pulmonary vein) the *artēria phlebōdes*, or "venous artery." For the next four hundred years, until the time of Galen, the dominant belief was that veins supplied blood to the body parts (hence the thick-walled arterial vein was so called in spite of its atypical structure) and arteries *pneuma* or airy spirit (hence the name *venous artery* for the thin-walled vessel between the lung and left ventricle).[40]

The claim that arteries contain *pneuma* rather than blood is not without empirical foundation: the arteries are in fact almost devoid of blood after death, having discharged most of their contents into the veins during the agonal stages. Since the heart was not thought of as a pump (but rather as a stove, where cooking took place and heat was supplied) the pulsation of arteries presented a puzzle, which was explained by the supposition that they contained an airy expansile spirit. To explain the discharge of blood from opened arteries, Erasistratus of Alexandria argued (according to Galen) that between the terminal branches of the arteries and veins were small passages or openings. These anastomoses (*synanastomōseis*) were open only under abnormal conditions, as when an artery was cut or punctured, releasing the *pneuma* and drawing blood into the arteries from the veins in accordance with Strato's doctrine of the *horror vacui*. In Galen's essay *On Phlebotomy: Against Erasistratus* (*Peri phlebotomias pros Erasistraton*), the theory is said to imply that fever results from the presence of an excess of venous blood making its way through the anastomoses into the arteries and thereby interfering with the distribution of heat and *pneuma*. Hence the efficacy of bloodletting in the treatment of fever. Galen states in his essay *On the Uses of the Parts of the Body* (*Peri chreias tōn en anthrōpou sōmati moriōn*) that the anastomoses of Eristratus seemed to have to useful purpose, but functioned only to produce fever and inflammation. In *Is Blood Normally Present in the Arteries?* (*Ei kata physin en artērias haima periechetai*), Galen attempted to show the logical inconsistency of the Erasistratean position. He concluded by asking how it was that intelligent men hold absurd beliefs and by replying that a double trap must be avoided by the lover of truth. He must neither reject what is plainly evident because of what is not yet known, nor accept what is not yet known on the basis of what is plainly evident: an observation should not be rejected simply because it cannot be explained, nor should an explanation be accepted simply because it explains an evident observation. To these remarks Galen casually appended the account of a crucial, but cruel, experiment that demolished Erasistratus's position: he had dissected out a segment of an artery in a living animal, tied it at both ends, excised it, and found that blood alone issued from a break in the wall made between the ligatures.[41]

We are now in a position to understand what Galen, and his followers down to the time of William Harvey, meant by a flux, that pathophysiological event that immediately preceded the development of a tumor in a part. The blood within the veins and the arteries was composed of a mixture of all humors, including "true" blood. Although we speak loosely of the Galenical or Aristotelian circulations, the fact is that Aristotle's model for the distribution of the blood was the one-way movement of water in a system of irrigation ditches, and Galen's model appears to be of the same character. The so-called tidal movement, to and fro, of the blood in the veins, often presented as an integral feature of the Galenical circulation, appeared on the historiographical scene only recently, as the result of a textual misinterpretation. Movement of the fluid within the vessels was determined not by the pumping action of the heart but by the physiological expulsive and attractive forces or powers (*dynameis*) of the various body parts. A pathological flux was simply a disproportionate movement of this kind involving one or more of the humors, either normal or altered by disease. The sole exception was Galen's "dry" inflammation, previously mentioned. In the normal course of events, the parts of the body were nourished by blood that was drawn out as needed from the vessels; it exuded like steam, vapor, or dew into the flesh (*sarxs*) or parenchyma (*parenchyma*) of the part. The inflammatory process differed from the normal in two ways, one quantitative and the other qualitative. The humoral mixture, i.e., the blood, accumulating in a part might, before reaching that part, contain abnormal components owing to the greater ability of the centrally placed, more "noble," parts to expel noxious matter. Alternatively, corruption of the humors took place at the local site. In either case the fluxed humors left the vessels and accumulated in the free spaces supposed to exist between the ultimate fibers of the parts. The extravascular fluid mass was then further altered or broken down (*diapltheretai*), either because it was improperly ventilated (*diapneisthai*) or because the part was unable to deal with it for some reason. Local concoction or ripening of the humors would have as its most successful outsome the disappearance or discharge (from a body surface) of the fully concocted *materia peccans;* if the local concoctive faculty (*peptikē dynamis*) were weak, an accumulation of septic putrefying residues (*sēpemenou perittomatos*) would ensure the persistence of the local tumor. The worst case (although Galen does not make the point), would seem to be the development of a cancer.[42]

What was the effect of the Harveian revolution on this imposing body of theory? We shall see that it was considerably less than might be expected. First, however, it is necessary to say something of Harvey's great achievement in physiological theory. Harvey received his degree in medicine from the University of Padua in the closing decade of the sixteenth century. Padua was, and had been for a good part of that century, at the center of a new interest in mechanics, scientific method, and anatomical investigation along new lines and the related problem of the movement of the heart and blood. Aristotle was the principal source of scientific method; and in his essay *Of the Manner and Order of Acquiring Knowledge*, written late in life as a preface to his book on generation, Harvey showed himself to be thoroughly Aristotelian in outlook.[43] Without detracting from Harvey's enormous merits, it is unlikely that he would have made his discovery had he not traveled to Padua for his medical education.

It was at Padua that Andreas Vesalius had prosecuted the anatomical studies leading up to the publication, in 1543, of his *De fabrica humani corporis;* it was also to Padua that Galileo, the foremost experimental physicist of the time, came in 1592 to lecture on mathematics. A reinterpretation of traditional ideas concerning the movement of the blood began to take shape at mid-century. Galenical doctrine allowed for the passage of an indeterminate amount of blood from the venous to the arterial side at three sites: the lungs, the peripheral parts of the body, and the heart. The movement was supposed to take place through the hypothetical anastomoses of Erasistratus. Galen said these anastomoses were too small to be seen by the naked eye; they "escaped the senses" (*ekpheugousi men tas aisthēseis hai synanastōmoseis*), but they were required by theory. Vesalius became increasingly doubtful of their presence in the muscular septum between the right and left ventricles on the (not entirely legitimate) grounds that they were not detectable. Realdus Columbus, Vesalius's successor at Padua, taught that the cardiac septum was impermeable and that blood passed via the pulmonary artery (the arterial vein) from the right ventricle through the lungs, where it was admixed with air, to the left ventricle via the pulmonary vein (the venous artery).

The chair in anatomy at Padua was next held, briefly, by Gabriele Falloppio; and, following his death in 1565, it was occupied until 1604 by Fabricius ab Aquapendente, the teacher of William Harvey. Beautifully illustrated studies of valves in the larger veins were published by Fabricius in 1574. Fabricius thought that the valves' purpose was to prevent excess reflux of a column of blood moving centrifugally toward the extremities; Harvey was later to demonstrate that their purpose was, rather, to prevent reflux toward the extremities of a *centripetally* moving column of blood. Work along these lines was proceeding elsewhere at the same time. Andreas Caesalpinus, botanist and professor of medicine at Pisa, stated in 1583 that the veins transmitted blood to the heart, and the arteries blood from the heart; he used the term *circulation* (*circulatio*) for the first time in connection with the movement of blood through the lungs. Somewhat later, he argued that the true explanation of the swelling of veins on the limb side rather than the heart side of a tourniquet was that centripetal blood flow was thereby hindered. And in France in 1553 Michael Servetus had already described how dark venous blood from the right ventricle was transformed into bright arterial blood by the addition of air or spirit during its passage through the lungs to the left ventricle.[44]

Thus, when Harvey arrived at Padua in the closing years of the sixteenth century, he must have been confronted by a mass of conflicting opinions regarding the motions of the heart and the blood. Some authorities followed Hippocrates and Galen in regarding the liver as the source of the veins and the heart as that of the arteries; others followed Aristotle and looked on the heart as the source of both the arteries and the veins. The movement of a quantity of blood through the lungs, allowed for by Galen, received new importance in the eyes of those who found no grossly visible pores, or anastomoses, in the muscular septum between the two ventricles. The actual amount of this blood, like that which according to Caesalpinus moved from the arteries to the veins in the rest of the body, was undetermined, although it was thought to be no more than a mere trickle. As for the existence of anastomoses in the cardiac septum and elsewhere, the adherents of Galen could point out to their adversaries that a failure to demonstrate passages regarded by Galen himself as too small to be seen hardly disproved their existence. In the discussion of unsolved problems and contradictions in the received dogma with which Harvey begins his *De motu cordis et sanguinis in animalibus,* he found it necessary to confute even the ancient Erasistratean belief that the arteries contained only air or spirit. Another point to which he called attention had to do with the movement of the so-called fuliginous waste vapors supposed by the Galenists to be generated in the left ventricle by a kind of combustion (compared by Galen himself to the burning of a candle). According to the accepted teaching, these vapors were transmitted from the left ventricle (not the right, as appears in some modern accounts) to the lungs for exhalation. Harvey observed that this would require the mitral valve—which separates the contents of the left ventricle from that of the left atrium and pulmonary vein—to be both competent and incompetent: incompetent (at least partly open) to allow for the passage of fuliginous vapors from the heart to the lungs; competent, when it functioned to prevent the reflux of blood passing from the lungs to the left ventricle.

After outlining the current situation, Harvey set forth his own findings. He accurately described the movement of the heart in several animal species, and inferred the direction of blood flow by placing ligatures between the great vessels and the heart on both sides (these experiments were performed on live fish and snakes). Next, he demonstrated that the contrary directions of blood flow in the arteries and the veins could be inferred from the effects of medium ligatures (which blocked venous flow only) and tight ligatures (which blocked arterial flow as well) placed around the human arm. In describing the pulmonary transit of blood he credited Galen with something of its recognition, but he vehemently denied the existence of pores in the cardiac septum or anastomoses elsewhere in the body, supposing instead that the blood "percolated" through the parenchyma like water through the earth. An estimate of the amount of blood discharged per minute by the heart into the aorta, made on the assumption that the left ventricular chamber emptied with each beat, led him to the conclusion that a quantity so large could not possibly be created anew and used up at the circulatory periphery; only if it were hypothesized that the blood moved, as it were, in a circle could the facts be accounted for.[45]

To the modern reader who has accepted Harvey's conclusion in advance and is unburdened by the Galenical schema, the *De motu cordis* seems to sweep to its conclusion with something of the inevitability of fate. The fact is that there are flaws in the perfection of the demonstration.[46] These flaws were presumably more obvious to Harvey's contemporaries, some of whom, moreover, saw that *De motu cordis* had implications for the whole of pathophysiology and therapy.

Perhaps the best-known and most respected of Harvey's opponents was Jean Riolan, professor of anatomy and botany at Paris.[47] Riolan saw that the Harveian doctrine of the circulation might reduce to nonsense not only the Galenical doctrines of the pathophysiology of fluxions and the production of *tumores praeter naturam* but the rationale of bloodletting as well. For if the blood moved rapidly and perpetually in a circle, and if (as Harvey claimed) it left the terminal branches of the arteries to percolate with equal rapidity through the parenchyma to reach the veins, how could a Galenical fluxion occur? And the therapeutic procedure of bloodletting, which in the old theory is equivalent to the draining of a sump or swamp, would no longer make sense. Riolan accepted that the work of Harvey and his predecessors necessitated at least some changes in the received doctrine, and he tried to reconcile the differences by compromise; his proposed circulation was, however, much closer to Galen's than to Harvey's. Riolan's chief divergence from the Galenical account of the movement of blood in the arteries and veins was his acceptance of the claim (first put forward by Caesalpino and later corroborated by Harvey) that venous blood moved toward, rather than away from, the heart. But he retained the Galenical arteriovenous anastomoses and permeable interventricular septum—the existence of which had been called into question by Vesalius and his followers, including Harvey. Only the blood in the larger vessels circulated (passage from arteries to veins being made possible by anastomoses between the larger vessels) and that at a snail's pace, once or twice a day at the most: "According to our doctrine only the blood contained in the larger channels of the vena cava and aorta moves through the arteries, descends or departs from the heart, and ascends or approaches to the heart by way of the veins, whereas the branches or offshoots of these channels contain blood which does not circulate in the channels, but flows about (*fluitat*) for the nourishment of the parts."[48] Riolan's view of the circulation permitted him to retain both the received Galenical theory of the pathogenesis of *tumores praeter naturam* and the therapeutic measure deemed most broadly effective against such tumors, namely bloodletting:

> Does the circulation of the blood interfere with the flux of impure humors in the ambit of the body, as in papules, macules, eruptions and effloresences? Not at all. The morbific humors in the lower vessels, which are offshoots of the larger channels, creep out under their own impetus or by natural vigor, or are propelled into the ambit of the body, but is it to be doubted that venesection can avert or retard that excretion? All practitioners agree that venesection draws the humors from the center to the periphery, but the circulation of the blood teaches the contrary, unless we say that when nature has been freed from the burden of corrupted humors she removes the remainder into the external parts. It is certain that depraved humors poured out in the lesser vessels made a path and exit to the skin or run back into the ambit of the body, whence they cannot be extracted unless a great evacuation of blood is carried out.[49]

A half-hearted acceptance of the theory of the circular movement of the blood is evident on the part of other writers of the time. For example, in the revised edition of Gregor Horst's *Medical Institutions* (1661), what purports to be the Harveian circulation is concisely described, but the more or less Galenical account of the pathophysiology of *tumores praeter naturam* proves to be inconsistent with the belief that the *whole* mass of the blood perpetually moves in a circle. We are told by Horst that an external acute inflammatory tumor may result from the irritation of an internal part by a plethora of blood, in consequence of which the excess blood is driven first from the larger to the smaller vessels and then to the extravascular parenchyma, where it occupies the space between fibers.[50] Harvey's account of the circulation was clearly incompatible with that part of the received Galenical doctrine that called for a shift of superfluous or corrupt humors from the center to the periphery (from the "noble" to the "common" parts, in the old phraseology), but the incompatibility could be glossed over by compromise or simply overlooked. On the other hand, Galen's belief that in the course of the inflammatory process blood became impacted in small blood vessels was quite in accord with the Harveian circulation. The model of silted-up branches in an irrigation system sluggishly dispensing a vital fluid had merely to be replaced by one of local blockage in the vascular channels of a dynamic circulatory system in which the blood was driven furiously in a circle by the pumping action of the heart.

Thus, with a few alterations, the traditional Galenical doctrine of fluxions—which not only explained the genesis and material nature of the *tumores praeter naturam* but also furnished a rationale for their treatment—was able to survive the Harveian revolution in physiology. Yet even Riolan—who seems to have been more aware than his contemporaries of the extent of the conflict between the old and the new understandings of the movement of the blood—failed to see all the implications. The heart remained, as Harvey said, the sun of the microcosm, but the mechanical force by which it drove the humors in a circle through the body now took the place of the Galenical retentive and expulsive forces, which had previously been thought to determine their movement.[51] A new account of the events leading to the production of inflammatory tumors (including scirrhous and cancerous forms) was called for but was not forthcoming until the second half of the nineteenth century, after neoplastic and inflammatory tumors had been placed in two separate categories.[52]

IATROCHEMICAL HUMORALISM

The first attack against the traditional doctrine of the four humors had been somewhat hesitantly launched in the sixteenth century by Paracelsus. In the following century, however, J. B. van Helmont, who is usually regarded as the founder of iatrochemistry, rejected the old humoralism in its entirety. Other physicians, such as Daniel Sennert and Gregor Horst, attempted to reconcile the conflicting doctrines put forward by the iatrochemists on the one hand and the Galenists on the other. The university schools of medicine were further divided by the opposition between adherents of traditional Arabic Galenism and proponents of new interpretations of Galen based on the original Greek texts. Paracelsus, who taught briefly at the University of Basel until his expulsion in 1528, is celebrated for having burned the *Canon* of Avicenna (representative, perhaps, of Arabic Galenism) in public a year earlier.[53] He was opposed to Galenism in general, however, and attempted to substitute for the four humors of the Greeks the three principles—salt, sulfur, and mercury—of the alchemists. Pagel argues that the modern concept of diseases as discrete entities owes something to Paracelsus:

"When you see Erysipelas, say there is Vitriol. When you see Cancer, say there is Colcothar. If you see Lupus, say there is Plumosum."[54] Thus the specificity of their chemical basis. But since colcothar is the residue, or *caput mortuum*, of distilled vitriol, we are not too far, conceptually speaking, from the received notions that erysipelas depends on the accumulation of fiery, hot blood, and cancer on melancholic dregs or residues. Pagel concludes that the views of Paracelsus were not in principle different from those of the old humoralists: chemical entities replaced the four humors, and, although Paracelsus's chemical terms were often vaguely stated in a context of "analogies and correspondences," nevertheless "there...[was]...an appeal to reality about them."[55] But it is to be doubted that the "appeal to reality" seemed convincing at the time; the orthodox contemporaries of Paracelsus had a very concrete representation of the four humors at their disposal.

By the sixteenth century the four Galenical humors were held to be visibly evident in drawn blood, especially when the blood was drawn off into a shallow basin in therapeutic bleeding. The following passage from a work (apparently for popular consumption) by the Dutch physician Levinus Lemmens (Lemnius, Lemnie), published in 1561 and translated into English in 1581, will suffice:

All the differences of humours, when a vein is opened (for it is not all pure blood that gusheth thereout) is plainly of all men to be perceived. First before it be cold it doth show and represent to the eye, an airy and foamy spirit, which by and by vanisheth away: then an exact and pure liquor of most perfect and excellent ruddiness, the which is pure and right blood: in which there swimmeth choler, and sometime tough clammy phlegm, sometime liquid and thin, according to the nature, condition and state of man. Last of all, if you turn up the whole mass or lump, you shall find melancholy, altogether of color black....And if a man were disposed by taste to have further knowledge in these humours, he may with his tongue and palate as well judge and discern the relish and tallage thereof, as he doth their color by the eye. For blood is sweet...choler is bitter, of the nature of gall; phlegm, unsavory as water, so long as it is not rotten, nor mixed with other humours, for then it is either salt or sourish. Melancholy is sharp, aigre and tart.[56]

J. B. van Helmont expressed himself along similar lines in a polemic against the Galenical humors contained in the *Ortus medicinae*, a work first published in 1648, four years after his death. Like Paracelsus, van Helmont was not a member of the academic establishment. He gives Paracelsus credit for being the first to laugh at the humors of the Arabists and Galenists, adding, however, that Paracelsus was not sufficiently fixed in his views and was prone to lapse into humoral categories (*ad humores labitur, et complexiones, nondum sat in suis thesibus funditus*).[57] Van Helmont says that the humors of the schools are mere fictions; he clearly does not accept their identification with the separated components of drawn blood:

> For they [the physicians of the schools] often observe the supernatant water and call it yellow bile or gall, because it is yellow and somewhat pale (although it does not taste bitter and lacks the essential property of gall). They call the sediment at the bottom, where it is heavier and darker, the black bile. And in the intervening space they observe red blood wherein they detect whitish fibers, the matrices of coagulation. These, they say, are phlegm (*pituitam*).[58]

Van Helmont's commitment to Neoplatonic light metaphysics, together with his peculiar use of such words as *Blas, archeus,* and *semen* (the last a relative cf the Stoic and Christian *logos spermatikos*), make his pathophysiology so idiosyncratic that it requires special interpretation.[59] To the extent that his ideas influenced the general course of medical thought, they were taken up and reformulated along more conventional lines. A physician schooled along Galenic and Aristotelian lines would have been able to make very little of what van Helmont had to say concerning the pathophysiology of cancer:

> For I have found that in luminous effects of this kind (*in huius modi actionibus luminosis*) there is a unitary connection at a point, to wit, of the occasional and efficient cause of our Archeus, through which they interpenetrate and radically unite, like lights, without any distinction other than that of relative terms. And now there shall be judgment concerning external, rabid poisons, likewise of carcinomata and others. For the formal virulent light (*lumen formale virulentum*) which springs up in our life is itself living, and hence just as the rabid Archeus takes up, ferment-wise, an external contagion, so also in cancer, going astray, it transports itself into rages, through which the flesh is damaged topically.[60]

Spagyrical or hermetic chemistry, brought by Paracelsus from the workshops of metallurgists and vintners to the physician's clinic, gradually replaced the traditional Aristotelian-Galenic "chemistry" of four qualities (*dynameis*), elements (*stoicheia*), and humors (*chymoi*), and, with the aid of Stahl's phlogiston theory, developed into an all-embracing system during the eighteenth century. The two outstanding chemists of the late seventeenth and early eighteenth centuries, Georg Ernst Stahl and Hermann Boerhaave, were in fact professors of medicine at Halle and at Leyden, respectively. During the transitional period several attempts were made to conciliate the rival doctrines of the Galenists and Hermeticists, the net effect of which was to facilitate acceptance by physicians of the new chemistry—wherein the model for physiological and pathophysiological processes was drawn from the brewery or winery rather than from the kitchen.[61] Of the conciliators the most industrious was Daniel Sennert, professor of medicine at Wittenberg, whose *De chymicorum cum Aristotelicis et Galenicis consensu et dissensu* was published successively in 1619, 1629, 1633, and 1655. Although Sennert stated that no one unskilled in the art of chemistry could lay claim to the name of a finished physician in his time (*elegantis medici nomen hodie vix sustinere potest, qui chymiae ignarus est*), his account of the genesis of tumors is, aside from a few references to acridities and such, hardly distinguishable from that of an orthodox Galenist.[62] Cancer, he says, is caused by adust, or black bile (*adusta seu atra bile*), a degenerated form of melancholy humor, which by itself is capable only of giving rise to a scirrhus. The adust bile adheres in the veins and is unable, because of its crassity, to issue from their tiny openings. The less acrid and hot form of adust bile causes latent and nonulcerative cancer. Adustion of melancholy humor can take place in the vessels or in the part affected.[63] Appropriately, the frontispiece of Sennert's *Practicae medicae* depicts Hermes and Hippocrates shaking hands.

Horst, too, attempted to conciliate the rival views of the Galenists and Hermeticists. His dissertation on "living and dead" anatomy (*de anatomia vitali et mortua*) will have a familiar ring to anyone acquainted with contemporary medical school debates between anatomically and chemically oriented physicians. The Hermeticists, says Horst, assert that physicians should not rest content with knowledge of the shape, make-up, and site of the parts of the body; they should go on to explore the inmost (i.e., chemical) principles of the body and the various properties deriving therefrom. There is an edge to Horst's tone when he remarks that: "*This*, certain of the moderns call *vital* and essential, *that*, local, material and dead; *this*, of the greatest necessity to the physician, *that*, they assert, least of all; *this*, the living properties of the living body, *that*, on the contrary, the accidents of the cadaver, thus they vaunt themselves in showing us."[64]

Nevertheless, Horst considers no irreconcilable conflict to be involved. The Hermeticists claim that generation of all kinds takes place by virtue of *seeds* acting in conjunction with the three spagyrical principles: salt, sulfur, and mercury. And by these terms, he says, they do not mean ordinary, but "philosophical," salt, sulfur, and mercury, where salt is the principle of solidity, sulfur the tempering principle, and mercury the principle of liquidity. When the Hermeticists issue forth with their new classification of diseases into sulfurous, mercurial, tartareal, and so on,

This spagyrical assertion (*assertio spagyrica*) can be brought into agreement with the ordinary assertion of the Galenists if we distinguish between that which primarily generates disease and that which produces disease through a mediating agent. The Galenists attribute morbific causes partly to the [solid] parts themselves, partly to the [fluid] contents and partly to the

driving forces (*impetum facientibus*). But the Hermeticists attempt to pene-
trate more deeply into nature; in the contents and containers [i.e., the solid
parts] they consider that which generates disease. The Galenists lay down
as the morbific cause bilious, melancholy, pituitous, or some other such
humor. The Hermeticists are not content; they go on further to enquire
precisely how that impurity, hiding in such a peccant humor, arises and
proximately serves to generate disease.[65]

More or less in this way, the spagyrical categories made their way into
the mainstream of medical thought. Aided by such outstanding iatrochemists or chemiatrists as Franz de le Boë (Sylvius) at the University of
Leyden and Thomas Willis at Oxford, the language of the chemists
became the language of the scientific physician, and of the so-called
empiricists as well; for example, Thomas Sydenham, whose writings
teem with references to fermentation, effervescence, volatile spirits, and
so on.[66] It is fair to say that, by the end of the seventeenth century, the
Galenical humors, while not forgotten, had begun to seem slightly quaint
to the scientific physician.

LYMPH

Discovery of Lymphatic Circulation

Harvey had denied the existence of anastomoses between arteries and
veins because he was unable to detect any connecting links between the
two systems of vessels in carefully examined boiled and macerated
preparations of liver, spleen, kidney, and lung.[67] In 1661, four years after
Harvey's death, Marcello Malpighi used a simple microscope to discover
that there was, indeed, a network of tiny vessels connecting the arteries
and the veins. Generalizing on the basis of a few observations, he induced
that circulating blood always remained within well-defined (but not
necessarily walled) channels; it did not, as Harvey had supposed, pour
out into the interstices of the parenchyma to percolate through to the
veins (*nec in spatia effundi, sed per tubulos semper agi*).[68] Meanwhile a new
system of vascular channels, containing a fluid that was later to assume
great importance in the pathogenesis of cancer and related diseases, was
coming to light. In 1628 appeared the posthumously published account
of Gasparo Aselli's discovery, made six years earlier, of certain milky
vessels (*vasa lactea* or *venae lacteae*) in the mesenteries of dogs and other
mammals.[69] In accordance with the Galenical scheme, Aselli believed
that these vessels were carrying nutrient material, or chyle, from the gut
to the liver. In 1651 Jean Pecquet described the *cisterna chyli* and its
continuation, the thoracic duct, which emptied into the great veins of the

neck. Between 1651 and 1653 Olaus Rudbeck independently described both of these structures and, more importantly, showed that a system of vessels containing a watery or milky fluid ran, via the lymph glands, from all parts of the body to form large trunks, which, like those in the mesentery, emptied into the thoracic duct. In his paper of 1653 Rudbeck refers to the mesenteric lymphatic vessels as watery hepatic ducts (*ductos hepaticos aquosos*) and to those elsewhere as serous glandular vessels (*vasa glandularum serosa*). At about the same time Thomas Bartholin of Copenhagen also involved himself in the study of the lymphatic vessels. In his first paper, *De lacteis thoracis* (1652), he held to the belief that the mesenteric lacteals ran to the liver. In 1653, however, in a paper entitled (provocatively, as it turned out) *Vasa lymphatica nuper Hafniae inventa* —the lymphatic vessels recently discovered at Copenhagen—he reversed his stand. Here we find the pathways in question referred to, apparently for the first time, as lymphatic vessels.[70]

Rudbeck had called the newly discovered system of vessels the *vasa glandularum serosa*, with reference to their association with lymph nodes (glands) and to their fluid content, which he considered to be derived from blood. Bartholin rejected the name *vasa serosa* on the grounds that the vessels did not contain serum. He suggested *vasa lymphatica, vasa aquosa,* or *vasa crystallina*—for, other than the mesenteric lacteals after feeding, the fluid in these vessels was watery and clear—and the first of these designations (lymph = clear spring or river water) became generally accepted. Bartholin believed that lymph was derived from blood through a process of straining or filtration: "Thus the water pre-exists in the arteries, although it is not pure and limpid, yet it keeps the state of water here and there. It is seen more pure and clear in the channels of the lymph because it has percolated through a tortuous route (*percolata fuit per viarum anfractus*), through the anastomoses of vessels, just as water in wells and streams runs sweet and clearer through sandy earth and stones."[71] The coarse red component of the blood (the "globules" which were described later in the seventeenth century by Antony van Leeuwenhoek) was of course separated out as clarification proceeded. According to the comparisons drawn by Galenists earlier in the seventeenth century, lymph would have consisted largely of phlegm and a variety of humoral breakdown products, with possibly an admixture of yellow bile. But with the diminishing credence accorded the four humors in the later seventeenth and the eighteenth centuries (when they began to assume a more figurative sense), and perhaps also due to the circumstances of discovery, the fluid contained within the lymph vessels was regarded as, in the main, a *succus nutricius,* or nutrient juice.[72] That the finer ramifications of the blood vascular system were continuous with the channels of the lymphatic system was the prevailing belief until about the middle of the nineteenth century. The belief in pores and percolation generally began to wane early in the eighteenth century as further work with the microscope and the use of injection techniques bolstered the view that the circulating fluids, lymph included, were always contained within well-defined channels. Anton Nuck, one of the first and perhaps the most skillful of the injectors, is said by Boerhaave to have prepared an injection specimen of the entire lymphatic system.[73]

Cancer "Seeds"

In the eighteenth century the importance assumed by the lymph in the pathogenesis of cancer was evident in the writings of Georg Ernst Stahl and Friedrich Hoffmann. Both men were appointed professors of medicine at the University of Halle near the end of the seventeenth century.[74] It is of interest to note that Stahl partitioned the components of the blood in light of the humoralism prevailing in his day, just as Lemnius and van Helmont had done when the four Galenic humors retained their validity. Stahl, who accepted both Harvey's circulation and his rejection of the capillaries, regarded the circulating blood as a composite of three primary fluids: (1) the true blood, a reddish mass consisting of a "diaphanous liquor" that contained "ruddy globules" (*globulos rubicundos*) or blood corpuscles (*corpuscula sanguinea*); (2) the useful nutritious lymph (*lympha utilis, nutritia*), a "gelatinous" fluid derived from the chyle, which contained corpuscles suitably proportioned for combination with the various solid parts of the body (*ad mixtionem singulis partibus proportionatam libero, et nondum varie connexo, seu jam firmiter mixto statu, praesto sunt*); and (3) the serum, a watery mixture of excrementitious saline, mucilaginous, oleaginous, etc., matter.[75] The "bile of the ancients" (*bilis veterum*) was, said Stahl, actually a composite of "salty serum and gelatinous lymph" (*salsuginoso sero et gelatinosa lympha*) mixed with a small amount of true blood. Trapped in the solid parts and undergoing further breakdown, this noxious fluid constituted a cancer.[76]

For Stahl, as for Hoffmann, cancer was simply the most unfavorable outcome of inflammation. Together with their more famous contemporary, Hermann Boerhaave, both men regarded circulatory stasis as the initial pathophysiological event of inflammation, regardless of the occasional external or internal causes. What happened in consequence of stasis depended in large measure on the structure of the part involved and the chemical constitution of the entrapped fluid. In the case of uncomplicated, exquisite inflammation the inherent protective forces of the body could, according to Stahl, break up the block and restore unimpeded flow. This, the most favorable outcome for the patient, Stahl called resolution. Less favorable outcomes were suppuration, sphacelation (necrosis), gangrene, scirrhus, and cancer: "Eminently and simply, at any rate, inflammation of course includes within itself the sanguineous stases; but whatever deviates from pure, well-mixed sanguineous [blood] taints and violates the purer genius of inflammation, so that something different and irregular in course and outcome arises..." Pure (phlegmonous or exquisite) inflammation, Stahl continued, occurs chiefly in parts of the body well provided with vessels and "pores" permitting the free flow of blood. Other parts, structurally suited for the passage of the more tenuous serolymphatic humors only, are likewise subject to the impaction (*infarctus*) of such humors; not only is this impaction more difficult to break up but, once broken up, it also yields acrid, ulcerative matter and tinder (*fomitem*) capable of damaging the surrounding healthy parts.[77]

According to Stahl, a scirrhus is a kind of tumor occupying a position midway between salutary inflammation (*inflammationem salutarem*), or mild solution of continuity in the solid parts, on one hand, and mortifying corruption (*sphacelosam corruptionem*) on the other. A scirrhus has, however, a perpetual disposition to undergo one or another form of corruption. Hence the wise counsel of Hippocrates to leave occult cancers untreated, for occult cancers are simply sanguineous scirrhous tumors located in glandular regions (*cancros occultos...sunt simpliciter tales in glandulosis locis scirrhi sanguinei*). A scirrhus consisted of humors like those in a cancer, the difference being that the "corruption" was potential in a scirrhus, and actual in a cancer.[78] Stahl's discussion of the archetypal form of cancer, that of the breast (which, he remarked, had given its name to tumors elsewhere in the body thought to be of the same nature although of different appearance) is worth noting. Although neither a spagyrical chemist nor an iatrochemist, and doubtful of the value of chemical studies to the physician, Stahl resorted to Paracelsian and van Helmontian "ferments" and "seeds" in his explanation of the poor results achieved by the surgical extirpation of breast cancers.[79] Surgical removal involves two dangers:

> ... First, of course, the true fermentative genius of the matter itself; if any of this still persists in the remaining whole part as residuum, nothing has been accomplished by the laborious resection of all the rest, so long as the actual ferment left behind does in fact not only propagate the residual like corruption, now more simply and wholly putrefying and mortifying, but also propagates it through the pectoral parts, simply rather the fleshy muscular parts. Hence, also, patients thrown to this Charybdis thereafter perish utterly, usually within a short space of time.

The true seed (*verum seminium*) or true root (*vera radix*) of this malady, according to Stahl, sits within distended, wholly or partially blocked sanguiniferous tubules. Further dissemination (*ulteriorem disseminationem*) of this matter into extremely minute branches lying beyond the apparent extent of the breast makes removal of entire lesions almost impossible. Even if this were to be accomplished, the patient would be exposed to a second peril: the development of a cancer in the remaining breast, possibly after the lapse of many years.[80]

Unlike most of his colleagues at the time, Stahl regarded the uncomplicated course of the inflammatory process subsequent to stasis as a reactive, protective physiological response on the part of the body to injury. Guided by the *anima*, which Stahl identified with the protective "nature" (*physis*) of Hippocrates, the body restored itself to normal. Hence Stahl's phrase "salutary inflammation" (*inflammatio salutaris*).[81]

Friedrich Hoffmann was one who looked askance at Stahl's teleological interpretation of the inflammatory process. In Hoffmann's brief book of aphorisms, *Fundamenta medicinae* (1694), he defines medicine as the art of rightly using physicomechanical principles for preserving and restoring health (*ars recte utendi principiis physico-mechanicis, ad sanitatem hominis conservandam et amissam restituendam*). His views regarding inflammation (in the broad sense) otherwise belong in the same category as Stahl's, although nowhere in his writings are they developed at such length. Hoffmann says that just as an abundance of blood may block flow in the arteries and the veins, so also excessive or overly tenacious lymph may retard movement in the lymph vessels and give rise to various diseases: when lymph does not circulate properly through the minute pores and tubules of glands and fleshy fibrous parts, it stagnates, distends its containing vessels, and may give rise to hard tumors in the testes, breasts, tonsils, salivary glands, and elsewhere. Stagnation of lymph may eventuate in suppuration; otherwise the end result is a hard tumor (*tumor durus*), or scirrhus. And if a gland becomes scirrhous under the action of corrosive matter (*a materia corrosiva*), the end result is a cancer.[82] Boerhaave, too, says much the same thing. Inflammation is in essence the stagnation of red blood in the smallest vessels; it can occur also in dilated terminal arterial vessels, or arterial lymphatic vessels (*in vasis lymphaticis arteriosis*) that have admitted red globules to which they are unable to give passage. Resolution and suppuration are the more favorable conclusions to the inflammatory process, but under unfavorable circumstances a hard, painless tumor called a scirrhus may be the outcome, most commonly in glandular parts. If the marginal vessels undergo inflammation a scirrhus may become malignant. It is then called a cancer, or carcinoma, because of its resemblance to a crab (*evadit malignus, et vocatur jam cancer, a similitudine, vel carcinoma*). Boerhaave includes among the precipitating causes of the cancerous change melancholy (*affectus animi tristes et biliosi*).[83]

We have seen that Stahl identified the seed of cancer as a ferment (*fermentum*). Implicit in this notion is the ability of a cancer ferment, like other ferments (in bread and wine, for example), to reproduce or replicate itself. A tiny portion of the cancer-ferment, left behind after surgical extirpation of a breast cancer, is thus able to revive the cancerous process in the adjacent parts. The importance ascribed to the seeds of disease in orthodox medical thought during the seventeenth and eighteenth centuries, a strand of which connects with the nineteenth-century development of bacteriology, probably owes something to those unorthodox physicians, Paracelsus and van Helmont. Pagel sees the entirety of van Helmont's work as a search for the seeds (*semina*) of living things, those "active principles in beings which are responsible for their *specific* form and function"; a "search for the *divine* spark in created beings." And to van Helmont a seed (*semen*), or at least a "seminal property," could be represented by a ferment.[84] Paracelsus likewise saw the divine seed or "word" (*logos*) that had informed the macrocosm reflected in the microcosm in the form of innumerable seeds convertible by alchemical transformation into concrete individual objects.[85] Both Paracelsus and van Helmont were drawing from the general fund of available notions in which the *logoi spermatikoi* ("seminal reasons") of the Stoics had been incorporated by early Christian theologians. And van Helmont's "search for the *divine* spark in created beings," as formulated by Pagel, is another version of the *tiqqun* in Lurianic Kabbalism, i.e., the search for the seeds, soulsparks, and soulroots scattered by the fall of Adam.[86]

Solidistic Lymphatic Theory

The seventeenth century having been, among other things, a time when many anatomical discoveries were made and the existing knowledge of the structure of the human body was considerably refined, we might reasonably expect an awakening of interest in the solid structure of tumors, heretofore regarded as intravascular or extravascular fluid or semifluid aggregates. Possibly due to a general lack of interest in the details of morbid anatomy on the part of medical investigators and theorists, relatively little information was forthcoming along this line until the beginning of the nineteenth century. Deshaies Gendron's little book of 1700 on the nature of cancer, which broke entirely with the school dogmas, furnishes an interesting exception.[87] In claiming that cancers were not tumors, i.e., that they were not inflammatory masses composed of fluxed humors, but solid structures derived from the transformation of nervous, glandular, and lymphatic vascular parts into a compact, uniform, cancerous substance inherently capable of destructive growth, Gendron departed from more than two thousand years of Western medical tradition. Partly as a result of this, the book exerted little effect on the course of medical thought in Gendron's time, and has remained almost unknown to later generations of physicians and compilers of historical medical bibliographies.[88]

Gendron's understanding of cancer purports to be based on experience rather than authority. After observing the clinical behavior of cancei.. and examining the substance of which they are composed, he says he reached the conclusion that cancers are not constituted of specific humors of one kind or another; instead, they are transformed solid parts. The actual cancerous mass represents the "transformation of nervous, glandular and lymphatic-vascular parts into a uniform, hard, compact, insoluble substance capable of growth and ulceration." This transformation is due to the collapse of normally present vessels and tubules and the resulting "cessation of filtrations" in the involved parts. Furthermore, it is an irreducible transformation (transformation irréduisible), i.e., there is no way in which the destroyed original structure of the part can be reconstituted. Scirrhous tumors have been incorrectly grouped with cancerous tumors; according to Gendron, a scirrhous tumor results from coagulation of fluid in the vessels of the involved part, and resolution (restoral to the original state) remains possible. Finally, Gendron attributed rupture and ulceration of the skin overlying a cancerous lesion to pressure exerted by the growing mass rather than to the effect of a corrosive acid present in the cancer. Therefore the search for therapeutic agents capable of neutralizing the supposed acid is in vain.[89] Gendron wrote that as a physician who could see with his own eyes and reflect on what he saw, he had come to doubt the existence of this corrosive acid (à douter de l'existence de cet acide corrosif). For what could be its source? Not the blood, since cancers usually took form while the patient was perfectly healthy; and not something at the site where a lymphatic humor had been extravasated (où il se sera extravasé quelque humeur lymphatique), since extravasations due to blows or compression were of common occurrence and resolved spontaneously.[90]

Gendron's remarks on the structure and growth of cancers have a very modern ring in comparison with those of his contemporaries. With reference to cancer of the breast, the paradigm of cancers, he states that the tiny tumor formed in the beginning represents a derangement of the structure of a few of the glandular particles (un dérangement de la structure de quelques grains glanduleux) that constitute the breast. The further increase in size of this tumor represents a successive transformation of the surrounding glandular substance, as its channels, and those of the neighboring blood vessels and nerves, become choked and compressed.[91] Gendron's attempt to draw parallels between the structures of cancerous tumors and those of animal horns and hooves, and human nails and "corns," will seem less than happy, however. If we agree that

> ...the nails of human beings, and the hooves of animals are merely the hardened and united ends of nerve fillets, which allow for the growth of nails and horns by admitting a nutrient lymphatic humor into the continuations of the fibers, there will be no difference of opinion, since the carcinomatous mass is formed solely by the collapse and union of an infinity of nerve fibers and lymphatic vessels, just as are hooves; the mass is nourished in the same manner, and since its fibers meet with no resistance, they will extend and enlarge themselves, compressing successively the other parts, in accordance with the absolute laws of nature, which are always uniform in their effects, and there will occur a new transformation in the contiguous glands and an increase in the size of the whole mass, without supposing the action of that purely imaginary corrosive acid.[92]

Aside from this rather bizarre, and to his contemporaries highly unorthodox, conception of the metamorphosis of nerve fibers and lymphatic vessels into a solid, cancerous substance, Gendron did not entirely avoid the preconceptions of his age. The only form of growth conceivable to him was that occasioned by the deposition of a fluid substance (the "nutrient lymphatic humor") on preexisting fibers. True, the "nerve fillets" are said to undergo elongation, but we are not told how this comes about. Nevertheless, his solidistic view of the nature of the cancerous substance is startlingly different from that of his contemporaries. It did not become generally accepted until more than a century later, when other physicians interested in the tumor problem employed, like Gendron, anatomical dissection in their studies. In this connection Stahl's explanation of the liability of breast cancer to recur after extirpation furnishes an interesting contrast with that of Gendron. For Stahl the seed (*seminium*) or root (*radix*) left behind after apparently complete removal of a breast cancer is humoral in nature; it is the ferment (*fermentum*) that continues to work its baneful effects. Gendron, on the other hand, has forgotten the chemically conceived seeds and ferments. Contrasting scirrhous and scrofulous tumors (which represent "simple excesses of humors coagulated in the vessels of the part" and can readily be cured by extirpation) with cancers, he writes:

> It is not the same likewise with the extirpation of the truly carcinomatous tumor (*la tumeur véritablement carcinomateuse*), since the chief induration does not represent the tumor in its entirety, and there are many filaments of the same substance as the tumor which are imperceptible to the touch but form part of the cancer. Being capable of growth and ulceration, and dispersed as they are in the neighboring parts, it is not surprising that they would come together after the extirpation and seem to form a new cancer, more dangerous than the one that was undertaken to be extirpated.[93]

Gendron does not condemn such operations entirely, since they were recommended by the ancients and were successful in some instances, but offers criteria of choice: "The observations which I have made on this subject have persuaded me that use should not be made of it [surgical extirpation] except in the case of cancers, those of the breast for example, which manifest themselves as a rolling tumor (*tumeur rollante*) without adherence at the margins, and which give no evidence to the touch of any induration in the remainder of the breast, so that there would seem to be no filaments spread by the cancer into the neighboring parts."[94] A pathologist of today might suspect that many of Gendron's "rolling tumors" were benign tumors, probably fibroadenomas.

Gendron appears to have been responsible for introducing the concept of cancerous degeneration into the context of tumor studies. Although this concept, like all of Gendron's ideas on the subject of cancer, was largely ignored by his contemporaries, it was widely used throughout the nineteenth century. In Gendron's book the terms *dégénéré* and *dégénérable* (but not the term *dégénérescence,* which was the nineteenth-century French equivalent of "degeneration") signify, respectively, the actual or possible transformation of a noncancerous tumor into a cancer. Transformation represents a change for the worse, a downgrading of structure characterized by the loss of features normally present in the family of parts to which the involved one belongs; hence that part is said to have degenerated. For example, a scirrhous tumor—which, according to Gendron, does not constitute a "derangement of the structure of the part" where it occurs, but is constituted instead by the plugging and distension of the normally present channels of the part by coagulated fluids—may "degenerate" into cancer. Gendron describes the process as follows: "A scirrhus becomes a cancer due to the tendency of the channels (*colatoires*) to undergo derangement of the order of their parts when their function is interrupted. The derangement primarily occurs in certain lymphatic vessels and nerve fillets, determining them successively toward a cancerous transformation which extends throughout the scirrhous tumor and forms that hardened, compact whole, capable of growth and ulceration, already described."[95] Other lesions capable of degenerating into cancers are scrofulous tumors (*écrouelles*), polyps (*polypes*), and sarcomas (*sarcomes*), the last term apparently signifying a class of benign soft-tissue tumors.[96] It should be added that, strictly speaking, the involved part rather than the benign tumor itself, viz., the scirrhus in Gendron's account, undergoes degeneration into cancer.

The essence of Gendron's revolutionary idea was that cancers were composed of a solid, structured substance of degenerate character that derived from the transformation of nervous, glandular, and vascular parts and were inherently capable of continued destructive growth. It was empirically based only to the extent that Gendron had by means of gross dissection satisfied himself that cancers were solid tumors with cordlike extensions into the surrounding parts. Otherwise it was as hypothetical as the conception of cancer it aimed to replace; that it was not accepted by his contemporaries is not surprising from this consideration alone. Furthermore, the humoralistic explanation of the genesis of cancer, part and parcel of humoralistic physiology and pathology, was strengthened by the promising new science of chemistry, whereas Gendron's explanation no doubt presented itself to his contemporaries as being of merely ad hoc character. Interest in pathological anatomy as a tool for the investigation of problems in pathology was slight in Gendron's time; almost a century was to elapse before it would have its day. Moreover, a theory of general anatomy, more solidly based on anatomical dissection than was the received doctrine of similar and dissimilar parts, would not be forthcoming until François Bichat appeared on the scene at the close of the eighteenth century.

Dominance of Lymphatic Humoralism in Eighteenth-Century Cancer Theory

The failure of Gendron's solidistic view of cancer to exert a lasting effect is evident in the two best-known treatises on the tumor problem written by French authors in the second half of the eighteenth century, those by Jean Astruc and Bernard Peyrilhe.[97] Both are in the traditional humoralistic vein. Astruc's two-volume treatise falls into the line of works stemming from Galen's *De tumoribus praeter naturam;* Peyrilhe's short book concerns itself solely with the problem of cancerous tumors. The first of Astruc's volumes deals with inflammatory tumors (in today's sense), and the second with scirrhous tumors, including cancers. Astruc tells us that the schools distinguish three classes of tumors: natural, nonnatural, and preternatural, or contranatural (*tumeurs...naturelles, non-naturelles et praeter-naturelles ou contre-nature*). Tumors of the first class are present in the body "by nature" (e.g., nose, breasts, superficial glands); those of the second class are normally but inconstantly present (e.g., a pregnant uterus); while those of the third class are abnormal. The third class divides into tumors produced by the displacement of a bodily part (e.g., an axillary tumor representing the dislocated head of the humerus) and those "bearing the name of humoral tumors" (*portent le nom de tumeurs humorales*), the latter being the subject of Astruc's treatise.[98] Astruc's subclassification of humoral tumors by (Aristotelian material) causes is revealing: "It is preferable, in accordance with the different causes of tumors, to divide them into tumors produced by blood, such as phlegmon and erysipelas, tumors produced by lymph, such as edema, tumors produced by separated and then reabsorbed (*récrémentielles*) humors, such as scirrhus, tumors produced by air, such as emphysema, and, finally, tumors produced by fat, such as the fatty tumors.[99] In the above scheme only phlegmon, erysipelas, edema, and scirrhus are humoral tumors, since neither fat nor air is a humor in any sense of the term. Astruc recognizes this implicitly when he points out that "emphysema, fatty tumors, and the other tumors which cannot be related to the four principal kinds" (*genres principaux*) must be discussed separately. He also states that the four principal kinds may occur in simple or compound form, and he supplies names for the twelve possible permutations (*phlegmon érésipélateux, oedemateux ou squirrheux,* etc.), leaving open the question of the difference between, say, an erysipelatous phlegmon and a phlegmonous erysipelas.[100]

Astruc accepts without question the view that tumors can arise only as a result of the accumulation of humors of one kind or another in the open spaces of the solid parts. In the case of scirrhous tumors, he says, the stagnant humoral mass undergoes hardening and corruption. Since blood is incapable of this alteration, and since scirrhous tumors show no evidence of accumulated blood when examined at autopsy and occur more often in the less vascular parts of the body, it is therefore plain "that scirrhus is caused by lymph or by the various recremental or excremental humors which are separated out in the various passageways and viscera."[101] The muscles and the fleshy parts generally are seldom subject to scirrhus. The tumor occurs more often in glandular parts, especially those in which the secreted humors are thick and viscid in character, such as the female breast, the uterus, the testis, and the liver. Unlike phlegmonous tumors, simple scirrhous tumors arise slowly, are painless even when touched or pressed, and are not associated with discoloration or increased local heat. As the name implies, they are extremely hard. In addition to the three combined forms (*squirrhe phlegmoneux,* etc.) and the simple (perfect, legitimate, or exquisite) scirrhus, Astruc recognizes a carcinomatous variant, *squirrhe carcinomateux.* This, the product of a scirrhus degenerating into cancer (*dégénérant en cancer*), is cancer itself.[102] Depending on the stage and manner of their development, cancers may be occult or open, i.e., ulcerated; some resemble fungi in these respects.[103] As for the degeneration of scirrhus into cancer, Astruc doubts that a corrosive acid is involved, for there is no evidence of such in the sanious lymph and blood from the ulcerated surfaces of cancers. He believes that the degenerative process is due instead to increased heat, which causes rarefaction of the matter composing the scirrhus.[104]

Bernard Peyrilhe's prize-winning doctoral dissertation was written in response to the question, "What is the nature of cancer?" posed by the

Academy of Sciences at Lyon.[105] His answer is in accordance with the humoral pathology of his time:

> The material or proximate cause of cancer is to be sought for in the fluid, which, according to the laws of the animal economy, is distributed to the organs we have just now spoken of. The experiments of Kaau, Boerhaave, Monro, and others, having sufficiently proved, that the lymph has a constant, and exclusive communication with the cellular texture, and with the generality of the glands. The lymph is therefore the proximate cause of cancer. We are not to listen to what antiquity says on this cause: we are to consider what she says of pituita, atrabilis, ferments, coagulating acids, etc. as pure fiction, founded wholly on the subtility of Galen's theory.[106]

Obstruction of the lymph flow, followed by inspissation of this seemingly harmless fluid, is the proximate cause of cancer due to the stagnant lymph's becoming subject to putrefaction and thus "ichorous." This "ichorous matter," says Peyrilhe, is the "true cancer virus," and it is capable of giving rise to secondary cancers within the body of the afflicted individual. Such secondary cancers " . . . are truly occasioned by absorption, and the virus thus carried by the lymphatics to those neighboring conglobate glands, irritates and determines them to a greater afflux of fluids, and thus produces the tumefaction and obstruction which follow."[107] It is worth noting that Peyrilhe takes account of Gendron's view of cancer, although he is of the opinion that Gendron mistook minute, obstructed lymphatic vessels for nerve filaments and thus failed to grasp the true nature of the roots of cancer.[108]

Hunter's "Coagulating Lymph"

In one form or another, the lymph theory of cancer had been part of the articles of medical faith for well over a century when John Hunter first addressed himself to the problem of its nature and origin.[109] While Wolff's claim that Hunter's version of the theory was essentially different from, and far superior to, the earlier versions is exaggerated, there are certain original features of Hunter's ideas on inflammation and neoplasia worth noting.[110] Among these are the distinction he drew between acute inflammation as a salutary physiological response to injury and the abnormal inflammatory process that results in tumor formation, and his introduction of the term *coagulating lymph* to characterize more precisely that component of the blood capable not merely of being coagulated by heat, alcohol, and so on but of spontaneously coagulating whenever the blood leaves its vessels. The coagulating lymph, thus distinguished from other and merely coagulable components of the blood, was given the name *fibrin* within a decade or two after Hunter's death.[111] As will be shown below, Hunter's enormous influence on his contemporary and succeeding generations, both in England and on the continent, led to the incorporation of his belief that the coagulating lymph represented the prototypical formative substance of healthy and diseased animal organisms into the blastema theory, which dominated pathophysiology in the first half of the nineteenth century and furnished the bridge to modern cell theory.[112]

In his *Lectures on the Principles of Surgery* Hunter states that the blood "when at rest" separates into "coagulable lymph, red particles and serum." The red particles, or "globules," are enmeshed in the coagulum, and the serum is "squeezed out" somewhat later.[113] The term *coagulable lymph* was an accepted one in Hunter's time, and it served to distinguish the lymph in the lymphatic vessels from the component of the circulating blood, to which it referred. The lymphatic vessels, as Hunter points out in the *Lectures,* were no longer thought to be the "terminations of the extreme ends of the arteries, not large enough to carry red blood but only serum and lymph," but rather a system of "absorbent" vessels.[114] John and William Hunter had been partly responsible for the anatomical studies on which the new view was based.[115] As already noted, the term *coagulable lymph* was to John Hunter a misnomer, since it failed to distinguish the merely coagulable part of the blood from that possessing an "inherent power of self-coagulation" made evident when the blood spontaneously clotted, whether in the vessels or after having been shed. Merely coagulable (by heat or chemical means) lymph was to be found in the serum extruded from blood clots; *coagulating* was a more appropriate term for the other component.[116]

William Harvey had believed that the blood was "prior to its receptacles," and in the *De motu cordis* he had quoted Leviticus 17:11 in support of his claim that life was primarily seated in the blood. The statement that blood was prior to its receptacles, i.e., that the solid parts of the body were formed from the blood, rested on studies of the chick embryo carried out (like those of his preceptor, Fabricius) with the naked eye. The *punctum saliens,* or "leaping point," is the first formed part in the chick embryo and marks the future heart, but, says Harvey, "blood is produced before the *punctum saliens* is formed."[117] In expressing a similar view, Hunter assumed (hardly more than a century after the publication of Harvey's work on generation) that his readers would find this view strange and paradoxical. Without mentioning Harvey he maintains that blood, far from being a "passive, inanimate moving fluid...deriving motion from the heart," is the "material out of which the whole body is formed and out of which it is supported."[118] "Life," says Hunter, is prior to "organization."[119] What this means is that the blood, or rather its formative component, the coagulating lymph, both generates the solid parts of the body in the course of embryonic development and maintains them in later life in accordance with need. Growth, regeneration, repair, and the daily nutritive requirements of all solid parts depend alike on the passage of required amounts of formative substance from the circulating blood to those parts.

Following the same line of thought, Hunter was able to assimilate pathological processes, in particular, inflammation and tumor formation, to physiological ones. Uncomplicated inflammation is "an action produced for the restoration of the most simple injury in sound parts that exceeds union by the first intention," i.e., immediate union. Inflammation in this uncomplicated form is a "salutary mode of action" and one of the "most simple operations in nature." In words reminiscent of Stahl's, Hunter states that "inflammation is in itself not to be considered as a disease, but as a salutary operation consequent either to some violence or some disease."[120] These statements, it must be remembered, refer to simple, healthy, or uncomplicated inflammation only. Hunter also recognizes various forms of unhealthy inflammation (usually involving suppuration or ulceration) due to the added action of specific irritating agents. There are as many kinds of unhealthy inflammation as there are of disease. Even here the inflammatory process may lead, in a roundabout fashion, to a cure, provided the disease is one in which it can "alter the diseased mode of action." But, adds Hunter, "where it cannot accomplish that salutary purpose, as in cancer, scrofula, venereal disease, etc., it does mischief."[121]

In the Hunterian scheme unhealthy inflammation is in essence a heightened stage of the physiological mechanism underlying all formative processes in animal organisms, whether adult or embryonic, perverted from its aims by certain poorly understood "principles" peculiar to specific diseases. Although Hunter's teleological interpretation of the uncomplicated inflammatory process involves a somewhat sharper distinction between tumors (in the modern sense) and inflammatory masses than any made by physicians before him, the same physiological mechanism remains responsible for tumor formation. Physicians generally mean by the term *tumor*, Hunter says, a "circumscribed enlargement in a part from disease, not strictly a disease of a natural circumscribed part, as a thickened diseased gland." Such enlargements "seem to depend on an accumulation of extravasated coagulable lymph, either in the adipose or cellular membrane, or both."[122] As will be shown in the following chapter, the "adipose or cellular membrane" is the eighteenth-century equivalent of the modern histologist's connective tissue in its generalized sense: a substance that surrounds, supports, penetrates, and binds together the organs of the entire body. According to Hunter, solid tumors of this kind are true new formations; they are composed of an

"entirely new-formed substance...of new structure." But he recognizes
as well two additional kinds of solid tumors, termed *warts* and *polypi*. A
wart is a solid tumor that forms on the skin and adjacent membranes
lining the body orifices, while a polyp is a similarly solid tumor on the
"inside membranes, or canals" of the body. Like tumors of the cellular
membrane, they commonly arise "from one fixed point, as a root." Hunter
does not say that they are likewise composed of an entirely new-formed
substance; in the case of warts, in fact, he states that they "appear to arise
from the true skin of the parts."[123] (The distinction is an important one;
only hinted at by Hunter, it was to become crucial in mid-nineteenth-
century disputes concerning the genesis of epithelial tumors, including
carcinomas.) He is similarly doubtful as to the status, in this respect, of
what he calls cystic tumors. These "commonly consist of a bag, or cyst,
filled with a substance softer and different from the surrounding parts,
although not necessarily so," and are of two kinds, "natural and acquired."
"Natural" cysts may arise from obstruction of the excretory duct of some
gland or from the retention of fluid or other matter in a preformed
space; "acquired" cysts present more of a problem, and Hunter is uncertain as to the uniformity of their origin. In some instances, as in the
case of hydatids, the cyst wall is formed of "thickened cellular membrane,
condensed by pressure"; in other instances Hunter is uncertain of its
constituents.[124]

Hunter was of the opinion that under the rubric *cancer* two distinct
forms of disease had erroneously been grouped together. The two forms
are "in appearance very different, and are probably very different in
their nature." He reserves the term *cancer* for hard circumscribed tumors,
arising most commonly in the breasts, uterus, pancreas, lips, and stomach
and tending to undergo a "species of suppuration" in the center and to
ulcerate on external surfaces. A tumor of this kind in its early, non-
ulcerated stage is termed a *scirrhus.* The second form of the disease is, like
cancer, incurable, but instead of eating away parts and undergoing only
a moderate increase in size meanwhile, its outstanding feature is its rate
of growth, which produces "a spongy fungus which cannot be kept down."
Hunter suggests the name *fungated ulcer* for this subclass of malignant
diseases.[125] Although he has little to say with respect to the genesis of
cancers and fungated ulcers, it is plain that he traced the former back to
an extravasation of coagulating lymph in the interstices of the connective
tissues. But he regards this lymph as different in nature from that capable
of giving rise to benign or scrofulous tumors. It has somehow been
contaminated by a "cancerous poison" and has become "coagulable lymph
which possesses the cancerous property." Persisting in its unorganized
form in the primary scirrhus it is capable of spreading from the primary
growth to produce what Hunter calls "consequent cancers" in distant

parts of the body, usually by way of the lymphatic channels, or "absorbents." In cancers of the breast the axillary glands, subclavicular glands, and glands along the internal mammary artery may be so involved, and the "consequent cancers" may not manifest themselves for several years after removal of the breast.[126]

Insofar as Hunter depicts the neoplastic process as a version, admittedly a perverted one, of the inflammatory process, he clearly remains within the confines of the pathophysiological theory enunciated by Galen sixteen hundred years earlier, although the four humors and their innumerable intermixtures and transformation products had long since lost their standing. In the sixteenth century their place had been usurped by the various mixtures of the spagyrical chemists. Insofar as cancer was concerned, black bile as the material cause or substance constitutive of the tumor had yielded to the corrosive acids and ferments of iatrochemical theory. These hypothetical acids and ferments had in turn lost their credibility. From the opening years of the eighteenth century their place in tumor theory—with Gendron alone dissenting—was taken by a new fluid, the lymph. Hunter's "coagulating lymph," however, is lymph with a difference. Not only is it a clearly demonstrable component of the circulating blood, varying in quantity in accordance with need, it is above all an "organizable" fluid substance. More than this, it is the fluid substance whose solid transformations account for *all* growth, restitution, repair, and maintenance of the solid parts of the body in both adult and embryonic life. And when Bichat, at the beginning of the nineteenth century, revived the old theory of the similar parts and gave it concrete embodiment in the form of tissue theory, Hunter's coagulating lymph stood ready to serve as a bridge between humoralism and solidism. In order to see how this was accomplished it will be necessary to revert to the dawn of interest in the solid parts of animal bodies.

2

TUMORS AND TISSUE THEORY, FIFTH CENTURY B.C. TO 1838

ANATOMICAL SCIENCE

Sources

Near the middle of the eighteenth century the erudite Swiss physician Albrecht von Haller offered the readers of his *Bibliotheca anatomica* an interesting account, buttressed with numerous citations from Greek and Roman authors, of the origins of anatomical science. He argued that the first human beings had been vegetarians. Hence, the rudiments of anatomical knowledge had not been acquired by hunters and butchers but by the priests and soothsayers who had officiated at ancient animal sacrifices and examined the entrails of the offerings for prognostication and other purposes. Citing Porphyry, von Haller claims that it was late in the history of humanity when the first mortal tasted sacrificial flesh, but thereafter not even the most stringent laws were able to restrain human beings—captivated by the agreeable taste of flesh—from ingesting that barbarous delicacy.[1]

Von Haller's account, based largely on myths and folk tales, is not without a grain of truth. Anthropologists tell us that the protohominids of several hundred thousand years ago were, like most anthropoid apes of today, mainly vegetarian in their diet. With the development of killing tools these early men were transformed into facultative carnivores. As hunters and butchers they became, ipso facto, practical anatomists, knowing where to strike in order to kill and how best to dismember their prey. At a later period of human evolutionary development the external parts of human and animal bodies were distinguished and named. Etymological evidence indicates that these parts were named along functional rather than morphological lines. The interior parts of animal bodies, hidden from the eye and less obvious in respect to function, were probably distinguished and named at a still later period. In any case, the first glimmerings of anatomical knowledge were on the gross level and largely concerned with those parts that are now called organs. Interest in the fine structure of the organs—the anatomy of what are now called the tissues—was a still later development, even though it antedated the invention of the microscope by nearly two thousand years. It is easy to imagine a primitive or early investigator inspired by the fibrous character of some animal parts to draw a comparison between woven or plaited artifacts and the handiwork of nature; but it seems that not until the flowering of Greek scientific thought did this actually take place.

Similar and Dissimilar Parts; The Ultimate Fiber

The Greek word *organon*, from which we derive our term *organ*, means a tool or instrument suited by virtue of its structure for one or more purposes. The application of the term *organon* to the internal as well as the external parts by Greek anatomists suggests that from the beginning they regarded the internal parts as functioning structures, or as structures with functions. Pure morphology, i.e., the study of form divorced from function, did not exist at the time; both the word and the idea are products of the nineteenth century. As for the fine structure of the organs, the absence of hard data at the microscopic level did not prevent Greek anatomists from devising a classification of similar parts in which a hypothetical *fiber* was the ultimate structural unit of living substance. In Plato's *Timaeus* the sinews (*neura*) are said to be formed of fibers (*ines*) present, at least potentially, in the circulating blood; flesh (*sarx*) represents the nonfibrinous component of the blood after it has left the vessels. Plato seems not to have known that defibrinated blood does not clot;[2] Aristotle, however, was aware of this fact.[3] Erasistratus is said by Galen to have believed in the existence of an invisibly small, simple fiber, perhaps an ultimate structural-functional unit.[4] Galen states that the solid parts of animal bodies are composed of fibers, membranes, and flesh (*sarx*).[5]

Aristotle's *De partibus animalium* requires careful study, for it is the fountainhead of Western anatomical knowledge. Aristotle's division of the parts of animal bodies into two categories, the similar parts (*homoiomerē*) and the dissimilar parts (*anomoiomerē*), remained current until well into the eighteenth century. The rationale of his procedure is not as straightforward as it at first appears, and it became the subject of considerable disagreement in later times. Present-day translators and commentators sometimes disagree on what Aristotle meant. For example, D'Arcy Wentworth Thompson remarks, in connection with a passage in the *Historia animalium* where the division is briefly set forth, that Aristotle derived the scheme from Anaxagoras and developed it (in the *De partibus*) into the doctrine of a three-stage synthesis of animal parts: first, the synthesis of the true elements, or *stoicheia* (i.e., the moist, the cold, the hot, and the dry); second, the synthesis of simple, or similar parts; and third, the synthesis of dissimilar parts (organs) from similar parts. The older sixteenth and seventeenth century European naturalists, Thompson continues, equated the *homoiomerē* with their own *partes similares s. simplices s. primae* and the *anomoiomerē* with the *partes dissimilares s. instrumentales s. organicae s. officinales;* hence, Bichat's division of the bodily parts into tissues and organs was along traditional lines. In his sixteenth-century anatomical treatise, *De differentiis animalium,* Edward Wotton writes that "the similars are numbered as follows: bone, cartilage, vein, artery, nerve, ligament, tendon, membrane, flesh, fat, nail, skin, and to these are added the humors, as the blood and the crystalline and vitreous humors of the eye."[6] Thompson says this passage gives a "very fair epitome of the tissues."

In his translations of Aristotle's *De partibus animalium* A. L. Peck correctly states that the Aristotelian term *part (morion)* includes both fluid and solid parts. Aristotle's *homoiomerē moria* and *anomoiomerē moria* cannot be equated with the tissues and the organs, respectively, of modern biology, because blood, serum, marrow, semen, bile, milk, and so on are not, according to current usage, tissues. Peck states that the term *organ* corresponds in current usage closely to what Aristotle called organic or instrumental parts (*organika merē*). The difference between Aristotle's two categories consists in each of the similar parts having a peculiar character as a *substance* (in the modern sense) and each of the dissimilar parts having a peculiar character as a *conformation.* The heart is the only part that falls into both categories; it is similar insofar as it consists of uniform flesh and dissimilar by virtue of its special configuration.[7] But Peck goes astray at this point. What Aristotle actually said was that *all* the viscera (*splanchna*) are uniform with respect to matter and nonuniform in respect of configuration. The viscera are composed of sanguineous matter; they are deposits left behind by the current of blood in the blood vessels, like mud deposited along the banks of a running stream. The heart, says Aristotle, should be composed of that form of nutriment from which it is seen to originate in the embryo.[8] (It is worth recalling that Aristotle's circulation—and Galen's as well—is linear rather than circular; it resembles a network of irrigation ditches, the more so since the smallest channels were not supposed to have distinct walls.)

In accordance with the scheme laid down in the ninth century by ibn Ishaq (Joannitius) and later adopted by Avicenna and other Arabic writers, the European authors of textbooks on the gamut of medicine (anatomy, physiology, pathology, hygiene, and therapeutics) opened their works with a discussion of the seven "naturals": the elements, the temperaments, the humors, the parts ·of the body, the faculties, the operations, and the spirits. The two outstanding sixteenth-century books of this kind are the *Universa medicina* (Paris, 1554) of Jean Fernel and the *Institutiones medicinae* (Basel, 1594) of Leonhard Fuchs. Of the two writers, Fuchs is more rewarding for the present purposes. Citing Galen, Fuchs makes the point that it is incorrect to define similar parts as those composed throughout of like particles; although this definition fits certain of the similar parts (e.g., fibers, membranes, flesh, fat, bone, cartilage, and nerve), it does not fit others (e.g., veins and arteries; which are in fact composed of both fibers and membranes. Galen's reason for calling veins and arteries similar is that each of their parts resembles any other part of the whole, i.e., the similarity is structural rather than compositional.

The instrumental parts (*instrumentariae partes*) of animal bodies, which the Greeks called *organika moria*, are composed of simple parts and include such structures as the head, hand, heart, brain, liver, etc. Fuchs says it is important not to confuse instrumental parts with organs (*organa*). An instrumental part is one that is merely composite, whereas an organ (*instrumentum*) is, as its name indicates, a part capable of performing an action or function. Arteries, nerves, and veins, however, are at once organs and similar parts, for they distribute vital spirit, blood, and sense and motion throughout the body and are more or less "similar" throughout. But they are not, properly speaking, instrumental or organic parts.[9] What Fuchs is apparently saying is that a similar part may function as an organ, although it is not composite in structure. The organic parts, on the contrary, are always composite.

The semantic confusion at this time was so profound that most authors attempted a clarification before proceeding to substantive matters. In the sixteenth century Gabriele Falloppio, who wrote an extended treatise on the similar parts that has been called the first separate treatise on histology, commented on the double difficulty presented by the obscurity of the subject matter and the disagreements and contradictions found in Aristotle, Galen, and the Arabic writers. Falloppio held that Galen had excluded the humors from the category of similar parts because the latter were supposed to lend shape and form to the body; on the contrary, the humors were confined and limited by the similar parts. Falloppio states that Avicenna followed Galen rather than Aristotle in this respect, and that he will do likewise. His list of similar parts comprises bone, cartilage, fat, flesh, nerve, ligament, tendon, membrane, vein, artery, nails, hair, and skin.[10] Most physicians followed Galen and Avicenna in excluding the humors from the category of simple parts; in the *Universa medicina* of Barthélemy Pardoux, blood, milk, semen, and the spirits are excluded from that category on the ground that a part coheres in a whole and participates in the common life. The spirits, humors, and various fluids of the body do neither; they "wander away" (*deerrant*) in vessels. Pardoux found several reasons in Galen why the similar parts are so-called: because they are divisible into similar particles (Galen, cap. 6, lib. 1, *Meth.*); because they are similar and uniform throughout; and because they are not composed of other parts (Galen, 8, *De placitis*). From one point of view the veins and arteries are similar parts; from another, they are dissimilar, since they are composed of villi, i.e., "fibers," and membranes (cap. 2, *De inaequali intemperie*).

Galen states further (cap. 6, lib. 1, *De nat.fac.*) that the heart, liver, and brain belong among the similar parts by virtue of their uniform composition, but among the organic parts by virtue of their structure. Pardoux and other medical writers, including Galen, emphasize a histogenic distinction between spermatic and fleshy, or sanguineous, similar parts. The spermatic simple parts are supposed to arise from the seed, or semen, alone; they are the solid parts *kat'exochēn*, for they confer form and stability on the body as a whole. The fleshy similar parts, on the other hand, arise from the blood; they surround the solid parts and fill out the spaces between the fibers. There are three kinds of fleshy (*carnosae*) parts: *caro simplex*, or flesh proper, which is found between the muscle fibers; *parenchyma*, the substance composing the viscera; and a third kind that is said to contribute to the growth of parts that vary in size but remain the same respecting their content of spermatical parts. The *"spermatic similar parts"* of Pardoux corresponds loosely with the modern category of postmitotic tissues, i.e., tissues composed in part or whole of cells that do not divide in adult life and are not replaced when lost or damaged. Citing Galen's *De semine* and *De constitutione artis*, Pardoux says that the spermatical parts as a whole are never replaced when lost, because the necessary material and formative power is not available (*quod desit illis materia et vis opifex*). According to him there are two classes of villi, or fibers, common to all body parts capable of action: they are, on the one hand, fibers present in voluntary muscles, and, on the other, fibers that are woven into (*intertextae*) the organs of natural movement, i.e., the viscera. Fibers of the second class, says Pardoux citing Galen's *De usu partium*, are of three kinds: straight, transverse, and oblique, which serve respectively to attract, expel, and retain.[11]

A convenient account of the matter of spermatical and fleshy similar parts is available to the modern reader in Robert Burton's *Anatomy of Melancholy*, in which the spermatical similar, or homogeneal, parts are described as "immediately begotten of the seed," in contrast to the "fleshy or carnal" parts derived from the blood. Burton lists "bones, gristles, ligaments, membranes, nerves, arteries, skins, fibres or strings and fat" among the spermatical similar parts, and cites in this connection Laurentius, the physician of Henry IV of France.[12]

The Galenical fibers (with their powers of attracting, expelling, and retaining) mentioned by Pardoux were lineal descendants of the fibers of Plato, Aristotle, Erasistratus, and the other Greek writers who antedated Galen by many hundreds of years. Pardoux's use of the term *interwoven* (*intertextae*) with reference to the disposition of Galen's straight, transverse, and oblique fibers has been noted; examination of certain viscera, e.g., the stomach, with the naked eye would furnish a considerable degree of empirical support for this classification. In his *De humani corporis fabrica* (1543) Andreas Vesalius alludes to the visibly present weave of fibers in certain of the parts.[13] Charles O'Malley has commented that Vesalius's belief in the existence of Galen's attractive, expulsive, and retentive fibers was so strong that in at least one instance he described their presence where none were to be found. The term *fabrica* in the title of Vesalius's book seems to imply that the intimate structure of the body was analogous to a woven fabric; O'Malley, however, preferred to translate it as "structure" rather than "fabric" or "workings."[14] Moritz Roth, the nineteenth-century German biographer of Vesalius, also wished to avoid the implications of the word *fabric;* he, too, translated *fabrica* as "structure" (*Bau*)[15]

The mid-seventeenth-century introduction of high-powered magnifying lenses into the study of the fine structure of plants and animals provided strong empirical support for the traditional belief in the essentially fibrous character of living matter. "The whole substance, or all parts of a plant," wrote Nehemiah Grew in 1671, "consist of fibers." Even the pulpy flesh of fruits and the soft, malleable pith of stems consist of threads or fibers "wrapped and stitched (though in divers manners) together."[16] And Robert Hooke had found a few years earlier that the fleshy substance of mushrooms was made up of an "infinite company of small filaments every way contexted and woven together so as to make a kind of cloth." Hooke also observed that tanned leather appeared under the lens to be a texture of filaments, or fibers; he suggested that just as in the case of plants, "texture in animal substance" was ultimately fibrous throughout.[17] Hooke's "discovery" of the cell, incidentally, is usually presented in a quite misleading fashion. Hooke's cell was neither a structural nor a functional unit; it was simply a bounded space. Since he supposed that some of these spaces were in communication, he occasionally used the words *pore* and *cell* interchangeably.[18]

Throughout the seventeenth century, advances continued to be made in microscopic anatomy by a number of investigators. One of them, Marcello Malpighi, has been called the founder of histology.[19] There is no question but that Malpighi—who described the capillaries, the Malpighian corpuscles of the kidney and spleen, and the Malpighian rete of the epidermis—was an outstanding microscopic anatomist. But to call him the first histologist is to blur the distinction between microscopic anatomy, which requires a microscope, and histology, which involves a doctrine of similar parts or tissues. If we trace the tissue concept back to the doctrine of similar parts, Aristotle becomes the founder of histology. He was not, of course, a microscopic anatomist.

TISSUE THEORY

"Cellular Tissue"

By the middle of the eighteenth century, the belief that plant and animal substance was a tissue composed of fibers had won general acceptance. Writers used the terms *cell* and *cellular* for grossly visible enclosed spaces of any kind. These terms were applied also to the spaces intercepted by fibers and membranes in a ubiquitous tissue thought to be distributed throughout animal bodies, namely, in the cellular tissue. Albrecht von Haller held that the ultimate structural unit of living tissues was a hypothetical fiber too small to be seen even under the most powerful microscope. For the anatomist, said von Haller, this hypothetical, sub-microscopic fiber was the conceptual equivalent of the geometer's line; it was the ultimate structural basis of all anatomical forms, figures, and textures. Following earlier writers, von Haller described both laminar and fibrillar fibers. In his account of the *tela* ("web") *cellulosa,* or "cellular tissue," we learn that it consists of an "infinite number of little plates or scales, which, by their various directions, intercept small cells and web-like spaces." The cellular tissue was all but ubiquitous; it circumscribed and penetrated the various organs and at the same time bound them together in a structural whole. He mentions that the term *tela cellulosa* has been used in this sense by anatomists before him.[20] And the following lines by Voltaire tell us that in the middle of the eighteenth century the term had moved beyond scientific circles of discourse:

> Dans quels recoins de tissu cellulaire
> Sont les talents de Virgile ou d'Homère?[21]

Cellular tissue was destined to achieve great importance in early-nine-teenth-century theories of tumor histogenesis.

Bichat

On the basis of clinical observations, Philippe Pinel argued in his *Noso-graphie philosophique* that in the classification of diseases account should be taken of the resemblances imprinted on pathological processes by the similarity of the parts in which they run their course. Inflammation, for example, had long been recognized as having certain features in common wherever it occurred in the body; and, said Pinel, the number of these features increased in proportion to the structural resemblances of the parts involved. He thus regarded it as trivial to separate the various phlegmasias according to their anatomical locale, as nosographers had done before him. Although the pleura, the arachnoid, and the peritoneum are located in different parts of the body, the similarity of the inflammatory state as it is manifested in each of these membranes should not be obscured.

Pinel divided all diseases into five categories, the fifth being "organic lesions, or changes in the intimate structure of the parts." Generalized organic lesions were those affecting, or capable of affecting, all parts of the body; for example, scorbutus, gangrene, cancer, syphilis, and phthisis. He offered no suggestions as to the histogenesis of cancer, and his ideas of the nature of cancerous disease appear to have been derived almost entirely from Laennec, Bayle, and Dupuytren.[22]

François Bichat's preliminary papers on the membranes (later termed the *tissues*) appeared in the Memoirs of the medical society of Paris. His *Traité des membranes* was first published in 1800. The 1802 edition, published after Bichat's death (apparently due to a wound infection acquired in the autopsy room) in July of that year, contains a brief biography and a eulogy. While acclaiming Bichat's treatise as the most outstanding French medical work since Théophile Bordau's papers on the glands and the mucous tissue, and noting that it contained the germs of Bichat's later work on the physiology of life and death and on general anatomy, the eulogist, Henri-Marie Husson, claims that science is more indebted to Pinel's clinical observations than to Bichat's anatomical investigations. Bichat himself freely admitted his debt to Pinel, with the reservation that many of his own findings were quite different from Pinel's.[23]

The *Traité des membranes* opens with a discussion of membranes in general. According to Bichat these organs (*organes*), disseminated through all other organs and contributing to the intimate structure of most of them, had never before been treated by anatomists apart from the organs of which they are constituents. Hence their analogous characteristics had been largely overlooked. The following chapters of Bichat's treatise are devoted to the mucous membranes, serous membranes, fibrous membranes, composite membranes, and contranatural, or pathological, membranes. The arachnoid membrane and the synovial membranes are dealt with in subsections. In keeping with established anatomical tradition, Bichat does not limit himself to structural considerations; his is a functional histology. In connection with each of the membranes, he examines "vital forces" (sensibility, tonicity, etc.), functions, and, briefly, diseases. Bichat states that although von Haller had exhausted every other aspect of anatomy he failed to establish lines of division between the various membranes. He had erroneously supposed that they were all of like texture (*texture analogue*), each being a modification of the cellular organ (*organe cellulaire*) from which they were derived.[24] Bichat is stricter than many anatomists in his use of the term *cellular tissue* (*tissu cellulaire*), or cellular organ; for some anatomists it was roughly equivalent to what is now called connective tissue. Bichat points out that it had originally been called cellular because of its potential spaces, which could be made actual by the insufflation of air. According to Bernhard Albinus, Bichat added, the mucous membrane of the stomach is underlain by a dense lamina of *tissu cellulaire*, called the nervous coat (*tunique nerveuse*) by the older anatomists; but the layer in question "exhibits no character similar to that which the name imports." Rather, it was of fibrous texture.[25] Bichat refers to the serous membranes (pleura, pericardium, peritoneum, arachnoid, synovia) as *séreuses lymphatiques ou cellulaires*, and it is not clear whether he supposes that they are *cellular* in the strict sense of the word (Bichat's translator notes that English anatomists never apply the term *cellular* to the serous membranes).[26]

The familiar three Galenic fibers reappear in a slightly different form in Bichat. He states that there are three fibers fundamental to the animal economy: the fibers of tendons, ligaments, and fibrous membranes; the nervous fibers; and the muscle fibers.[27]

In his discussion of pathological membranes (*membranes contre nature*) Bichat briefly touches on questions of histogenesis, although without using that term. The "contranatural membranes" include cysts, scars, pyogenic membranes (as Bichat calls them elsewhere), and tumors. Bichat supposes that cysts arise when fluid collects in one of the cells of cellular tissue. As the fluid accumulates, the wall of the expanding cell becomes thickened by the incorporation of the walls of adjacent cells, and a large, closed sac is gradually formed. A fully grown cyst possesses an interior secretory lining and a fibrous wall. According to Bichat, a tumor is merely a cyst turned inside out; its secretion is directed outward and its cavity is obliterated. Although he was aware of the tentative and insufficient character of these suggestions, Bichat was convinced that cysts and tumors grew in accordance with laws analogous to those governing normal tissue growth. As for the precise mechanisms involved in the origin and continued growth of "contranatural membranes," he writes only: "Let us stop where first causes begin."[28]

This notion of the limits of histological knowledge seems rather narrowly drawn in the *Traité*. Bichat's scepticism concerning the microscope's value in anatomical investigations is also evident in this work.

Bichat observes that he cannot confirm the findings of Johann Lieber-
kuehn's "vaunted microscopic experiments" on the intestinal villi, and
adds that the microscope is an instrument "from which physiology and
anatomy do not seem to me...ever to have derived any great assistance,
because when we view an object obscurely, everyone sees it in his own
light, and according as he is affected."[29] One of the attractive features of
Bichat's *Traité* is its nondogmatic character; he is at least as concerned
with raising new questions as with answering old ones.

Bichat's most important work, the treatise *General Anatomy Applied to
Physiology and Medicine*, was published in 1801.[30] Here, too, Bichat made
no use of the microscope. He relied, as before, on the knife, naked eye,
and a few simple chemical reagents as tools sufficient for his analysis of
the parts and their function in health and disease. A contemporary of
Bichat, the histologist Jean-Baptiste Montfalcon, stated in 1821 that Bichat
"had a great and happy idea when he applied analysis to anatomy, when
he separated our organs and distinguished their elements. He showed
that these elements or simple tissues...have everywhere the same properties, whatever the composition formed by their union. After having
made this important discovery, he described the character of each tissue
in detail; he compared it with others, indicated its specific differences in
organization, described its form and function, and submitted it to various
known reagents. Such is the aim of general anatomy."[31] It is hard to
believe that Montfalcon was unaware that the "important discovery" he
attributed to Bichat was as old as Aristotle and had been part of medical
dogma ever since his time. The second part of Montfalcon's eulogy is,
regarding the source of Bichat's enduring fame, somewhat more enlight-
ening. It reveals that Bichat's concept of the tissues was based on functional and chemical as well as purely anatomical data. Thus, while he
cannot be called the father of histology—still less that of microscopic
anatomy—Bichat can, with considerable justification, be called the founder
of histochemistry, histophysiology, and histopathology.

Bichat's list of twenty-one tissues is in many respects reminiscent of
the lists of similar parts discussed above; in a sense Bichat was the reviver
of a time-honored anatomical scheme that had fallen into disuse in the
eighteenth century (it plays no role in von Haller's anatomy and physiology, for example). Bichat's twenty-one tissue systems are: (1) cellular;
(2) nervous, governing "animal" life; (3) nervous, governing "organic"
life; (4) arterial; (5) venous; (6) exhalant; (7) absorbent; (8) medullary;
(9) cartilaginous; (10) osseous; (11) fibrous; (12) fibrocartilaginous;
(13) muscular, governing "animal" life; (14) muscular, governing "organic" life; (15) mucous; (16) serous; (17) synovial; (18) glandular;
(19) dermoid; (20) epidermoid; and (21) pilous.[32] The similarity of this
list to the older lists of similar parts is obvious. Bichat follows Galen

rather than Aristotle and excludes fluid parts from his list of tissues. Most of Bichat's twenty-one tissues can be subsumed under the four categories generally accepted by contemporary histologists; epithelium, connective tissue, muscle, and nerve. Four of Bichat's tissues fall under the heading of epithelium (epidermoid, mucous, serous, and synovial); six under connective tissue (dermoid, fibrous, fibrocartilaginous, cartilaginous, osseous, and cellular); two under muscle; and two under nerve —the distinction between nervous governing "animal" life and nervous governing "organic" life corresponds with that between the voluntary and involuntary nervous systems. The arteries and the veins, long sources of contention, are classified today as compound tissues. The absorbents and the exhalants (which Bichat thought to be open-ended vessels) have dropped out or been replaced by the lymphatics. His medullary system has no counterpart among the present-day tissues.

Bichat's "general anatomy" has even less in common with the discipline of histology than might be supposed. Aside from his lack of concern with microscopic anatomy, Bichat embraced many aspects of theoretical medicine and physiology:

> I will make but one remark upon the experiments contained in this work; amongst them will be found a series upon the simple textures (*tissus*), which I subjected successively to desiccation, putrefaction, maceration, ebullition, stewing, and to the action of the acids and alkalis. It will easily be seen that it was not the object of these experiments to . . .give a chemical analysis of simple textures; for this purpose they would have been sufficient; but their object was to establish the distinctive characters of these simple textures, and to show that each has a peculiar organization, as each has a peculiar life . . . .The different reagents that I used were only to assist me where the scalpel was insufficient.[33]

Besides illustrating Bichat's chemical procedures, this passage, with its reference to the "peculiar life" of the individual tissues, calls attention to a resemblance between the current concept of the cell and Bichat's concept of the tissue. Today the cell is believed to be the unit locus of independent life; Bichat accorded the tissue that place. According to Bichat, the fundamental vital properties of irritability and contractility were resident in the tissues, each of which was alive and responsive in its characteristic fashion. Unlike his vitalist predecessors, Bichat does not refer life to a generalized vital principle, or *archeus*. Although he was not the first to conceive of a separate life of the body parts, a *vita propria*, he seems to have been the first to locate it in the tissues rather than in the organs or in the body as a whole.

Alternative classifications were soon forthcoming. In his 1821 review of French lists, Montfalcon mentions Hippolyte Cloquet's list of tissues (cellular, membranous, vascular, osseous, cartilaginous, fibrocartilaginous, ligamentous, muscular, tendinous, aponeurotic, nervous, and glandular); Anthelme-Balthasar Richerand's and Guillaume Dupuytren's eleven tissues (cellular, vascular, nervous, osseous, fibrous, muscular, erectile, mucous, serous, epidermoid, and parenchymatous); and his own list of three "fundamental" tissues (cellular, vascular, and nervous), which, he claimed, composed the others.[34] In Italy in the first decade of the nineteenth century, four tissues were distinguished by Giacomo Tommasini and seven by Stefano Gallini. In Germany, eleven tissues derived from embryonic cellular tissue were described by Philipp von Walther. In 1809 Karl Rudolphi followed Bichat's procedure and divided the tissues along structural, functional, and chemical lines into eight systems — *tela cellulosa, tela ossea, tela cartilaginea, fibra v. tela tendinea, tela v. fibra cornea, fibra arteriosa, fibra muscularis,* and *fibra nervea.* In his physiology textbook of 1821 Rudolphi revived the old terminology and defined *similar parts* as structures present throughout the body, and *simple parts* as simple but not ubiquitous tissues.[35]

A "cellular tissue" appears in all of these lists; as Burkard Eble pointed out in 1836, Bichat had to some extent revived von Haller's "cellular tissue." In the latter part of the eighteenth century a number of observers (including Caspar Friedrich Wolff, Georg Prochaska, and Johann Blumenbach) had denied that von Haller's fibers, plates, and intercepted cells existed as such in the living state.[36] The description of the *tissu cellulaire* in Bichat appears to have been taken almost verbatim from von Haller; it is described as an aggregate of soft, whitish filaments and plates intertwining and interlacing to create a large number of irregularly shaped, intercommunicating cells of various sizes, which serve as "reservoirs of fat and serosity." Like von Haller, Bichat stated that the cellular tissue surrounds the body organs and penetrates into their depths, at once separating and binding them together.[37]

The younger Meckel, Ignaz Doellinger, and Karl Rudolphi joined the ranks of those who denied the existence of von Haller's cellular tissue, and they continued to deny it after Bichat's work had become well known. These anatomists held that the so-called cellular tissue was actually an amorphous, semifluid ground substance, perhaps containing an admixture of small globules. In 1821, Rudolphi wrote that the cellular tissue was an amorphous semifluid substance in the living state; only after death did it coagulate into the "fibers and plates that were formerly regarded as the basic constituents of the organism." He stated that he would have prefered, following Théophile Bordeu, to call the tissue in question *mucous tissue (Schleimgewebe, tissu muqueux)* but the term *mucous* had already acquired a fixed meaning. Rudolphi added that although the term *cellular tissue* was poorly chosen its meaning was well understood, and he mentioned the "old and correct observation" that if all other body components were removed, outlines of the body and its contained organs would still be visible.[38]

Not only are there no *cells* (in either the current or in von Haller's sense of the term) in the cellular tissue of the eighteenth- and early-nineteenth-century investigators, there may indeed be no *tissue*. Unless this is understood, statements made by biologists of that time prove extremely puzzling. Early in the nineteenth century we find J. B. Lamarck, for example, claiming that protozoa are gelatinous, translucent organisms, devoid of structure and composed only of a *"masse de tissu cellulaire variée"*[39] A few years later Hippolyte Royer-Collard stated that the *tissu cellulaire primitif,* of which protozoa consist, was the equivalent of that "matter which has been termed *plastic lymph."*[40] In 1833 Johannes Mueller stated, in his textbook of physiology, that cellular tissue (*Zellgewebe*) was composed of minute fibers. He rejected the claim of Bordeu and Wolff that it consisted of an amorphous mucus, or *Schleim,* and added that certain investigators had reached the "fantastic conclusion that in the embryo all organs are generated from cellular tissue," whereas he himself believed them to be generated from an amorphous blastema.[41] But it is obvious that the objective referent of Mueller's "blastema" and the generative "cellular tissue" of the unnamed investigators was one and the same.

TISSUES AND TUMORS

Tissu Cellulaire

Bichat ascribes unique reproductive powers to his ubiquitous cellular tissue. It has the faculty of "throwing out a kind of vegetation, of elongating and reproducing itself, of growing when it has been cut or divided." And it is upon this faculty that the formation of cicatrices, tumors, and cysts depends.[42] The tumors of which he speaks are not mere inflammatory swellings or infiltrations of the tissues by extraneous substances, but overgrowths of the *tissu cellulaire.* Like the normal organs of the body, the various kinds of tumors—spongy fungoid growths, fleshy sarcomatous tumors, cancers, and polyps—have, according to Bichat, a vascular and cellular nutritive base, which is the part of the lesion where true growth occurs. "All tumors, then, are cellular," writes Bichat. Tumors differ from one another only with respect to the character of the matter deposited in the cellular base in consequence of "morbid alterations" occurring therein.[43] Even tumors of muscular, tendinous, or cartilaginous character begin as overgrowths of cellular texture. The characteristic matter is later deposited in the nutritive base: "Examine the tumours that appear in the muscles, the tendons, the cartilages, etc.; you will not see there an expansion of fleshy, or tendinous fibres, or of the cartilaginous substance, etc.; the cellular texture alone goes from the organ and is spread in the tumour."[44]

Bichat's theory of the histogenesis of tumors is a theory of the histogenesis of the stroma of tumors, i.e., of the nutritive base of tumors, as presently understood. Further insight can be gained from what Bichat has to say on the structure of cysts. A cyst is a "membrane, in the form of a sac without an opening, which is accidentally developed, and which, containing fluids of different nature, has been on this account divided into many species." Cysts, like tumors, are basically overgrowths of the cellular texture and differ only in the nature of the fluid or semisolid substances accumulating within them during their growth. Bichat says that a tumor "throw[s] from...[its]...external surface the fluid that is separated there," whereas a cyst "exhales this fluid by its internal surface."[45]

One might have expected Bichat to give additional attention to the histogenesis of tumors in his lectures on pathological anatomy delivered in Paris shortly before his untimely death in 1802. However, the only account we have of these lectures adds nothing to the subject and is, in any case, of questionable validity. These lectures, which were first published in 1825, derive from a manuscript by P. A. Béclard, and it appears that Béclard did not reach Paris until long after Bichat's death.[46] In the lectures, diseases are divided into two classes, functional and organic, the same distinction made by Matthew Baillie in his *Morbid Anatomy* (1793). However, Bichat deals with lesions of tissues, whereas Baillie deals with lesions of organs.[47]

The French School

According to Jean Cruveilhier, Guillaume Dupuytren delivered a course of lectures on pathological anatomy at Paris in 1803.[48] Cruveilhier wrote that Dupuytren "established the species, genera, orders and classes of organic lesions, elevated pathological anatomy to the rank of a science and gave it an appropriate code of laws." Afterward, Dupuytren's ideas were elaborated by Gaspard-Laurent Bayle, René Laennec, and others. The only record of Dupuytren's views at this time is in an 1805 article, presumably written by Dupuytren himself, in the bulletin of the medical school at Paris, in which Dupuytren is given priority over Bichat in moving from organ to tissue pathology. He divided anatomic lesions into four categories: (1) those composed of "analogous tissues"; (2) those "without analogues in the normal tissues"; (3) those differing in accord-

ance with the nature of the parts in which they have developed; and
(4) malformations, which subdivides into two groups—those due to
"defects in the organization of the germ" and those that develop after
conception. The transformation of one kind of tissue into another falls
under Dupuytren's first category: cellular, adipose, fibrous, bony, and
cartilaginous transformations are mentioned. The second category includes "inflammation . . . white degeneration, encysted tuberculous affection . . . scirrhous, cancerous and carcinomatous affections . . . hydatids,
etc."[49]

René Laennec, who is better known as a clinician and as the inventor
of the stethoscope than as a pathologist, was one of Bichat's pupils. In
1812 he contributed an important article on pathological anatomy to the
Dictionnaire des sciences médicales.[50] The article requires careful reading to
be correctly understood; Laennec employs the term *organic* as an equivalent of *structural* or *visible* when it qualifies *lesion*, and he often uses *organ*
where we would use *tissue*. Laennec says that the novelty of Bichat's
approach to pathological anatomy lay in his claim that "every type of
lesion always presents the same manifestations in all organs [read *tissues*]
belonging to the same system, whatever the difference of form and
function between the parts [read *organs*] into the composition of which
these organs [read *tissues*] enter." This new way of regarding lesions
changed the face of pathology, says Laennec. But in the end it led Bichat
into error by inclining him to believe that "every system of organs [read
tissues] had a large number of lesions found in it alone." Hence his
erroneous claim that "tubercles were peculiar to the tissue of the lungs,
serous cysts to the cellular tissue, ossification to the fibrous system, and
so on." Eventually Bichat concluded, according to Laennec, that there
were only two lesions common to all tissues, namely, inflammation and
cancer (scirrhus).[51]

Contrary to Bichat (and anticipating present-day opinion), Laennec
contended that all varieties of lesions would eventually be found to occur
throughout the organs and the tissues.[52] However, he followed Bichat in
dividing diseases into two classes: *maladies organiques* and *maladies nerveuses,* characterized, respectively, by the presence and the absence of
visible lesions. Laennec defined pathological anatomy as the study of
visible alterations produced by disease. Neither he nor any other pathologist of his time regarded anatomical lesions as other than products of a
disease process, i.e., they did not take the static view of disease so often
imputed to them by later writers. As pathologists they recognized the
existence of diseases that pathological anatomy could not explain by an
underlying visible lesion. In such diseases the symptoms were thought to
be functional or nervous in origin. To call a disease nervous (as opposed

to organic) did not necessarily imply that emotional disturbances were involved, either as cause or as consequence; it simply meant that the body's physiological workings were deranged in the absence of a visible anatomical lesion. Apparently physicians diagnosed the *maladies nerveuses* largely by exclusion. Laennec states, for example, that if a patient complains of difficulty in breathing, and if his physician can find "no signs indicating pulmonary pathology, heart disease, aneurysm of the great vessels, or any other organic affection of the parts contained in the thorax, then it may be concluded that the disease is nervous."[53]

Laennec rejected all purely anatomical classifications of organic diseases, whether based on the organs (G. B. Morgagni, Matthew Baillie) or on the tissues (Bichat) involved, in favor of a scheme of his own. The basis of his classification was partly functional, partly structural, and partly etiological. Organic lesions were grouped under four headings: (1) hypertrophic and atrophic changes brought about by increased or decreased tissue nutrition, respectively; (2) alterations of texture, (3) alterations in the form or position of organs; and (4) parasitic productions, i.e., living foreign bodies. Tissue lesions or textural alterations resulted from either trauma, the local accumulation of some naturally occurring substance, inflammation, or the accidental development of a tissue or local accumulation of a substance not normally present at that site. In the last category Laennec included both varieties of accidental tissues, or substances, i.e., those with and those without analogues in normal tissues.[54] He separated inflammatory from true tumors, although he was willing to grant that the inflammatory process was sometimes the "occasional cause of the formation of many accidental tissues and morbific substances."[55]

Laennec stated that he preferred to follow Morgagni's procedure in the study of anatomical lesions, i.e., the "successive examination of all alterations in each organ." In the study of textural alterations or tissue lesions, however, he found this procedure repetitious. He pointed out that such lesions presented the same features wherever they occurred in the body.[56] This idea of Laennec's has often been ascribed, erroneously, to Bichat. Rudolf Virchow may have been the first to do so when he claimed (in 1895) that Bichat's desire to base pathological anatomy on the doctrine of the tissues had failed to reach fruition because his pupils returned to the older doctrine of organ pathology.[57] If we are to believe Laennec, however, it was precisely Bichat's position that each system of tissues had its own characteristic set of lesions and only inflammatory and cancerous lesions were found in all tissues. Laennec held, on the contrary, that most lesions presented the same features regardless of the tissue in which they occurred, and further, stated that inflammatory lesions sometimes presented *different* features in the *same* tissue. In the skin, for example, inflammatory processes due to "insect-bite, the inoculation of anthrax or the virus of small-pox" differed in appearance.[58]

Accidental tumors, tissues, and textures often resembled one or more of the normal tissues of healthy organs. Such lesions could, wrote Laennec, readily be classified in accordance with the normal tissue or tissues they most closely resembled. But the classification of accidental tumors composed of tissues or of substances without normal analogues constituted a knottier problem. Such lesions were prone to "change continually, both in nature and appearance," and to undergo self-destructive changes at one point while continuing to grow at another. Lesions of this kind, so-called cancerous lesions, included tubercle, scirrhus, melanosis, and encephaloid.[59]

What were the criteria for the recognition of cancerous lesions at this time? Or, as Bayle and Jean-Baptiste Cayol asked in 1813, how could lesions arising variously on the skin and mucous membranes, in the bones, viscera, and soft parts generally, and appearing randomly as ulcers, tumors, excavations, excrescences, indurations, and softenings, be grouped under the common designation of cancer? Bayle and Cayol replied that a cancerous lesion (1) spreads gradually, inevitably, and destructively; (2) is ultimately fatal if left untreated, even though it may lie dormant for many years; (3) is prone to return after removal, either in the original location or elsewhere in the body; and (4) causes a nutritional disturbance leading ultimately to cachexia. The clinical behavior of a lesion is therefore the ultimate criterion of its cancerous nature. (Bayle and Cayol give a graphic description of the course of untreated cancer of the breast in their *Dictionnaire* article.[60])

In the absence of modern cell theory and relying almost exclusively on observations of the naked eye, the histopathologists of the first four decades of the nineteenth century had no means of distinguishing between the truly neoplastic part of a tumor mass and its accessory supporting tissues. Indeed, they had great difficulty in distinguishing the tumor mass from adjacent or included normal tissues. Laennec states, for example, that scirrhous cancers arising in the stomach are almost always accompanied by hypertrophy of the gastric musculature;[61] he was probably misled by the diffuse manner of spread characteristic of that form of cancerous growth. In general he looked on tumors as composite growths, i.e. as made up of several "accidental tissues" in close combination.

Laennec was not even certain that the term *tissue* was properly applicable to all tumor components. Was the encephaloid or cerebriform matter, which at times made up the bulk of a cancerous tumor, a tissue in the literal sense? Like the other components of cancers, this matter underwent a series of changes over the course of time. At the height of its development, writes Laennec, it is "homogeneous, milk-white, and almost like brain substance...cut into thin slices it is delicately translucent; when examined in slightly thicker pieces it is opaque." In gastric cancers the same matter was at times diffusely present throughout the stomach wall or present as a local accumulation with a "centrally placed, irregularly circular or ovoid depression...the surface of which is rather flat and often smooth"—an appearance somewhat resembling that produced by "a blow of a hammer on a mass of lead."[62] In discussing the spread of tumors from the stomach to the liver, Laennec commented on the characteristic central depression, or umbilication, of the exposed surfaces of the secondary deposits.[63] From Bayle and Cayol's criteria for cancerous growths, it is clear that pathological anatomists were well aware of the tendency of cancer to involve distant organs in its spread.

The term *degeneration* as used by Laennec is important enough to warrant special consideration; he sometimes refers to cerebriform degeneration rather than cerebriform matter. As ordinarily used by physicians, *degeneration* designated "a change in the nature of some object or other...a passage from the original state to one lower or worse." Thus physicians would speak of a simple tumor degenerating into a cancer or, perhaps, refer to the degeneration of a scirrhus into a cancer. In Laennec's opinion, however, when a tumor of osseous, tuberculous, or scirrhous character arose it did so not as a *transformation* of the organ or tissue involved but as a *new formation.* It represented a "new creation,...an accidental production, foreign to the usual state of the animal economy and in no way a 'degeneration' of one of the constituent parts."[64] His notion of the mechanism of new formation is as follows: a morbid substance is deposited in the meshes of the normal tissue, "somehow infiltrating and compressing" the tissue.[65] One of Laennec's definitions of *degeneration,* namely, the "deposition of an accidental substance in the interstices of normal tissue," would serve equally well as a definition of what today is called *infiltration.*[66]

Apparently, Laennec was trying to distinguish between the transformation and the mere infiltration of a tissue. He states that the transformation of lymph nodes or of the parenchyma of a viscus into tuberculous or cerebriform matter represents degeneration. On the other hand, the term ought not be applied to a "tuberculous mass developed in the lung" or to a "cerebriform tumor" arising in the cellular tissue.[67] How then can a distinction be made between degeneration, i.e., transformation, and infiltration? Laennec has a rather subtle criterion: a degenerative process leaves no demarcation between normal tissue and morbid substance (or tissue); in an infiltrative process a rim of normal tissue may be identified before complete replacement by the infiltrating mass has occurred. Laennec admits that the distinction is not easy to employ in practice. It is difficult for the pathologist to ascertain whether the total conversion of an organ or a part of an organ into a particular morbid substance "results from successive deposits of that substance in the interstices of the original tissue...or from the development of a unique tumor which, due to continual pressure, has entirely destroyed the organ whose place it occupies."[68]

Laennec's attempt to distinguish infiltration from transformation (degeneration), with the relatively limited technical and conceptual means available to him, can only be admired. The distinction itself remains valid and important today. Laennec's description of a tissue undergoing transformation with "no addition of foreign matter" — namely, the transformation occurring in the mucosal tissues of a prolapsed vagina or rectum when the mucous membranes are seen to "take on the color and the greater part of the characteristics of the skin" — is readily recognized as the tissue change known today as keratinizing squamous metaplasia.[69] Laennec's concept of degeneration was partly coextensive with his concept of accidental tissue formation; he describes accidental cartilage as cartilage present "where it ought not, in accordance with the usual laws of nature, be present."[70] Little or no progress was made beyond this point in the structural analysis of tumors and tissue transformations until the microscope and the cell theory appeared on the scene some three decades later.

The Third Version of Humoralism

It will be recalled that classical humoralism rested on the Hippocratic corpus and the writings of Aristotle. Systematized by Galen and the Arabic medical writers, it was taught in the universities of Europe up to the middle of the seventeenth century. By the end of that century it had become almost obsolete; other than at Paris and a few other strongholds of Galenism, its place had been taken by a second version of humoralism, the creation of such sixteenth- and seventeenth-century iatrochemists as Paracelsus, van Helmont, Sylvius, and Willis, which spoke of fermentation, putrefaction, acidity, acridity, and other features of spagyrical chemistry. But this second version of humoralism, too, lost its credibility at a rapid rate. Toward the end of the eighteenth century, it received its death blow with Antoine Lavoisier's reformulation of chemical language and theory.

The decline of the second version of humoralism was probably hastened by the rising interest among physicians in pathological anatomy following the work of Morgagni. Another feature of late-eighteenth-century medical thought was the emphasis on the role of the nervous system in disease. Here, too, attention was directed toward the solid rather than the fluid parts of the body. An important principle in the neural pathology of this time was irritability: in William E. Horner's treatise on pathology (1829), the old is combined with the new to create such chapter headings as "Irritations of Cellular Tissue," "Irritations of Pulmonary Tissue," and so on.[71]

Writing in 1841, the French pathologist August Chomel stated that the first three decades of the nineteenth century had been characterized by an almost exclusively solidistic approach to the pathogenesis of disease. He claimed to have been one of the first to raise his voice against this approach.[72] Chomel counted himself among the proponents of the third incarnation of humoralism, the roots of which sprang from the late-eighteenth-century thought of John Hunter and William Hewson.[73] The new humoralism (which survived Lavoisier's reform of chemistry) shifted the emphasis toward chemical changes demonstrable in the blood and other body fluids during the course of disease. As examples of such changes Chomel cites the "decrease of albumen in the blood in Bright's disease and its appearance in the urine; the change in composition of the blood relative to its content of fibrin and globules in inflammatory disease," as well as other chemical changes in milk, urine, and saliva, as accompaniments of disease.[74] The new humoralism had started as a revival of the doctrines of Hunter and Hewson and had gone on to develop them further. The plastic lymph (later to be termed *blastema*) was thought to be a fluid, formative substance carried in the circulating blood and distributed to the tissues; it was supposed to constitute the material basis for the maintenance, growth, and repair of the solid parts. Chomel's remarks reveal that by 1841 the third form of humoralism had taken on features familiar to today's physician.

One of the most influential proponents of the new doctrine of humoralism was the German chemist Justus Liebig. Liebig's book on organic chemistry as applied to physiology and pathology was published in 1842.[75] As noted above, the generally accepted belief, to which Liebig also subscribed, was that a "plasma" or "blastema" consisting chiefly of albumen and fibrin derived directly from ingested foodstuffs circulated in the blood and was distributed to the tissues. There it became incorporated into the solid parts of the body.[76] Liebig stated, as had Aristotle two thousand years earlier, that a wooden rod stirred in freshly drawn blood would pick up soft, elastic fibers. He supposed these fibers, representing the fibrin of the blood, to be similar in most respects to muscle fibers. The serum remaining behind after the fibers had been removed contained a substance that formed, upon heating, a "white elastic mass...called albumen and identical in all its properties with egg white." Liebig concluded that proteinaceous substances move in a great metabolic or nutritive circle from food to blood to tissue and back again to food. "Albumen and fibrine, in the process of nutrition, are capable of being converted into muscular fibre," he writes, "and muscular fibre is capable of being reconverted into blood...these facts have long since been established by physiologists."[77]

Liebig could discern no chemical difference between plant and animal fibrins and albumens. The blood proteins derived from plants were necessarily the "starting point of all other animal tissues"; hence the name *protein*, "from *prōteuō*, 'I take first rank'," a term first used by the Dutch physician and biochemist Gerard Mulder.[78] Mulder had shown in 1838 that albumen, fibrin, and casein were modifications of a single substance having the chemical formula $C_{40}H_{31}N_5O_{12}$. In its natural state this substance was variously combined with sulphur, phosphorus, and other elements.[79]

A German-born pathological anatomist, J. F. Lobstein, attempted the first account of tumor histogenesis in light of the new version of humoralism.[80] Lobstein held that the first step in the formation of an accidental tissue—whether homeoplastic, i.e., with a normal tissue analogue, or heteroplastic, i.e., without a normal analogue—was the movement of a "substance capable of organizing itself," a "coagulable lymph," from the blood to the tissues. By *organization* he meant the transformation of an amorphous fluid exudate into a structured, solid tissue, whether homeoplastic or heteroplastic in character.[81] The phenomenon of organization (explained today by the growth of tissue into an exudate, rather than by the transformation of an exudate into a tissue) was real enough. Lobstein saw that it could not be accounted for by the principles of solidist physiology and pathology, namely, sensibility, irritability, and contractility. Lobstein argued for the existence of a plastic force (*force plastique*) resident in the body, a force of unknown nature and mode of operation, but somehow capable of transforming amorphous exudates into structured tissues. The *force plastique* first manifests itself in the sequences of embryonic development and remains operative throughout the life of the organism, preserving the body parts in their original form and regenerating them, within limits, after injury or disease.[82]

Did a similar *force plastique* determine the growth of homeoplastic and heteroplastic accidental tissues, and did the formation of these tissues require merely an abnormality of the exuded coagulable lymph? Or was the coagulable lymph normal and the *force plastique* somehow deranged? Lobstein suggested the second alternative for homeoplastic accidental tissues and the first for heteroplastic accidental tissues. Normal (euplastic) coagulable lymph, he said, had a counterpart (kakoplastic lymph) that formed the substrate of lardaceous, fungus-medullary, and scirrho-cancerous new formations.[83] Homeoplastic growths reflected excessive or accelerated tissue nutrition; heteroplastic growths, with respect to their substance, were anomalous as well. To a degree, Lobstein agreed with François Broussais and other believers in the inflammatory pathogenesis of cancer, but he argued that "aberrations of pathologic nutrition," and the consequent new growths of heteroplastic accidental tissue, were too varied in character to result from ordinary inflammation.[84]

Formative Molecules

Lobstein may have been the first to draw a strict analogy between embryogenesis and the genesis of tumors. But it was inevitable, once tumors had been recognized as constituent parts of the body rather than independent parasites, and as organized aggregates of tissues rather than abnormal accumulations of humors, that someone would do so. Lobstein develops the comparison as follows:

> Once the initial *molecule* of each of these heteroplastic growths is deposited in an organ, it grows and develops therein exactly as the organs themselves grow and develop. In the cellular tissue of an embryo Nature deposits a *molecule* of organic matter corresponding to the larynx. Little by little this *molecule* changes into the thyroid body. Likewise, the germ of a fibrous body deposited in the uterus grows and develops in accordance with a life-process. The primitive natural organs form without the aid of inflammation. No doubt the same may be said of those engendered by disease, since it is more rational to explain organic alterations by means of the laws of life than to devise a new physiology for the disease state.[85]

If *cell* were read for *molecule,* the above passage would fit the current notion of the development of metastatic tumors. By *molecule* Lobstein meant a small but visible mass. Georges Buffon, in the eighteenth century, had spoken of "organic molecules" as hypothetical, ultimate living particles characteristic of plants and animals. In 1828 Robert Brown called attention to certain active or elementary "molecules" visible under the highest powers of the microscope. They were, he supposed, the "elementary molecules or organic bodies, first so considered by Buffon and Needham...and, very recently by Dr. Milne Edwards, who has revived the doctrine."[86] And as late as 1863 John Hughes Bennett (in his *Lectures on Molecular Physiology, Pathology, and Therapeutics*) was concerned with the "visible molecules of the histologist" rather than the "hypothetical molecules of the chemist."[87] Thus Lobstein's hypothesis, as fanciful as it may seem to a modern biologist, had an empirical basis.

In trying to account for the origin, growth, and maintenance of embryonic and adult tissues, Lobstein adopted as his model the development of solid tissue from fluid blood. He equated the fibrinous fibers of clotted blood with muscle and tissue fibers, an equation that subsequently found support in the results of chemical analysis. The commonplace observation that exudates of various kinds—on the surfaces of ulcers, between the edges of incised wounds, between inflamed loops of gut, and so on—underwent transformation into solid tissues offered additional support to Lobstein's hypothesis.

Lobstein's account of scirrho-cancerous new formations is illustrative of his approach to the study of tumor structure. Seen under the magnifying glass, he writes, such tumors consist of intermingled horny translucent and fibrous opaque substances. He supposes that the opaque substance is "fibrous and cellular tissue" and the interpenetrating translucent matter, albumen. As the tumor increases in size a third component becomes evident, which, because of its resemblance in appearance and consistency to the brain, he called cerebriform matter. Chemical analysis of one such scirrho-cancerous tumor of the breast revealed that its chief constituents were albumen, fibrin, and gelatin.[88] Lobstein was able to find blood vessels in the tumor mass of a cancer of the breast only after the development of cerebriform matter. He interpreted this observation —which, because of its reliance on the naked eye or a low power lens, was faulty—to mean that in the first stages of their growth heteroplastic lesions consisted entirely of abnormal matter. Later, heteroplastic tissue might be changed into homeoplastic tissue in the course of natural healing.[89]

While pathological histologists of the premicroscopic era invariably refer to homologous or homeoplastic tumors as tissues, they often refer to heterologous or heteroplastic tumors as substances. This reflects some uncertainty whether heterologous lesions are tissues in the proper sense, i.e., composed of fibers. Cancerous lesions often contained varying quantities of fluid or semifluid matter intermixed with fibers. No special attention or significance was given to the semifluid component until Jean Cruveilhier argued in 1827 that the only difference between scirrhous cancers and cerebriform cancers was the greater amount of semifluid in the latter. Christening this component "cancer-juice", Cruveilhier describes it as a "grayish gruel...peculiar to cancerous tissue." It represents the truly cancerous component.[90] In his essay of 1816 Cruveilhier does not mention cancer-juice, but states that scirrhous cancer is "apparently formed of a fibrous and cellular tissue permeated by albumen."[91]

Andral

Another important member of the early-nineteenth-century Paris school of pathological anatomists was Gabriel Andral. His treatise on pathological anatomy was translated into English shortly after its publication in France in 1829.[92] Despite Andral's attempts to eliminate the concept of cancer as a disease or lesion *sui generis,* his views on the subject hardly differ from those of Lobstein and Laennec. Cancer, according to Andral, is not a separate kind of lesion but an end-stage of a number of lesions, chiefly characterized by spreading ulceration and necrosis: "This quite metaphorical expression signifies only the common termination of alterations greatly differing from each other." *Cancer,* like *inflammation,* "belongs to the infancy of science."[93]

In Andral's opinion, lesions involving hypertrophy, atrophy, or transformation of tissue were ultimately due to disturbances of nutritive and secretory processes at the tissue level. The literal meaning of *hypertrophy* is overnutrition, and the visible result of overnutrition, according to Andral and others, was an increase in the mass of the organ or tissue involved. Andral held the term hypertrophy to be solely applicable in instances where the normal structure and organization of the part involved was preserved, although he allowed for a certain degree of structural distortion resulting from the hypertrophy of a single component in a composite organ. In the case of the *tissu cellulaire*—the most ubiquitous of all tissues and the one most prone to undergo hypertrophy —the visible result of such overgrowth might appear variously as "striations, whitish layers, tumors of various sizes and shapes...composed of cellular tissue that has become increasingly condensed, and terminating by resembling...now the cut surface of a turnip, with dull white lines streaking a grayish parenchyma, now lard, now imperfect cartilage of the kind to be seen in the earliest stages of fetal life."[94]

The *tissu cellulaire* was also the most frequent site of tissue transformation, according to Andral. "In this same cellular element, the common framework of all embryonic tissue," he writes, "all tissues may undergo accidental development."[95] Malignant or cancerous lesions, however, involved something more than the hypertrophy or even the transformation of preexisting tissues. Andral believed that a nutritive-secretory disturbance, which led to the production of a morbid secretion, was at the root of the cancer process. Andral divided these secretions into those capable of developing into solid structures and those lacking this capability, including among the latter pus, tubercle, and gelatinous and fatty matter. *Scirrhous cancer, encephaloid cancer, sarcoma, fungus hematodes,* said Andral, were mere names, arbitrarily imposed on different kinds of more or less organized morbid secretions. Scirrhus and encephaloid are,

in fact, "nuances of the same morbid alterations"; they represent hypertrophy of the *tissu cellulaire* in combination with one or more products of
morbid secretion.[96]

ENGLISH AND SCOTCH INVESTIGATORS

At the beginning of the nineteenth century in England the Society for
Investigating the Nature and Cure of Cancer formulated a series of
thirteen questions in regard to the character of that disease. "Does any
alteration in the structure of a part take place, preceding that more
obvious change which is called cancer; and if there be an alteration, what
is its nature?" was the second of these questions.[97] In 1804 John Abernethy
attempted to answer that question and in doing so put forward a classification of tumors based on gross anatomical structure, pointing out that the
study of tumors was properly a part of morbid anatomy.[98] He made the
important proposal that the term tumor should be limited to "such .
swellings as arise from some new production, which made no part of the
original composition of the body."[99] Abernethy subscribed to the belief
that tumors were formed by the organization of exuded coagulable lymph.
"The coagulable part of the blood being either accidentally effused, or
deposited in consequence of disease," it then becomes "an organized and
living part, by the growth of the adjacent vessels and nerves into
it....Thus an unorganized concrete becomes a living tumour...though
it derives a supply of nourishment from the surrounding parts, it seems
to live and grow by its own independent powers; and the future structure
which it may acquire seems to depend on the operation of its vessels."
Although the structure of a tumor often resembled that of the adjacent
parts, there were many instances in which this was not true. Hence, "we
seem warranted in concluding, that in many cases the nature of the
tumour depends on its own actions and organization; and that, like the
embryon, it merely receives nourishment from the surrounding part."[100]
Abernethy's investigations of tumor structure antedated the transmission
to England of Bichat's concept of tissues; consequently, his gross anatomical
classification of tumors lacks a histological basis.

Abernethy gave a concise and satisfactory answer to the question of
the need for an appropriate morphological classification of tumors. "An
arrangement of tumours once made, so that the history of each species
could be particularly remarked," he observes, "we might perhaps be
able...to form a probable opinion of the nature of the tumour and of the
mode of treatment which it would require; and, by adverting to the
structure of the removed tumour after an operation, we might determine
whether it would be right to remove or leave the contiguous parts."[101] He

suggested that when an organizable coagulum, or plastic lymph, was not deposited locally in consequence of injury or inflammation, a similar deposition might result from the "diseased action" of the surrounding vessels, in which case the only hope of cure would lie in a surgical excision wide enough to include not only the tumor but also the abnormally acting vessels.[102] The concept of diseased actions of vessels was probably derived from John Hunter, whereas the observation that unencapsulated poorly defined tumors are apt to recur after local excision had long since been made by surgeons.

Proceeding in the systematic manner of an eighteenth-century nosologist, Abernethy divided the class of local diseases into several orders. The order of tumors was, in turn, subdivided into genera and species. "Sarcomas or sarcomatous tumours," which receive their name from their "firm and fleshy feel," constitute one of these genera, says Abernethy, "encysted tumours" a second, and "osseous tumours" a third. Abernethy's genus of sarcomatous tumors contains eight species, including a "carcinomatous sarcoma." A common tumor of the female breast, it had been called scirrhus before it underwent ulceration and carcinoma thereafter; Abernethy favored his own term because not all of these tumors were significantly hard or indurated. Such tumors rapidly extended to the adjacent axillary lymph glands and frequently reached the glands along the internal mammary vessels.[103] Abernethy's genus of encysted tumors also includes a number of different species, which occur both on the surface and in the interior of the body. Some contain "steatomatous, atheromatous and melicerous" matter, others, especially those occurring in the ovary, contain hair. Abernethy thought that tumors of this genus were curable by simple excision, with the exception of the lesion William Hey called "fungus haematodes."[104]

A brief discussion of this interesting tumor will illustrate some of the terminological and classificatory difficulties faced by oncologists at the time. In 1800 John Burns separated out a category of inflammatory lesions that he called *spongioid*, in consequence of their spongy, elastic feel (according to Burns *all* lesions of the tissues are inflammatory in nature). Aside from the spongioid variety of inflammation, he recognized the simple, the phagedenic, the scrofulous, and the cancerous. A spongioid inflammation began, said Burns, as a small subcutaneous mass, which ultimately broke through the surface of the skin. If left untreated it spread to the neighboring lymph glands.[105] A few years later William Hey applied the term *fungus haematodes* to several tumors that he had encountered in the breasts of middle-aged women. These tumors were irregularly multicystic, and the constituent cysts contained gelatinous or brainlike material intermingled with a substance resembling clotted blood.[106]

In 1809 James Wardrop described several additional instances of what he regarded as spongioid inflammation, or fungus haematodes. But in Wardrop's patients, the lesions were found in the eye, kidney, and liver. Wardrop pointed out that tumors of this character had also been called soft cancer or medullary sarcoma in the past. He was of the opinion that such tumors, unlike cancers, occurred more frequently in young patients and involved organs often spared by cancerous disease. None of the proposed names were satisfactory, Wardrop concluded, and even his own preferred term, *fungus haematodes,* suffered from the drawback that cancers, too, often had a fungous or cauliflowerlike appearance.[107] Bichatian histology had not reached Burns or Hey, but its influence on Wardrop is patent. The question that "naturally suggests itself" in regard to fungus haematodes is, according to Wardrop, from "what particular system or texture of the organs" did the lesion originate—the vascular, absorbent, cellular, or nervous texture? Given the destructive character of fungus haematodes, Wardrop was led to suggest that it was constituted of "morbid matter *sui generis"* and was without an analogue among the normal tissues of the body.[108] The clinical distinctions he drew between fungus haematodes and cancer broadly resemble those presently drawn between sarcoma and carcinoma.[109] In his day, *sarcoma* signified no more than a fleshy tumor, usually benign in its clinical course.

Hodgkin's Generative Membranes

The eminent English physician Thomas Hodgkin set forth his views on the histogenesis of tumors in 1829, several years before his account of the disease that bears his name.[110] In spite of his skill as a microscopist, Hodgkin carried out his work in tissue pathology at the gross level alone. He took for granted the assumption that tumors were in some way a result of "an anomaly in the function of nutrition," and he adopted the histological approach of the Bichatian school. Hodgkin had studied in France under Laennec in 1822, and refers to him as "my late and valued preceptor."[111] It is likely that Hodgkin was also influenced in his views on tumor histogenesis by the work of embryologists (particularly those in Germany) on the so-called generative membranes of the early embryo. Hodgkin's underlying idea, clearly derived from Bichat, was that the same laws of tissue formation applied to solid and to cystic tumors.

Whether the adventitious new formations were obviously cystic or apparently solid, each one was generated by a serous membrane. Among the serous membranes found in animal bodies as adventitious new formations were true parasites. Hodgkin pointed out that the distinction between true parasites, such as hydatids and acephalocysts, and pseudo-parasitic new formations had at times been overlooked by investigators of the tumor problem.[112] He divided nonparasitic adventitious cysts into two varieties: cysts with walls composed of "condensed cellular membrane" enclosing foreign bodies (e.g., bullets or accumulations of pus) and cysts with membranous walls that not only enclosed but *produced* the contained matter (including subcutaneous cysts that contained "sebaceous, meliceritous or atheromatous" material).[113] Cysts of the second variety could be subdivided in accordance with their tendency, or lack of it, to grow, multiply, and spread. The first subvariety, which included adventitious synovial bursae and a variety of solitary cysts found in the lungs, breast, ovary, and choroid plexus, showed little inclination to grow or spread. The second comprised new formations that displayed the "very remarkable property of producing other cysts of a similar character...or morbid growths, which, if they do not present, strictly speaking, the character of cysts are nevertheless referrible to the same mode of formation."[114]

In support of his thesis that solid as well as cystic new formations arise from generative membranes, Hodgkin presented evidence from his painstaking dissections of tumors. He found his paradigm for the process of new formation in the structure of those membranous, multicystic tumors of the ovary known today as mucous or serous cystadenomas. Hodgkin described in detail the pedunculated secondary cysts and the broad mass of solid tumor tissue often found within the larger cysts of such ovarian growths; he inferred that the membranous walls of the cysts were truly generative membranes that gave rise to the secondary growths.[115] Hodgkin pointed out that the structural similarities between cystic tumors of the ovary and apparently solid tumors elsewhere were not revealed by the pathological anatomists' usual procedure of dissection, namely, of making gross cuts through alcohol-hardened tissues. He found that more careful dissection revealed that even the apparently solid tumors were built up of tightly infolded membranes. And from the interior surfaces of these membranes arose numerous pyriform, pedunculated bodies; in larger tumors there were often several such "enclosed packets of pedunculated bodies." Nourishing blood vessels entered through the peduncles, hence the liability of such tumors to undergo strangulation of their blood supply. Hodgkin states that vascular strangulation accounts for the "disposition to central softening or decay" so common in heterologous adventitious tumors. The basically membranous structure of solid tumors may be further obscured by the secondary organization of fluid matter secreted by the generative membrane.[116]

The precision of Hodgkin's naked-eye observations on tumors is shown by a passage in which he explains why the "indurated cellular membrane," i.e., the dense connective tissue, extending from advanced breast cancers into the surrounding fat is itself of malignant nature. In the dissection of such fibrous prolongations he had found scattered throughout certain "small and delicate pedunculated cysts, some of which scarcely exceeded the size of a pin's head." It was to the proliferation of such cysts that he attributed the spread of cancer.[117]

Hodgkin's group of apparently solid but in reality membranous heterologous new-formations comprises only two members: the true scirrhus, and the tumor variously called fungus hematodes, medullary sarcoma, and cerebriform cancer. Hodgkin regarded the melanotic tumors described by Laennec and Dupuytren as variant forms of medullary sarcoma.[118] Noting that the "question of malignancy is almost constantly agitated with reference to individual tumours," Hodgkin gave an analysis that is still pertinent today of the meaning of the word *malignancy.* A definition by intension being impossible to devise, the physician must content himself with a list of features concurring in whole or greater part in "cases to which the appellation of malignant has by common consent been applied." These features are: (1) the gradual appearance in the immediate neighborhood of the tumor of tissues resembling those of the tumor proper; (2) a peculiar kind of ulceration characterized by elevated edges and a depressed center "bathed by an unhealthy secretion, to which the name of pus can scarcely be applied"; (3) enlargement of the "absorbent glands situated in the course of the lymphatics leading to the part...by a deposit having very much the same characteristic possessed by the original tumor"; (4) similar "secondary depositions" in distant lymph nodes and organs, especially the liver; and (5) signs of a constitutional affection, such as a sallow complexion, fever, loss of appetite, etc.

In modern terms Hodgkin's first four criteria of malignancy would be invasion, metastasis, and a characteristic form of tumor ulceration. But there was no means in Hodgkin's day for distinguishing the invasive and metastatic substance in cancer from that in inflammatory disease. Hence he was forced to admit that similar changes in neighboring lymph nodes and distant organs could also occur in "scrofulous, venereal and common inflammations." Worse yet, all the characteristic features described might be lacking in certain tumors that competent judges recognized as malignant.[119]

Carswell

Robert Carswell's book on pathological anatomy requires attention at this point. Beautifully illustrated with color drawings from his own hand, it was published (in twelve separate fascicles) in London between 1833 and 1838.[120] Carswell, like Hodgkin, had studied in France, and while there had taken up the new discipline of histopathology. His book has eleven chapters, devoted to inflammation, analogous tissue new formations, atrophy, hypertrophy, pus, mortification, hemorrhage, softening, melanoma, carcinoma, and tubercle. In the second chapter Carswell distinguished clearly between analogous accidental tissue and analogous transformations of preexisting tissues, a distinction Andral had blurred somewhat. In Carswell's opinion, the range of possible transformations of a tissue under pathological conditions corresponded precisely to the range of transformations displayed by that tissue "in different periods of fetal life and in different animals." Cellular tissue underwent direct transformation during fetal life into "serous or fibrous tissue, and this into fibro-cartilaginous, cartilaginous and osseous tissues in succession." Such changes could, therefore, occur in adult life under the appropriate abnormal circumstances. But the direct transformation of cellular tissue into muscle or nerve did *not* occur in the embryo; it was therefore not to be met with in the adult under any circumstances.

In accordance with the generally accepted view, Carswell stated that analogous new formations took origin from plastic lymph derived from the circulating blood. He cited the transformation undergone by stagnant blood within vessels as an indubitable instance of the development of fibrous tissue from plastic lymph. Carswell suggested that the blood vessels that made their appearance in organizing intravascular clots arose within the clots and then connected with the blood vessels of adjacent normal tissues. Laennec, on the contrary, had held that the newly formed vessels grew in from the periphery.

In the writings of the French school of histopathologists and their followers in England, benign tumors appear under the headings of analogous tissue transformation, of analogous new-formation, and of hypertrophy. Carswell's work is no exception. For example, he places the "fibrous tumours...most frequently found in the parietes of the uterus, where they vary from the size of a pea to that of a child's head, or even larger" among analogous tissue transformations rather than, as might be expected, among analogous new-formations. In modern terms, the lesions referred to would pass for leiomyomas. In discussing a fatty tumor in the intestinal submucosa and a fatty tumor of the pleura (described by Andral and Laennec, respectively) Carswell placed both in the category of analogous new formations. But he states, rather inexplicably, that "lipomas" occurring in adipose tissue belong under the heading of hypertrophy.[121]

Carswell was generally unsympathetic to the views of Hodgkin on the histogenesis of tumors. In discussing adventitious cysts he does agree with Hodgkin in finding that "heterologous formations, especially the carcinomatous...exist as pediculated tumours" within membranes re-flected over the surface of the tumor and back to the pedicle. But Carswell rejects Hodgkin's claim that such tumors, indeed any tumors, are gener-ated by cyst walls, and he traces all tumors, including cystic ones, back to the organization of effused plastic lymph.[122] He finds, moreover, that the cystic structure regarded by Hodgkin as an intrinsic feature of all tumor growth is absent in tumors of the lungs, kidney, brain, lymphatic glands, and spleen. Its occasional occurrence must be regarded as "mere co-incidence, or as the consequence of the disease." To the views of Abernethy on heterologous tumors Carswell raised the objection that many of Abernethy's tumors were "not *tissues,* as he believed, as they were described at about the same time by Laennec, but amorphous masses." Finally, Carswell rejected Cruveilhier's double claim that the *tissu cellulaire* was the primary site of "organic transformations and degenerations (as he calls them)" and that all other tissues were capable only of hypertrophy or atrophy.[123]

Hodgkin's Amplification

In 1836 Hodgkin published an amplification of his views on the histo-genesis of tumors.[124] What was implicit in 1829, namely, the analogy between embryonic and neoplastic membranes, was now set forth openly. Hodgkin stated that the serous membranes "present themselves to our notice in Nature's earliest processes for the formation of an animal." Even before the embryo is visible, its generating membranes, "which bear the strongest resemblance to, if they are not absolutely identical with, the serous" have already taken form.[125] Since Hodgkin followed John Hunter in believing that the embryonic membranes themselves ultimately originated from a primary form of coagulable lymph, his views on tumor histogenesis are not too far removed from those of his colleagues. Whereas other pathologists assumed a two-step process in-volving the transformation of coagulable lymph or blastema into tumor tissue, Hodgkin assumed a three-step process: coagulable lymph, gener-ating membrane, and tumor tissue.

Aside from the embryological argument, Hodgkin, as already noted, found support for his views in the well-known and generally accepted cystic structure of certain adventitious tissues: the structure of serous cysts of the ovaries had furnished him with a "key to the formation and development" of tumors.[126] It is possible that he derived additional support from the structure of parasitic cysts. Nevertheless he was far from believing, as had some earlier theorists, that cancerous growths were parasites in the true sense of the word.[127]

In the closing chapter of his *Lectures* Hodgkin assessed the opinions of his contemporaries on the genesis and nature of cancer. Laennec, he stated, had held that cancers were "produced by a sort of epigenesis," whereas Dupuytren had regarded all so-called accidental tissues, including cancers, as "nothing more than the result of the transformation of natural tissues" and had characterized those of heterologous structure as degenerations. Broussais and Gilbert Breschet (he might have added Andral) had blurred the distinction between inflammation and cancer. Finally, Hodgkin took issue with Carswell on the origin of blood vessels in adventitious tissues. He was "sceptical as to the production of new and independent vessels, except in the case of an embryo," and believed that the blood vessels of tumors were prolongations of surrounding normal vessels.[128] Hodgkin's own theory of tumor histogenesis was presented to North American physicians in 1839—the year Schwann's book on the cell was published—in what was probably the last work on Bichatian gross histopathology.[129]

Hodgkin's failure to employ the microscope in his study of tumors warrants comment. Unlike other oncologists, he was well acquainted with its use. In 1827 Hodgkin and Joseph J. Lister published a paper on the microscopy of the blood and certain animal tissues.[130] Using Lister's newly devised lenses, they demonstrated the artefactual character of the globular structure of tissues described by observers from Leeuwenhoek's time up to Milne Edwards's. According to Hodgkin and Lister, the finest structural elements of the tissues are fibers. The so-called globules are nothing more than artefactual rings produced by uncorrected lenses around tiny particles—some of which, of course, may actually have been cells.[131] In 1836 Hodgkin repeated that he was convinced of the "absolute fallacy of the globular theory"; the belief (evidently still current in the 1830s) that the minute fibers composing tissues were themselves in turn composed of "globules, arranged like strings of beads" had its sole foundation in optical illusion.[132] The inability of one of England's outstanding pathological anatomists, in collaboration with one of the foremost optical experts in Europe, to find a use for the newly improved microscope in the study of tumors illustrates the limitations of a technical advance unaccompanied by an appropriate conceptual advance. With their corrected lenses Hodgkin and Lister could only confirm the ancient doctrine of the ultimately fibrous structure of living matter.

GERM-LAYER THEORY

Embryology is concerned with the genesis of form in developing organisms, oncology with the genesis of newly formed abnormal tissues in partially or fully developed organisms. Thus it is not surprising that relations were established between the two fields of investigation almost as soon as oncologists reached general agreement that tumors were structured host tissues rather than foreign parasites or accumulations of abnormal matter. Since oncologists borrowed from embryological theories, in particular from the germ-layer theory, a brief historical comment on the germ-layer theory will be appropriate here.

Germ-layer theory was worked out long before cell theory. Its beginnings even antedate the new interest in tissues signaled by Bichat's studies. According to the germ-layer theory in its most general form, the structure of living organisms is derived from the folding and transformation of one or more membranous or leaflike primitive structures. Credit for this idea is usually given to Caspar Friedrich Wolff. Wolff stated that the organs of plants arose from the various transformations undergone by leaflike primordia, and he showed that the intestinal canal in the chick embryo likewise arose from the folding of a primitive membrane.[133]

Goethe, too, is well-known for his work on the metamorphosis of plants. His *Urpflanze* is, however, an ideal type rather than an embryonic primordium. In quoting from J. F. Meckel's translation (1812) of Wolff's book on the embryogenesis of the gut (*De formatione intestinorum* [1768]), Goethe seems to accept Wolff's priority in the discovery of plant metamorphosis.[134]

The germ-layer concept was worked out early in the nineteenth century by Christian Pander, a pupil of Ignaz Doellinger at Wuerzburg. Pander's findings in the chick embryo were generalized by his friend Karl Ernst von Baer to include the embryonic development of all vertebrates.[135] Whether or not Pander or von Baer drew inspiration from Wolff is an open question, but it seems unlikely that either man would have been unacquainted with the relevant studies of Wolff or, for that matter, those of Goethe.

Pander's short but profusely illustrated monograph on the embryology of the chick was published as an inaugural dissertation in 1817.[136] Although he had a compound microscope at his disposal, his essential findings were made with the naked eye and a small hand lens. The few comments on fine structure in Pander's monograph suggest that he was an adherent of the globule theory (his microscope, of course, had uncorrected lenses). Pander states that the germinal disc "consists of an assemblage of small grayish-white globules (*Kuegelchen*)" and that the germinal membrane (*Keimhaut*) is, in the unincubated egg, a "simple layer of granules (*Koerner*)."[137] A short time after incubation has commenced, Pander continues, the primary germinal membrane becomes overlain by a second membrane consisting of a "very delicate, dense and more uniform layer composed of granules" that are less distinct than those in the primary membrane. After twelve hours of incubation the germinal membrane consists of "two quite different lamellae, the inner thick, granular and opaque, the outer smooth, transparent and thinner." Pander called the outer layer the serous leaf (*Blatt*) and the inner, the mucous leaf. Toward the end of the twentieth hour of incubation a third layer, the vascular membrane, arises between the serous and mucous leaves. At this point, according to Pander, the foundation for the entire future structural development of the chick embryo has already been laid. What takes place thereafter amounts to nothing more than a "metamorphosis of this membrane and its leaves." As they undergo metamorphosis the three layers interact: "In each of the three layers a specific kind of metamorphosis begins to take place; each layer hastens toward its goal but none are independent enough to accomplish by themselves that for which they are destined; each one requires the help of its fellows, hence all three work together until they have reached a certain level, although they are destined in the beginning for different ends."[138]

Von Baer, who generalized and somewhat modified Pander's concept of the germ layers, likewise carried out his embryological studies almost exclusively at the gross level.[139] Incidentally, he regarded Pander rather than Wolff as the founder of germ-layer theory.[140] Unlike Pander, however, von Baer distinguished not three but four germ layers. The germinal membrane, he says, undergoes division into superior and inferior layers. The former give rise to "animal" parts, the latter to "plastic body parts." The inferior layer is composed of two closely united leaves (*Blaetter*), the mucous leaf and the vascular leaf. The superior layer likewise consists of two leaves, one of which gives rise to skin, and the other to bone, muscle, and nerve. Von Baer calls the second of these leaves the flesh-layer (*Fleischschicht*). He continues: "Thus the differentiation of the germ into layers yields the mucous membrane (the membrane of interior, open cavities), further, the layer for the trunks of the vascular system, the flesh-layer, the skin-layer and, in vertebrates, the nerve-layer (the layer for the central part of the nervous system)." Both nerve-layer and skin-layer are derived from the superior surface of the embryo, i.e., from what is today called the ectodermal layer.[141] In 1837 von Baer termed the superior layer the *Hautschicht* ("dermal-layer"). He noted, however, that this term was not entirely appropriate for a layer that gave rise to the central nervous system as well as to the skin. The inferior, or inner, layer von Baer termed the *Schleimhautschicht* ("mucous-membrane-layer"). Lying between the superior and inferior layers was a third component derived from both whose upper layer constituted the *Fleischschicht*, its lower the *Gefaessschicht* ("vascular-layer"). When the inner and outer layers proceed to roll up into tubes the embryo begins to take shape.[142]

Von Baer distinguished three phases in the course of what he called the separating-out or differentiation of the originally homogeneous germ. The first phase consisted of the differentiation of heterogeneous germ layers from the homogeneous primary germinal membrane. The next phase, called by von Baer a "histological separating-out" (*histologische Sonderung*), involved the differentiation of blood, bone, cartilage, and muscle. The third phase (morphological) had to do with the development of external form: "The neural tube divides into sense-organs, brain and spinal cord, the mucous membrane tube into oral cavity, esophagus, stomach, gut, respiratory apparatus, liver, urinary bladder, and so on."[143] In von Baer's opinion the increasing heterogeneity of structure found in the developing organism was not so much the result of new-formation (*Neubildung*) as of transformation or metamorphosis (*Umbildung*). In other words, growth in mass does not by itself lead directly to the production of a new part. On the contrary, a new part, whether tissue or organ, always differentiates out of a less heterogeneous mass. Where nerve tissue is to be formed, for example, one does not find a hiatus or open space which in time fills up with nerve tissue, but "rather a common mass which separates into nerve and not-nerve."[144]

In the second part of his monograph, which was published in 1837, von Baer pointed out that his three modes of differentiation were not strictly sequential. The first in point of time was, of course, the differentiation of the germ layers or leaves from the undifferentiated germinal membrane. The leaves then folded into tubes, the most primitive organs. Superimposed on the latter process—and taking place before the layers generated by the primary separating-out (*Sonderung*) had become completed tubes—was morphological differentiation. The organs of the adult organism are, he says, formed through "modified growth," i.e., differential growth that produces appropriate alterations in length, thickness, etc., in the primordia of the future organs. Histological differentiation generally followed the completion of morphological differentiation, although partial overlapping occurred.[145]

The term *leaf* in the writings of Pander and von Baer is not merely metaphorical. In the mind of Wolff (and possibly also of Goethe) an embryonic leaf, whether of a plant or an animal, constituted a primordial organ. According to Goethe, a flower was a folded, differentiated leaf. So also, according to Pander and von Baer, were animal organs.

Thus, germ layer theory, including the notions of histological and morphological differentiation, was at its inception independent of the cell theory and of microscopic anatomy. Like students of tumor genesis, embryologists had microscopes at their disposal but were unable to use them effectively. As Rudolf Virchow would say of pathologists in 1855, oncologists and embryologists had not yet learned to "think microscopically" (*mikroskopisch denken*).[146] Two years before the appearance of Theodore Schwann's book on the cell, all that von Baer could say of the fine structure of the developing embryo was that it consisted "of an almost completely homogeneous mass, composed partly of a light, coagulated, and otherwise formless mass."[147] And although von Baer had clearly described the cleavage of the frog egg yolk four years earlier, he did not conceive of the process as involving successive cell division.[148]

3

CELL THEORY AND THE GENESIS
OF CELLS IN TUMORS, 1838-52

USE OF THE MICROSCOPE

Although simple and compound microscopes had been in use since the middle of the seventeenth century, they had contributed very little to the understanding of pathological processes by the early eighteen hundreds.[1] The failure of investigators to utilize the microscope was due, it has been suggested, not only to the relatively imperfect lenses then available but also to a degree of ideological opposition on the part of certain theorists, which began with Sydenham and Locke.[2] Furthermore, the microscope — unlike the telescope, which was fruitfully used during the same period — opened up an entirely new world, one in which the visual objects had not been adequately conceptualized. Like once-blind men newly restored to sight the early microscopists were confronted with the difficult task of learning to see. To discriminate accurately between objects and non-objects (artifacts) would have been difficult enough even if corrected lenses had been available. Moreover, the imaginations of some microscopists operated with a minimum of restraint. The result was widespread scepticism on the part of more sober minds as to the value of the microscope.[3]

"Illusory micrography," as Bruno Zanobio has recently called it, continued to play an important and confusing role in the early years of the nineteenth century.[4] In the 1820s, however, optically corrected microscope lenses were manufactured by William Tulley in England, Giovanni Amici in Italy, and Charles Chevalier in France.[5] J. J. Lister's paper of 1830 on the design of achromatic objectives signaled the end of the period of trial-and-error procedures.[6] It has been noted that in the hands of Lister and Hodgkin the improved lenses contributed to the overthrow of Milne Edwards's revival of the globule theory of fine tissue structure, although Lister and Hodgkin remained adherents of classical fiber theory. In the hands of other microscopists the new lenses soon led to the identification of cells as the ultimate units of structure and function in normal animal tissues. And, almost immediately thereupon, cells were identified as the fundamental units of tumor tissue.

Globules and Cells

Some of the globules described by early microscopists working with uncorrected lenses were, no doubt, cells in the modern sense of the term. Corrected lenses, however, made it possible for the skilled microscopist to draw a sharp line between globular optical artifacts and the globules, spherules, and corpuscles, as they were variously called, that were later designated cells. One of the first passable descriptions of cancer cells may be found in a brief note submitted to the Academy of Sciences at Paris by Gottlieb Gluge in 1837. Gluge writes of certain "globular bodies" (*corps globuleux*) visible under the microscope in fluid expressed from encephaloid, i.e., soft cancer. He observes that the globules "do not have like volumes; the smallest are larger than pus globules, measuring about 0.008 mm. in diameter; their shape, although it approximates the spherical, is far from regular."[7] Strongly contrasting with these accurate observations are those made by Everard Home in 1830. Under the microscope a purportedly cancerous tumor proved, according to Home, to be composed of uniform small spheres, or lymph globules. The illustration accompanying Home's report is quite unconvincing.[8]

Mueller

Johannes Mueller preceded Gluge in the study of tumors under the microscope; Mueller's preliminary findings on the subject had been submitted on two occasions in 1836.[9] Unlike Gluge, Mueller used the term *cell* (*Zelle*) in his account of the fine structure of tumors. But he used it only in reference to certain membrane-bounded structures all or for the most part visible to the naked eye. Mueller's cell is no more than the standard eighteenth-century cell of cellular tissue (*Zellgewebe*). But his use of the term can easily confuse the modern reader. When he states, for example, that the "fat cells" (*Fettzellen*) of fatty tumors are spherical in shape, "as in normal fatty cellular tissue" (*Fettzellgewebe*), we may at first suppose that he is referring to modern, or Schwannian, cells. We find instead that he is describing membrane-bounded compartments similar to those found in normal fatty subcutaneous tissue. At times Mueller's use of the term is clear enough; thus he describes "cellular membranous compartments visible to the naked eye" in tumors of cartilaginous nature. And the membranous cells of certain carcinomas are said to average two or three lines in diameter (1 Paris line = 2.256 mm.). Like Gluge, in describing what can be safely identified as Schwannian cells, Mueller used the terms *globe* (*Kugel*) and *globule* (*Kuegelchen*). Mueller notes, for example, that a certain "albuminoid fibrous tumor" (*eiweissartige Faser-*

geschwulst) consists of "interwoven microscopic fibers, among which are strewn a large number of globules." And in the tumor entity described as "reticular carcinoma" he observed numerous "round to oval globes, larger than blood corpuscles," scattered throughout a finely fibrous meshwork background.[10]

In this preliminary report (soon followed by a monograph on the fine structure of tumors) Mueller stated that no one had yet determined whether the microscope would be useful in distinguishing benign (*gutartig*) from malignant (*boesartig*) tumors.[11] His own work on the fine structure of tumors encouraged him to believe that the microscope would be of help in this respect. Whereas Gluge had merely commented in passing on the variation in size of the *corps globuleux* found in encephaloid cancer, Mueller was of the opinion that this feature had practical diagnostic value.[12] Once again, however, it should be borne in mind that Mueller's report did not anticipate the forthcoming cell theory. Mueller's cells were mere tissue compartments, and he did not at this time consider his globes and globules to be living structural and functional units.[13]

SCHWANN'S PAPERS OF 1838 AND THEIR RECEPTION BY MUELLER

Among botanists, however, the traditional belief in the ultimately fibrous nature of plant substance had already been replaced by the hypothesis that plants were aggregates of more or less autonomous living units, so small as to be visible only under the microscope. No later than the first quarter of the nineteenth century the term *cell* had been applied to these living units. It was no novelty, therefore, for Matthias Schleiden to state, in 1838, that plants were aggregates of cells (*Zellen*) and that each cell, in addition to participating in the life of the whole plant organism, led an individual life of its own.[14] But Schleiden's account of the manner in which "that peculiar, small organism, the cell" reproduced itself was new.[15] Schleiden, presumably making use of the newly improved microscope in his studies, had concluded that the cell nucleus, or *Kern* (a small, inconstantly present body lying on the cell wall), was the reproductive organ of the cell. This body, incidentally, had been discerned only seven years earlier by Robert Brown, an English botanist.[16] Schleiden supposed that new cells were generated from nuclei within mature cells, in a manner described below.

Following an informal exchange of views with Schleiden, Theodor Schwann, one of Mueller's pupils, conceived the idea that in animals, too, the cell was the unit of structure, and its nucleus, the reproductive organ.[17] Schwann's three preliminary papers on cell theory appeared in the early months of 1838. They were entitled, appropriately, "On the Analogy in the Structure and Growth of Animals and Plants."[18] A question is: was his adoption of the belief that animal cells were "autonomous" due *solely* to the similar belief held by Schleiden and other botanists with respect to plant cells? In any case he did not hesitate to apply it also to animal cells.

Schwann began by pointing out that botanists considered plants to be aggregates of more or less independently living cells (*Zellen*), each one of which had derived somehow from an original simple, or single, cell. Schleiden, he said, had shown that plant cells reproduced themselves *only* from within, and that the reproductive organ of the cell was a parietally placed body—the nucleus, or *Kern*, of Robert Brown. Schwann's summary of Schleiden's account of the visible changes accompanying the formation of young cells within brood, or "mother," cells is as follows. The first step is marked by the appearance within the mother cell of a small, spherical, parietally placed body, the nucleus, which contains one or more smaller bodies, the corpuscles or nucleoli (*Kernkoerperchen*). The next step is the gradual appearance of a blister, or vesicle, which arises from the surface of the nucleus. (As Schleiden had said, the vesicle sits on the surface of the nucleus like a watch-glass [*Urhglas*] on a watch.) The vesicle continues to expand until it has reached the size of a mature cell. The nucleus persists for a time in the cell wall. The final step is the absorption and disappearance of the nucleus and the mother cell. (The reader will note that in Schleiden's account of cell reproduction there are several features reminiscent of the process of endosporulation in certain kinds of fungi.)

After summarizing Schleiden's findings, Schwann suggests that "all these phenomena...can be demonstrated in animal structures" and that "all animal tissues might be referable in origin to cell formation of an analogous kind." This is largely supposition on his part. He himself had seen within the microscopic cells of notochordal tissue a "flattened nucleus provided with one or two nucleoli," or even "one or more round, young cells." His strongest statement with respect to the steps in cell reproduction described by Schleiden is that he had seen them in developing cartilage tissue and in the extremely thin-walled cells—"previously discerned by Professor Mueller"—of frog notochord.[19] However, this statement is not backed up by a description of the series of changes in question.

Schleiden's *Uhrglas* theory never achieved general acceptance, neither among zoologists nor botanists, as an exclusive mechanism of cell reproduction. It was almost immediately discarded by Schwann and, soon after, by Schleiden himself. But the belief that animals, like plants, were structured aggregates of more or less autonomous cells proved much more durable.

Schwann also had to contend, however, with microscopically visible
constituents of mature animal tissues that bore little resemblance to the
rounded or multilateral objects most readily identifiable as cells. Under
the microscope a bewildering variety of finer constituents of tissues
presented themselves to the observer. Were cells only one form of
structural-functional element or were all elements, whatever their appearance, derived from cells? Schwann adopted the latter view, cautiously
advancing the working hypothesis that as growth and development in
the embryo proceeded the constituent cells underwent far-reaching
structural changes. For example, the lens of the eye in an adult organism
did not appear to be composed of cells, but in the fourteen-day-old chick
embryo the lens was clearly made up entirely of "extremely transparent
cells."

It was by pursuing the genesis of tissues in each instance to their
embryonic origins that Schwann obtained supporting evidence for his
idea, appropriated from Schleiden, that animal organisms were aggregates of cells—i.e., aggregates of *transformed* cells. In embryonic connective tissue, for example, he had seen "hosts of corpuscles marked
within by one or two dark points...very similar to nuclei and their
nucleoli." Despite the eminently noncellular appearance of muscle and
nerve tissues in adult organisms, Schwann wrote that they could be traced
to clearly recognizable cells in the embryo. He called attention to Jacob
Henle's demonstration of a year earlier that the flattened, platelike
squames that form the outer layer of animal epidermis begin their lives
as round, nucleated cells in the Malpighian layer below.[20]

Schwann was familiar with the gross, or tissue, embryology of his day,
and, just one year after the publication of part two of von Baer's study of
that subject, he took the first step in the development of cellular embryology. According to Schwann, the primary tissue (*Urgewebe*) of an
animal organism consists of a germinal vesicle and a germinal membrane.
All tissues of the adult organism can be traced back to some component
of the *Urgewebe*. The germinal vesicle (*Keimblaeschen*) is a single cell,
containing a nucleus and nucleolus. This germ cell gives rise to the
germinal membrane (*Keimhaut*) and its several layers, or leaves.

Schwann initiated cellular embryology with the statement that the
serous leaf of the germinal membrane in a twenty-four-hour-old chick
embryo consists of regularly arranged, angular squamous scales, or
platelets (*Schueppchen*), which contain nuclei with enclosed nucleoli and
strongly resemble epidermal epithelial cells. Again citing Henle's observation of 1837, Schwann states that the same is probably true of the
germinal membrane, especially since cells on its margins are in fact still
spherical and have similar, parietal nuclei. The mucous leaf of the

germinal membrane is likewise composed of cells, some of which contain "daughter" cells. It thus appeared to Schwann that the embryo not only originates from a single cell but is also, at this stage of its development, composed exclusively of cells.[21] Does this mean that Schwann had anticipated by almost two decades Rudolf Virchow's 1855 aphorism, *omnis cellula a cellula* ("Every cell arises from a preexisting cell")? Not at all. For Schwann also tells us that he has seen, at a later stage of embryonic development, cells arising *de novo* from the "gelatinous, structureless mass" constituting the bulk of embryonic connective tissue.[22]

Since the history of the origins of cell theory continues to be characterized by conflicting claims regarding priority, it is worthwhile noting Mueller's reception of Schwann's three papers in 1838. After having reviewed Henle's work on epithelium, Barthélemy Dumortier's investigation of cell genesis in the molluscan liver, and Alfred Donné's and Pierre Turpin's studies of vaginal epithelium, Mueller added that by far the most important work along this line had been that of Schleiden and Schwann. Schleiden's discovery of the "origin of new plant cells from nuclei in mother cells," Schwann's confirmation of a like mode of origin of new cells in animal tissues, and his claim that animal tissues were also aggregates of more or less transformed cells called for a new theory of "life, generation and development," wrote Mueller; one in which the cell would function as the cornerstone. Mueller noted that Turpin had already compared the squames found in vaginal fluid to plant cells and referred to them as "living vesicles."[23] Apparently both Schwann's conception of cells in animals as living units (rather than membranous boundary layers) and his analogy between plant and animal cells were not entirely new.

What distinguishes Schwann from his contemporaries is, Mueller recognized, his designation of the cell as the fundamental and exclusive unit of ontogenesis, embryogenesis, and histogenesis in animal organisms. Today, when the word *cell* is uttered it carries with it this corpus of beliefs; hence we are prone to read them into the word wherever it appears. It is easy for a historian of science, if at all tendentiously motivated, to commit this error. No doubt nineteenth-century investigators other than Turpin regarded some animal cells—regardless of the designations they may have employed—as living entities, comparable to plant cells. And it is unlikely that Schwann's hypothesis that all microscopic structural units of animal tissues are transformed cells, formerly globular, or spherical, in shape, was not independently entertained, at least for a time, by one or more of his contemporaries.

Schwann suggests, in the closing paragraph of the first of his three papers, that the cell concept will prove equally fruitful in the study of tumors. "Supported by my observations," writes Schwann, "Dr. Mueller

has investigated enchondroma and alveolar cancer...and found a like
formation of cells...he has also observed cellular structure in another
kind of cancer, where the formative globes (*Bildungskugeln*) appeared to
be cells enclosing other cells."[24] At the end of Schwann's third paper are
some verbatim remarks by Mueller on the presence of cells in tumors.
Here, for the first time, Mueller uses the term *cell* in the Schwannian
sense. He states that nucleated cells of the kind described by Schwann are
to be found in a number of benign and malignant tumors. Further, he
identifies certain tailed bodies (*geschwaenzten Koerper*)—elongated microscopic bodies described by him in several kinds of tumors—as transformed cells.[25]

REVISION OF MUELLER'S THEORY

Later in 1838 the first fascicle of Mueller's "On the Finer Structure and
the Forms of Morbid Tumors" appeared, a monograph in which he
greatly expanded and revised his earlier studies in the light of Schwann's
cell theory.[26] Using a Schieck microscope equipped with corrected lenses
magnifying up to 500 diameters, Mueller found that tumors, whether
benign or malignant, were composed of "fibers, granules, cells with or
without nuclei, tailed and spindle-shaped corpuscles (*Koerperchen*) and
vessels." The granules (*Koerner*) were considerably smaller than the
smallest cells and were both intracellular and extracellular in position.
The tailed corpuscles often contained nuclei. Mueller repeated his earlier
claim that the tailed corpuscles were Schwannian cells halfway transformed into fibers. In tumors, in contrast to what Schwann had described
in normal embryonic connective tissues, the "formation of fibers does not
progress beyond the embryonic form of cell-fibers," insofar as these
tailed corpuscles are concerned. Reiterating what had become a commonplace among oncologists, Mueller remarks that embryonic formations
are repeated in tumors in a most striking way.[27]

Mueller's "Cells"

Mueller's use of the term *cell* in his monograph, together with his claim
that he had already "recognized the microscopic cellular structure of
several tumors in the year 1836," requires comment. There is little doubt
that he was reinterpreting his observations of 1836 in the light of
Schwann's findings of 1838, for Mueller's "cells" and "cellular structures"

were, at the earlier date, grossly visible, membrane-bounded compartments. Alternatively, we may assume that Mueller's formative globes
had become, in his newly acquired terminology, cells. The matter is
actually somewhat more complicated and less clear, for even in the
monograph of 1838 Mueller sometimes uses the term *cell* in its older
sense. In reference to certain cancerous tumors, for example, he describes
"microscopic cells that have not fused together...the cavities of which
are recognizable from a smaller cell or several corpuscles contained
therein." The smallest of these "cells" measured from 0.00014 to 0.0012
Paris inches (4 to 32 microns), hence we can provisionally accept them as
Schwannian cells. But a little later in his text Mueller develops the
notion of cell wall fusion to the point where the Schwannian cell—a
minute living organism—is merged with the traditional membrane-
bounded compartment constitutive of eighteenth-century cellular tissue.
Alveolar cancer is said to consist of cells of various sizes, the largest being
"visible to the naked eye." Large cells are formed by the repeated fusion
of the walls of microscopic cells. "In *carcinoma alveolare,*" writes Mueller,
"the mother cells continue to grow, reaching two, three or more lines in
size [1 Paris line = 2.256 mm.]; the walls of the cells fuse with each other
and with the wall of the mother cell." In many tumors "cellular formation
is so marked that cells are visible with the lowest magnifications or even
with the naked eye." But in *carcinoma simplex,* "fusion of cells does not
occur, and the cells do not continue to grow." Instead, they persist as
"microscopic formative globes" lying within the "meshes of a fibrous
background or *stroma.*"[28] The last-cited passage proves that Mueller had
identified his "formative globes" (*Kugeln*) with Schwannian cells. Similar
reservations must be stated with respect to Mueller's claim that he had,
before 1838, identified the tailed corpuscles as Schwannian cells.[29]

  Nevertheless, Mueller openly professed his indebtedness to Schwann.
The aim of his study of the fine structures of tumors had been, he wrote,
to find out whether the "new discoveries of Schleiden concerning the
development of young plant cells from the nuclei of mother cells, and
those of Schwann concerning the structural correspondence between
plants and animals, the composition of all embryonic tissues from cells...
and, finally, the subsequent transformation of cells into tissues" were
applicable to tumors.[30] To a considerable extent, Mueller concluded,
Schwann's findings were applicable to tumor tissue. But Mueller's attempt
to derive membrane-bounded compartments visible to the naked eye—the
"cell" of the older histologists—from microscopic cells by means of the
assumption that the walls of Schwannian cells regularly underwent fusion
to form the walls of larger, eventually visible, cells, cannot be traced to
Schwann; it seems, rather, to have been an effort to reconcile his earlier

observations of tumor structure with the subsequent studies influenced by Schwann.

Mueller's Cancer "Seeds"; Return to the Blastema Theory

Mueller convinced himself that at least some new cells in tumor tissues arose from nuclei within preexistent cells in the manner described by Schleiden and confirmed by Schwann. "Young cells in enchondroma and in alveolar cancer," he wrote, "take form exactly as they do in cartilage and chorda dorsalis, and my observations make it seem very likely that the same mode of formation occurs in several kinds of cancer and in cellular sarcoma."[31] Whereas Schwann regarded the germinal vesicle as a single cell, he did not derive all other cells of the embryo directly from that cell. Mueller, similarly, did not derive all tumor cells in a given tumor directly from a single, original tumor cell. Nor did he derive the original tumor cells directly from normal cells: "The germinal cells of carcinomas arise not from already present fibers but independently from a true *seminium morbi* which develops between the tissue components of an organ." Perhaps what Mueller meant to say was "not from already present cells." Or he may have intended a passing emphasis of his belief that fibers arise from cells rather than cells from fibers. In either case, his point is that so-called cancerous degeneration is not the *transformation* of existing tissue but the *new formation* of cancerous tissue. Admittedly, a growing cancer brings about a state of cancerous degeneration in the adjacent muscles, nerves, glands, bones, and other tissues. But the initial state, or "primary manifestation," consists "not in the mere transformation of already present healthy tissue into cancerous degeneration but in the development of the formal elements of cancer between the tissue components of an organ."[32] This same point had been made several decades earlier by Laennec, although within a quite different theoretical context.

Mueller fails to express himself with full clarity on this matter, but in accordance with the above-cited remarks he must have believed that cancer cells arose *de novo*. For if they arose from a preexisting normal cell, the cancerous process would have to be described as a *trans*formation, rather than as a *new*-formation. Even when he writes elsewhere that the disease-seed (*seminium morbi*) of cancer may, at an early stage, consist of a cluster of "fine, spheroidal cells," this must not be supposed to represent the earliest stage. Once cancer cells have been formed they may give rise to other cells in the manner described by Schleiden and Schwann. Even so, Mueller did not find the watch-glass phenomenon of sufficiently frequent occurrence to justify the belief that all tumor cells arise in the manner described by Schleiden. It is Mueller's opinion that, even in well-developed tumors, new tumor cells arise outside of preexisting cells as readily as within, perhaps more so. In either event, they develop from granules (*Koernchen*), which can arise independently of cells, although their presence may point to the rupture or dissolution of preexisting cells. Mueller also argues that tumor cells, whether they arise within or without preexisting cells, take origin from nuclei.[33] Mueller appears to be glossing over a fundamental difference between his view of cell formation and that of Schleiden and Schwann. What he is in fact proposing is simply a new version of the blastema theory: the "cell," rather than the "fiber," is the first fully formed structural tissue unit to arise from the amorphous granular blastema, cell formation being preceded by the formation of intracellular or extracellular "nuclei." The *seminium morbi* of cancer would be represented at its inception by an abnormal blastema or a normal blastema subject to appropriately abnormal influences. Despite this (to us) backward step, Mueller's work on tumors placed the cancer cell at the center of oncological interest, a place it still occupies.[34]

Schwann had stated in his papers of 1838 that some cells in animal organisms arose from nuclei within preexistent cells, in the manner described by Schleiden, while other cells arose in an unspecified manner from a "gelatinous, structureless mass," i.e., extracellularly. He had also stated that "all animal tissues might be referable in origin to cell formation." Here are two tentative claims, the first bearing on cytogenesis, the second on histogenesis.

In 1839 Schwann's full-scale study of normal histogenesis, together with some remarks on cytogenesis that reveal Mueller's influence, appeared under the title "Microscopic Investigations of the Correspondence in Structure and Growth of Animals and Plants."[35] Schwann presented a large amount of evidence in support of his histogenetic thesis, which he concluded was in fact applicable to all animal tissues. Calling it his cell theory (*Zellentheorie*)—for Schwann did not use the term *histogenesis*—he states it as follows: *"there is a common developmental principle for the most different elementary parts of organisms . . . this developmental principle is cell formation."*[36] (A complete theory of histogenesis would have had to account for the ordering of elementary parts into structured aggregates, i.e., tissues, as well as to identify, as Schwann's did, the elementary parts as transformed cells.)

Schwann then presents his theory of cytogenesis. "The basic phenomenon," he writes, "through which the productive force in organic Nature everywhere expresses itself is, accordingly, as follows: *There is present at first a structureless substance, which lies either within or between already present cells. Cells are formed within this substance in accordance with prescribed laws, and these cells develop in manifold ways into the elementary parts of organisms."*[37]

Schwann adds that under the heading of "theory of cells" (*Theorie der Zellen*) he distinguishes all conclusions that can be drawn concerning the forces underlying these phenomena.[38]

TISSUES REDEFINED IN THE LIGHT
OF SCHWANN'S CELL THEORY

Bichat had transformed the ancient doctrine of "similar parts" into the new doctrine of tissues; in both the new and the old doctrines, structure was specified empirically at the macroscopic level alone. Bichat's general anatomy, as he proposed to call it, was general macroscopic anatomy and—aside from its functional, or physiological, aspect—nothing more. Schwann now proposed that the foundations of general anatomy be reconstructed at the microscopic level, in the light of the cell concept. "Since the underlying form of all organic structure is the cell," he wrote, "the most scientific arrangement of general anatomy would obviously be one based on the greater or lesser degree of development that cells must undergo in the formation of a tissue."[39] In effect, he substituted the concrete, observable cell for the hypothetical ultimate fiber of von Haller. From a purely theoretical standpoint, what occurred was the replacement of *fiber* by *cell* in von Haller's previously cited statement to the effect that the fiber was to the anatomist as the line was to the geometer. The tissue concept thereby loses its autonomy. Not only do Schwannian microscopic "tissue" patterns (which are now cell patterns) displace Bichatian macroscopic tissue patterns, but the structural characteristics of the transformed cells constituting the elementary units of the new patterns become decisive in the identification and classification of tissues.

In accordance with this proposal, Schwann divided the tissues (*Geweben*) into five classes, each defined by the nature and arrangement of its component cells. Class I includes tissues in the Aristotelian sense only, i.e., composed of detached cells and distinguished by virtue of the characteristics of these cells. Blood and lymph are normal tissues of class I; pus is the representative pathological tissue. Class II includes the crystalline lens of the eye, the chorda dorsalis, and all epithelial tissues. Here the constituent cells, while still discrete, are closely bound together into a structure of higher order. Class III comprises cells similar to those in the preceding class, but with "fused walls"; Schwann includes cartilage, bone, and teeth. In class IV he places all tissues composed of "fibrous cells," whether loosely or tightly bound together, such as loose connective tissue and tendons. Class V, like class III, includes tissues composed of cells with fused walls, but the constituent cells are further characterized by the presence of intercommunicating cell-cavities (*Zellenhoehlen*). Nerve, muscle, and capillary vascular tissue belong in this group.[40]

Schwann's remarks on the subject of epithelium are worth considering, not only because they reveal the looseness of his classificatory procedure but also in view of the importance that epithelium acquired in later discussions of the histogenesis of carcinoma. "It is very difficult to determine," Schwann writes, "what is to be understood by the term epithelium." The flat, polyhedral cells that form the outer layer of the chorda dorsalis in the larval frog look like epithelium and constitute a covering layer, but they cannot be so classified because they are clearly flattened cells of the same type as the round cells that compose the bulk of the chorda dorsalis.[41] But he accepted the flat cells of the outer epidermis as epithelium, even though Henle had shown that the round, nucleated cells of the Malpighian layer epidermis are "probably the young epidermal cells."[42] The serous leaf of the germinal membrane in the early stages of embryogenesis is also revealed under the microscope to consist of a layer of flattened cells. But Schwann adds that the serous leaf "cannot be regarded as epithelium, although it has the same structure." He gives no reason, but it may be because earlier writers had not applied the term to the serous leaf. Frankly admitting the difficulty of framing a definition of epithelium that would not include the serous leaf, Schwann says that he will not engage in a dispute over words and abruptly drops the subject.[43] He then describes the cellular structure of tissues customarily designated epithelium, including the interior lining of blood vessels.[44] Schwann's grouping of the tissues is more a matter of convenience than a classification carried out in accordance with strict rules.[45]

Schwann's tentative solutions to the problem of the cytogenesis of the cells composing the tissues of the above five classes reveal how far he had moved from his position of the previous year. Lymph corpuscles (*Lymphkoerperchen*) in which nuclei can be demonstrated by treatment with acetic acid, he writes, "probably take form in the lymph-fluid constituting their cytoblastema," although it is unknown whether nuclei are present from the beginning.[46] Mucous corpuscles, likewise, take form from the mucus that constitutes their cytoblastema. Pus corpuscles arise in a "cytoblastema of anomalous composition exuded in large amounts during inflammation." Here, too, it seems likely that nuclei form first.[47] The same mode of formation occurs in epithelium, the most important member of class II. Schwann's studies of the development of epidermis in the fetal pig more or less confirmed those of Henle. The first step is the formation of naked nuclei at the dermal-epidermal junction, where no cells are as yet visible and the "nuclei lie very closely packed together, with a small amount of finely granular intermediate substance." The second is the formation of a cell about the nucleus. Only very rarely does a young epithelial cell form *within* a mother cell: "The majority of epithelial cells in all vertebrates definitely do not form as cells within cells, but outside of cells in a minimum of cytoblastema, which is exuded by the cutis."[48] Of the tissues in class II only the chorda dorsalis and the crystalline lens display intracellular cell formation; in the case of the chorda, Schwann no longer believed that its cells arise from nuclei or cytoblasts.[49]

Class III includes cartilage, the tissue that, Schwann had claimed in 1838, best illustrated the formation of young cells within mother cells as described by Schleiden. But, after having reinvestigated cell genesis in the gill cartilages of larval frogs, he found that the new cells arise "in the cytoblastema, not in the cells already present." Schwann identifies the intercellular substance (*Intercellularsubstanz*), in which the cartilage cells lie, with the cytoblastema.[50] Class IV includes the loose form of connective tissue traditionally known as cellular tissue or texture (*tissu cellulaire, Zellgewebe*). Here too, according to Schwann, the "transparent, structureless, primary substance (*Ursubstanz*) of gelatinous character that we term, provisionally, the cytoblastema" is found. Although difficult to discern, especially where the fibers, i.e., the transformed cells, are closely packed, the cytoblastema "probably persists, throughout the course of life, between the fibers of cellular tissue." The cytoblastema, he supposes, is a primary substance from which all "corpuscles"—nucleoli, nuclei, and cells—take form.[51]

Of the mode of genesis of the class V cells, Schwann has little to say, although he does suggest that embryonic muscle cells form in a cytoblastema. Subsequent fusion of their walls results in the production of multinucleated adult muscle cells.[52] Schwann's cytoblastema resembles the plastic lymph of the humoral theorists of the preceding decades, the only difference being that the concrete cell has replaced the hypothetical fiber.[53]

But if new cells arose, in the manner described by Schwann, from an amorphous blastema or cytoblastema, how was their orderly metamorphosis into epithelial, connective tissue, muscle, and nerve cells to be understood? Were all such cells identical when first formed, and their subsequent differentiation the result of local factors? Were they different from the beginning in consequence of a special feature of the formative cytoblastema? Or were factors of both kinds operative? (Lobstein and Andral had postulated a "plastic force" to account for the metamorphoses of the plastic lymph under normal and pathological conditions.) Schwann would have by-passed some aspects of the problem had he remained with Schleiden's initial hypothesis that new cells formed within old. That is, he could have supposed that in the adult organism all cells gave rise only

to like cells.[54] That (admittedly partial) solution was now no longer
available to him. Schwann recognized the problem, but made no attempt
to deal with it. His sole comment on the subject occurs in a passage
discussing the "matrix" of dermal tissue underlying the epidermis. He
writes: "But whether the cytoblastema exuded from the matrix has a
specific character, or whether the horn cells take form for the same
reason that muscle cells and cellular tissue cells arise elsewhere in the
body, namely in consequence of the overall organismal plan, cannot as
yet be decided."[55]

CELL THEORY; GENESIS OF CELLS IN TUMORS

Championed by Schwann and Mueller, the view that both normal and
pathological tissues were structured aggregates of transformed cells,
developed for the most part *de novo* from an amorphous cytoblastema
ultimately derived from the circulating blood, became widely accepted.
Throughout the 1840s and the early 1850s this was the ruling presup-
position of almost all work on the cytohistogenesis of tumors. To the
investigators of that time it seemed to rest on a firm, if incomplete,
observational base. Within the confines of dogma there was room for
numerous differences of opinion with respect to the possibility that the
cell-generative behavior of blastemas, normal and abnormal, was determined by their intrinsic chemical constitution, and with respect to the
question of the precise sequence and nature of the events that culminated
in the formation and transformation of cells arising in such blastemas.
The possible roles of local and general factors remained an open question.
Aside from a rare dissenter, physiologists, physiological chemists (notably, Justus Liebig), pathologists, and biologists joined in confessing to
the new belief. But, despite this show of unanimity, its rule was brief; the
blastema theory was abandoned in Germany in the mid 1850s and in
England and France a decade later.[56]

Vogel

A review of the cytohistogenesis of abnormal tissues by Julius Vogel,
published in 1842 in Rudolf Wagner's encyclopedia of physiology and
pathology, illustrates the degree to which the stated assumptions were
shared at that time.[57] According to Vogel the cytohistogenesis of abnormal
tissues was precisely like that of normal tissues. In both instances the
constitutive cells arise from an "amorphous formative substance, or
cytoblastema." Obeying the "general laws of organic development," nuclei

take form in the cytoblastema, and cells then enclose the nuclei. The resultant nucleated cell undergoes appropriate structural transformations to yield one or another of the elementary components found in abnormal tissues. Vogel's comment on the troubling question—Why do normal tissues develop under one set of circumstances, and abnormal tissues under another?—is couched in the Aristotelian terms that had long played an important role in embryological thought: *potentiality* (*dynamis*) and *actuality* (*energeia* or *entelecheia*). The developmental potentiality of a given cytoblastema, he says, is inscribed in the nature of the substance composing it, whereas the "transition of *potentia* into *actus*" is dependent on external factors such as temperature, available water and oxygen, and so on. Vogel also mentions the possibility of a "life-force" (*Lebenskraft*) inherent in the organism and its parts, which influences the development of cytoblastemas. (Since he drops the subject at once, this seems no more than a gesture in the direction of discarded romantic biology.) Vogel phrases the chief question very clearly: "Does a given cytoblastema have only a general capacity for development, or does it have a tendency to develop into a specific tissue; and is or is not the nature of the tissue arising therefrom determined by the nature and chemical composition of its cytoblastema?" Vogel was unable to ascertain any crucial chemical differences between those cytoblastemas yielding normal, and those yielding abnormal tissues; hence he was inclined to believe that extrinsic factors were more determinative in this respect.[58]

In addition to benign and malignant tumors, Vogel included scars, tissue hypertrophy, and tuberculous or scrofulous masses under the heading of tissue new formations (*Neubildungen*). He denied that a sharp distinction could be drawn between localized tissue hypertrophy and benign tumors.[59] He also opposed the practice of classifying tumors as benign or malignant on the basis of their liability to recur after extirpation, offering instead a criterion based on histology and histogenesis. So-called benign tumors were those in which the formative blastema had advanced, via cell genesis and transformation, to become a persisting and more or less normally formed local mass of tissue. The formative blastema of a malignant tumor, on the other hand, either failed to reach the point of cell genesis (as in tuberculous or scrofulous tumors) or, if it did, the cells broke down in the course of a destructive process that usually involved the surrounding normal tissues. Accordingly, Vogel subdivided malignant tumors into: (1) unorganized (scrofula and certain other tuberculous lesions); (2) organized, with persisting cells (medullary carcinoma, certain tuberculous lesions); (3) organized, with both persisting cells and fiber formation.[60] As for benign tumors, Vogel proposed a subclassification "in accordance with histological principles." He mentions lipomas, enchondromas, vascular tumors, benign pigmented (melanotic) tumors, and "fibrous" tumors. The last group includes smooth muscle as well as fibrous tissue tumors.[61]

Vogel's essay represents the first attempt to treat pathological histology from the standpoint of a cell theory—admittedly, one more or less "Schwannian" in character, based on the belief that cells arise *de novo* from amorphous blastemas. In 1845 he elaborated his views on this pre-Virchovian manifestation of cellular pathology in a systematic treatise.[62] By this time Vogel had moved further in the direction of classifying tumors on the basis of histological, rather than clinical, criteria. He argued that purely clinical criteria of malignancy in tumors—such as the tendency to recur locally after surgical removal—were contradictory and unworkable unless histological criteria were added thereto. "The malignity which forms the grand principle of division between these two classes of tumors," writes Vogel, "is connected with the very nature of the tumor itself, and depends on its histological elements."

Adapting a concept introduced by gross histopathologists (notably Lobstein) to the cell era, Vogel stated that from a histological point of view tumors fell into two great categories, one comprising tumors composed of cells and tissue *homologous* to those normally present in the body, and the other comprising tumors composed of more or less *heterologous* elements. Mueller had rejected this concept on the ground that under the microscope both kinds of tumor proved to be composed of precisely the same elements. Vogel did not return to it because of his belief that cancer cells were identifiable under the microscope as heterologous elements (as did some of his colleagues), but because, in his opinion, cancerous cells and tissue *en masse* were so identifiable. The practical value of the division of tumors into heterologous and homologous depended on the empirical evidence that most heterologous tumors were clinically malignant, and most homologous tumors benign, in the sense that the former did and the latter did not tend to recur after extirpation. A further complication, Vogel pointed out, was that the common scirrhus was composed of both homologous and heterologous tissues, i.e., of histologically "non-malignant and malignant elements."[63] Vogel thus broadened the ill-defined concept of malignancy to embrace certain features of histological structure, which entails an end to purely descriptive histological characterizations of tumors. Hereafter, they will be predictive as well, and thus, in practice, involve an element of uncertainty.

That malignant tumors, the so-called pseudoplasmata, "take their origin from an amorphous cytoblastema is indubitable," Vogel says, and "it is no less indisputable that this cytoblastema is furnished from the vascular system."[64] The reader who forgets that observational data are seldom given other than in the context of accepted theory will find

Vogel's confidence in the existence and role of the (now mythical) cyto-blastema rather puzzling. In order to lend a semblance of reality to this cytoblastema, it will be convenient to begin with Vogel's account of the lesion then known as "tubercle," regarded by him and others as a form of malignant tumor with little or no organization to its formative cyto-blastema.

A tubercle was a tumor or new-formation characteristic of a "specific disease or morbid tendency—tuberculosis." In this disease, nodules composed of a grayish or yellowish, opaque or semitransparent, more or less homogeneous substance were found scattered throughout the body but most commonly present in the lungs. Under the microscope such lesions revealed themselves to be composed of an intermixture of imperfectly formed cells and nuclei, an amorphous substance that "per-fectly resembles coagulated fibrin and micro-chemically reacts like it" (i.e., soluble in acetic acid and alkalis), and minute granules of "modified protein," insoluble in acids and alkalis. Sometimes no cells are present and sometimes the "whole mass of the tubercle appears to consist of cells and cytoblasts." Admittedly, the tuberculous cytoblastema is not seen in its original, fluid state, but Vogel can conceive of no other source for the solid substances actually visible than the circulating plasma of the blood. The formative cytoblastema is "secreted from the capillary vessels" and "fills up all the interstices of the tissues." This pathological process falls under the rubric inflammation. The cytoblastema is an exudate. The underlying mechanism of the development of inflammatory pseudo-tumors and true tumors, or neoplasms, is thus one and the same.[65] In the case of the latter, a similar amorphous substance could often be discerned, intermingled with cells and fibers, and was "to be regarded as the solid cytoblastema of cancer."

Certain cancers (e.g., encephaloid) were composed almost entirely of cells. Others, scirrhus in particular, contained a large proportion of fibers, thought by Vogel to be derived directly from the cytoblastema as well as by way of cell transformation. Unlike simple inflammatory tumors and benign tumors generally, cancerous tumors possessed an "innate capacity for augmentation." Cancer cells arise not only directly from the cytoblastema but also, secondarily, from already formed cancer cells, some of which "contain in their interior young cells...capable of a similar mode of increase." "Clearly," says Vogel, "there is no limit to the increase of cancer cells."[66]

In his 1842 essay Vogel had commented briefly on the character of intrinsic and extrinsic factors that possibly govern the direction of cyto-blastema development. He elaborated these ideas somewhat in 1845, but added nothing essentially new. Leaving aside possible chemical differ-ences in the composition of blastemas (of which, Vogel admitted, nothing was known), it appeared that the more rapidly a formative blastema was exuded from the blood vessels to accumulate locally, the less capable it was of organization. Presumably this was because the "influence of the surrounding histological elements" was diluted or otherwise hindered. On the other hand, "small exudations repeatedly occurring" could be fully integrated into the histological structure of the site of their occurrence, as in the case of "simple hypertrophy," which was merely a heightened degree of the normal process of nutrition. That the subsequent course of development of an exudate, i.e., of an extruded cytoblastema, was more or less influenced by the histological character of the surrounding parts seemed a well-attested observation. This presumed regularity Vogel designated the "law of analogous formation." The more complex the structure of the tissue in which the new formation occurred, the less perfect was the analogy between the two. Thus, bone and connective tissue were readily reproduced, nerve and muscle tissue less so, and brain and lung tissue not at all. In the case of heterologous new formations, however, the "law of analogous formation" seemed to be inoperative. Here, Vogel said, one might have to fall back on the views of the humoral pathologists, according to whom the peculiar structural features of scirrhus, encephaloid, tubercle, etc., depended on a corresponding chemical peculiarity of the formative blastema involved. Alternatively, the view of the solidary pathologists, who sought for an explanation in terms of a changing "nervous influence," might be adopted. In the absence of conclusive evidence, Vogel supposed that both "changes in the cytoblastema" and "changes in the physiological properties of the tissues" were conjointly at work in the production of heterologous neoplasms.[67]

Rokitansky

Vogel's cautious response to the question of the chemical specificity of blastemas contrasts strongly with that given at about the same time by Karl von Rokitansky, holder of the newly created chair in pathological anatomy at the University of Vienna. Rokitansky, the acknowledged leader in the field of gross pathological anatomy in German-speaking lands, was the author of a three-volume *Handbuch* on the subject that was published between 1842 and 1846.[68]

In writing the first volume (which appeared last) Rokitansky, whose experience with microscopy seems to have postdated the publication in 1842 of the third volume of his treatise, rashly attempted to work out the laws of pathological histogenesis in the light of both the new cell theory and the humoral doctrines of *crasis* and *dyscrasis.* Like Vogel, he held that the blastemas for new growths were derived from the blood plasma and that, after having been exuded from the capillaries, they underwent development into granules, nuclei, cells, and fibers, the direction of development being partly determined by the structure of the tissues at the site of exudation. This was orthodox enough, but Rokitansky also claimed that in the case of pathological new formations a "native anomaly in the blastema" was "practically demonstrable." Indeed, the blastemas responsible for such new growths contained "protein compounds...in various states of oxydation."

With a rather free hand, Rokitansky proceeded to create a corpus of chemical dyscrasias, each of which was presumed to be the source of the particular pathological-anatomical alteration characteristic of a given disease.[69] He agreed with Schwann that the normal sequence of tissue formation from the cytoblastema was nucleus to cell to fiber, but he believed (like Vogel) that fibers sometimes arose directly, without passing through the cell stage. Again like Vogel—and contrary to the opinion expressed by Mueller eight years earlier—Rokitansky supported the old concept of heterology or heteroplasia, claiming that in many malignant new growths the cells, fibers, and tissues were morphologically and chemically different from normal (homologous) structures. The "grade of malignancy" of such a tumor was "directly proportional" to the "degree of its heterogeneous nature."[70] With respect to the overall classification of tumors, Rokitansky held that the existence of transitional forms made either purely chemical-clinical or purely microscopic-morphological criteria unworkable, and hence they had to be used in combination.[71]

Virchow

In 1846 Rokitansky's system of humoral pathology, as set forth in the *Handbuch*, was subjected to a devastating critical analysis by Rudolf Virchow, another former pupil of Johannes Mueller. Among other things, Virchow pointed out that Rokitansky had offered absolutely no empirical evidence in support of his claim that oxidised proteins and pathological albuminates were the determining features of the various blood dyscrasias (and presumably of the abnormal blastemas derived therefrom). Virchow had words even less kind for Rokitansky's applications of the microscope and cell theory to general pathological anatomy, remarking that Rokitansky's working principle seemed to be that "for God nothing is impossible." And, while professing to follow Schwann, Rokitansky had described no less than four ways for cells and fourteen ways for fibers to arise from blastemas.[72] Virchow's attack, supported by Johannes Mueller, apparently reached home;[73] in the 1855 edition of the *Handbuch*, Rokitansky omitted the section on blood dyscrasias. But by 1855 Virchow, along with others of the Berlin circle, had come to the conclusion that cells arose only from preexisting cells. Hence Rokitansky's work once again proved unacceptable to Virchow.[74]

Throughout the eighteen forties, however, Virchow remained a convinced adherent of Schwannian cell-blastema theory. In 1847 he set forth, in two long papers, his views on the histogenesis of tumors in the light of that theory.[75] These papers also bear on a number of important methodological problems. For this reason, and because of Virchow's key position with respect to the subsequent development of oncological theory, they merit detailed consideration. From one of them we learn that doubt about the value of the microscope in the study of pathological processes had begun to reassert itself (at least among medical practitioners) after only a decade or so of enthusiasm. Virchow observed that skepticism of this kind was not limited to the older generation of physicians, those reared on a diet of gross pathological anatomy, but was met with in younger physicians as well—clear evidence, according to Virchow, that the true significance of microscopic studies for general pathology had never been grasped by them.[76] On the other hand, he added that it was unreasonable to expect two thousand years of clinical experience to yield precedence overnight to little more than a decade of experience (much of it of questionable validity) with the microscope.

As a conceptual error contributing to the prevailing skepticism, Virchow put his finger on the vice of "ontologizing" prevalent among microscopic pathologists, i.e., creating entities out of transitory developmental stages in pathologic processes. Johannes Mueller's greatest contribution to the understanding of the cancer problem, according to Virchow, had been the recognition of the "law of the identity of embryonal and pathological development" and its corollary that the various histopathological lesions, or "pathological products," discerned by medical microscopists could not be considered as "given, ontologically complete things but merely as *tissues in stages of development.*" Unlike normal tissues, however, the pathological tissue of a cancer never achieved a stage of completion and relative stability, but broke down and ended as a fibrous scar. With a hint of Hegelian dialectic, Virchow called this end-stage the "negation of cancer." Instead of designating as "finished, given ontologies," i.e., as distinct entities, what were no more than developmental stages, histopathologists should direct their attention toward the factors responsible for the organization of blastemas or exudates into malignant tumors. Further, to those who understood "Mueller's law" the search for absolute differences between cancer cells and normal cells was a vain endeavor.[77]

Virchow was fully convinced of the role of blastemas. "All organic formation," he stated, "takes place from an amorphous substance; nutrition and new formation, embryonal and pathologic, are in essence the differentiation of a formless, solid or fluid substance."[78] Under the microscope this substance could be readily seen. It appeared, said Virchow, as a yellow-, brown-, or red-tinged "gelatinous mass" containing few if any formed elements; it was most evident in the case of colloid cancer, in which the proportion of jellylike amorphous blastema far outweighed that of cells and fibers. It was also abundant, in a more solid form, between the cells and fibers of bone cancers. The chemical nature of blastemas, said Virchow, was as yet not understood, and the unsubstantiated claims of Rokitansky, Vogel, and Henle were alike unacceptable.[79] The latter two investigators had claimed that the essential constituent of blastemas was fibrin, or an abnormal variant thereof. In spite of his skepticism in this matter, Virchow himself believed that he had seen cancers arise from fibrin coagula within large veins, under circumstances that permitted the exclusion of an exterior origin. Hence, his remark that the cancerous metamorphosis of *extravascular* fibrin masses was "not improbable" in principle, even though it had not been demonstrated unequivocally.[80]

In the second paper, Virchow promulgated four laws governing the development and organization of tissues, whether normal or pathological: (1) "All organization results from the differentiation of a formless substance, a blastema"; (2) "All blastemas first pass out of the vessels in a fluid state"; (3) "All organization commences with cell formation"; and (4) "Cells are transitory formations, and beyond a certain point nothing more can become of them."[81] The first two laws are independent of cell theory; they apply equally to the "fiber-era" blastema theory. Evidently Virchow wanted to emphasize the continuity of scientific thought. He had already acknowledged that many students of the tumor problem, himself included, were returning to the "path marked out by the best observers before the time of the cell-theory." They were attempting, as Lobstein, Carswell, Cruveilhier, and others had done before them, to understand cancerous growth as a consequence of a disturbance of the nutritive process (*Ernaehrungsprocess*).[82] The third of Virchow's laws shows that he, unlike Vogel and Rokitansky, did not allow for the direct formation of fibers, or of any other structural elements, from blastemas. The *cell* was the primary and indispensable morphological unit, and all other units took origin from it. (This might be paraphrased as *omnis structura a cellula*). Virchow called this, "Mueller's law"—not, as might have been expected, "Schwann's law."[83] It is worth noting that by 1847 the formation of new cells within mother cells was regarded as such a rare occurrence in normal tissues that Virchow found it necessary to point out that the intracellular formation of new cancer cells was not a constitutive feature of that lesion.[84] Nevertheless, as far as Virchow was concerned, there was no difference, in principle, between intracellular and extracellular formation of new cells. Distinguishing two modes of cell genesis seemed trivial; in one instance, the new cell arose from cyto-blastema contained within the boundaries of a previously formed cell; in the other, it arose from "free," i.e., extracellular, cytoblastema.[85] Ob-viously, the notion of the cell as a mere container of cytoblastema was still present in Virchow's mind, together with the notion of the cell as the fundamental unit of life (in the absence of any conflict between the two).[86]

While recognizing the validity of Mueller's claim that all tumors, homologous or heterologous though they might appear at the gross level, were composed alike of cells, fibers, and granules, Virchow favored the retention of the traditional distinction, although in a somewhat altered sense. The "heterology" of cancer, tubercle, sarcoma, and so on did not lie in the ultimate morphological constitution of the tumors in question, but rather in the course of development undergone by their formative blastemas. The task of the pathologist, said Virchow, was to determine why organization took place now in one direction, now in another.[87] For Virchow, the terms *homologous* and *heterologous* were not synonymous with *benign* and *malignant.* Homologous organization of a blastema yielded tissues appropriate to the site; heterologous organization did not. According to Virchow, this was the crux of the matter.[88] What were the factors determining organization? Impressed by the influence of the surrounding tissues on the organization of blastemas, Vogel and Henle had emphasized the law of analogous formation. But this "law" had numerous exceptions: regardless of their site, large exudates tended to undergo heterologous development; and not all normal tissues were capable of appropriately transforming regenerative exudates, e.g., muscle, whereas some abnormal tissues were capable of so doing.[89] In this con-nection Virchow called attention to the tendency of pathological blastemas, i.e., exudates, to repeat the same pattern of structural organization regardless of where they might be deposited in the body of a patient with a given disease. That is, in a patient with the cancerous diathesis all exudates tended to undergo cancerous organization; in a patient with the tuberculous diathesis, tuberculous organization, and so on.

Exudates could be said to possess "memory" (*Gedaechtniss*) in that they retained the ability to produce one and the same organizational pattern in different parts of the body. Rokitansky had attempted to account for this phenomenon by assuming that the circulating blood plasma (from which all blastemas were ultimately derived) was, in such cases, marked by a generalized chemical dyscrasia of the appropriate kind—cancerous, tuberculous, etc. But Virchow objected that clinical observations proved that cancer and tuberculosis could coexist in one and the same patient; hence, it would follow that two different states of mixture could coexist in the same plasma, which was absurd.[90] The reader may wonder why Virchow did not attempt to resolve the problem by assuming that specifically abnormal cells—rather than blastematous exudates mysteriously endowed with "memory"—were disseminated via the blood stream to various parts of the body, there to develop into foci of cancer, tuberculosis, etc., in accordance with the nature of the specific cells concerned. The answer seems to be that this would have involved "ontologizing," i.e., he would have had to accept cancer cells, tubercle cells, and so on, as specific entities; whereas he believed that they, and all cells, were merely transitory formations derived from blastemas.

DEBATES OVER THE SPECIFICITY OF CANCER CELLS

Mechanism of Metastasis

Metastasis, in its medical sense, is now used almost exclusively in reference to the development of new tumor tissue in a part of the body in consequence of the dissemination, via the blood or lymph, of specific cells derived from tumor tissue elsewhere in the body. Originally, however, the term referred to the shift or displacement, from one part of the body to another, of the internal and external manifestations of *any* disease. Dunglison's medical dictionary of 1842 defines metastasis as a "change in the seat of a disease; attributed by the Humorists, to the translation of the morbific matter to a part different from that which it had previously occupied; and by the Solidists, to the displacement of the irritation."[91] The clinical phenomena in question were familiar to the Hippocratic physicians, to whom we owe the term.[92]

Mueller himself was not averse to the idea that the spread of tumors in the human body might be due to the dissemination of a *seminium morbi* in the form of a fluid blastema. But he expressed much more clearly the possibility that the *seminium morbi* in such instances consisted of already formed cells or germ-nuclei (*Keimkerne*), capable of generating new cells. Mueller couched his idea in the terms of a venerable medical metaphor, that of the seed, the sowing, and the soil (already implicit in the Latin *seminium morbi*). "Once cells with a productive tendency have arisen," he states, "it can readily be seen how the uptake of germ-nuclei into the circulation can lead to their spread via the circulation to a soil suitable for their development, and thus give rise to secondary tumors."[93]

In 1840 Mueller's former pupil Jacob Henle—in an essay that breathed new life into the somewhat discredited notion of "seeds of contagion" (as found in the writings of Girolamo Fracastorius and Athanasius Kircher in the sixteenth and seventeenth centuries) and foreshadowed the approaching era of bacteriology—suggested that the spread of cancer might be due to the transmission of "germs (*Keime*) of the pathological formation" via the blood stream from the primary focus of cancerous disease to distant parts of the host body. Although Henle did not state explicitly that the "germs" in question had to be, or even could be, cancer cells, something of the sort is implied.[94] To Henle, however, the spread of cancer by the dissemination of cells within the body of the host represented only a special instance of a general case, e.g., he states also that if "tubercle cells" are carried by the blood stream to sites distant from the primary focus, "tubercles" will develop in those sites.[95] Henle remarked on the resemblance of such "germs" or cells to fertilized egg cells, insofar as they had the capacity for independent growth and development.[96] This comparison has already been met in earlier writings on the subject of cancer.

Mueller's monograph on the microscopic structure of cancer in the light of Schwann's cell theory appeared in an English translation in 1840. In the same year his ideas and findings were disseminated in France by Louis Mandl.[97] Mueller's work was given further currency in the English-speaking world by Walter Walshe, whose superb review of the cancer problem was published in England in 1841 and in the United States three years later.[98] Walshe appears to have relied almost entirely on the findings of Mueller, insofar as the microscopic structure and the genesis of tumors were concerned. But whereas Mueller had simply suggested that dissemination via the blood stream of germ-nuclei or cells derived from primary cancerous growths might give rise to secondary cancers elsewhere in the body, Walshe—without offering any new evidence—was somewhat more positive in his manner of expression. "The micrography of cancer shows," he writes, "that the translation and deposition of a few cells only from the original nidus might lead to the development of the largest mass; each cell is in itself *the possible embryo of a tumor.*" He admits, however, that the actual translation and deposition of "cancerous matter" has never been seen.[99]

In retrospect, it is apparent that Mueller—with Henle and Walshe in his wake—did little more than reformulate the traditional medical doctrine of the *materia peccans* ("peccant matter"), according to which the shifting clinical manifestations of a given disease within an afflicted body correspond to the shifting of a noxious substance (*materia peccans, materia morbosa, materies morbi*) from one part of the body to another. At the time that Mueller wrote, the *materia peccans* was defined as the "matter or material which is the cause of disease."[100] It was not the disease itself that was transmitted, from this point of view, but the *cause* of the disease, a distinction that Henle emphasized in his essay on miasmas and contagions.[101] Reformulating the old doctrine in the light of Schwann's cell theory, Mueller conceived of the *materies morbi* in cancer as the "disease-seed," or "germ" (*seminium morbi, Keim*)—perhaps a cell, endowed with the power of independent life and reproduction. In Henle's case the underlying idea was subjected to still further generalization; some of the "germs" were wayward cells derived from the body's own stock, e.g., his "tubercle cells" and, possibly, cancer cells, while others were "germs" from the outside world, *contagia animata,* that had made their way into the body.

In contrast to these speculations of Mueller, Henle, and Walshe, a young *Privatdozent* at Goettingen, Bernard Langenbeck, brought forward some rather impressive, but by no means conclusive, empirical evidence in favor of this explanation of metastasis in cancer.[102] In the course of two autopsies carried out on women with uterine cancers Langenbeck found aggregates of "cancer cells" within the pelvic veins, right heart, and pulmonary artery. The cells in question were not described by Langenbeck with a high degree of precision; he mentions "large carcinoma cells...five or six times the size of blood corpuscles" and, in passing, "smaller cancer cells."[103] Continuing with his dissection, Langenbeck found a number of subpleural nodules, and on opening the tiny pulmonary arterial branches leading to them he discovered aggregates of similar cancer cells. In some instances the coagula were fused with the subpleural nodules.

In interpreting his findings, Langenbeck asked, could the tumors have been primary in the lung and secondary in the uterus? Langenbeck was well aware that cancers in other parts of the body almost invariably preceded the development of lung cancer. Primary carcinoma of the lung was so uncommon that Bayle had seen only one case, Jean-Baptiste Bouillaud two, and Andral none whatsoever.[104] Langenbeck knew that if a tumor primary in the lungs were to spread by way of the veins to the uterus, the component of the tumor acting as the "seed" of the disease would have to move against the current. He called attention to the well-known finding that carcinomas originating in the organs drained by the portal vein gave rise to secondary tumors in the liver, which suggested that the "seed" had been carried by the portal flow to a point of impaction in the first set of capillaries reached, i.e., within the liver.[105] What was the nature of that "seed"? "If my observations on the development of cancerous tumors from simple cancer cells were correct," he wrote, "I had every reason to believe that the *seminium morbi* consisted in these cells alone, and that only through them was the dissemination and transfer of carcinomas possible."[106] In drawing this conclusion Langenbeck went far beyond his evidence, a point that should not be overlooked simply because he was right.[107]

In Langenbeck's opinion there were only three ways in which the spread of cancer could be accounted for. The first was that a fluid cancer matter (*Krebsstoff*) somehow developed in the circulating blood, and cancer cells then took form and subsequently became seated in various parts of the body; thus *all* tumors were secondaries. On the other hand, if the cells constituting a tumor arose primarily in some organ or tissue rather than in the blood, there were two possibilities: either a cancer-juice (*Krebssaft*) or cancer cells gained access to the blood stream and sowed the disease elsewhere in the body. Langenbeck postponed judgment on the first two of these possibilities until such time as he could publish further observations bearing on the matter.[108] While he did not claim that the third possibility (that of the dissemination of cancer cells derived from the primary tumor) was the sole mechanism of metastasis, he does seem to have thought that his autopsy observations of the two women with uterine cancers pointed clearly in this direction.[109]

If living cancer cells were in fact the *seminia morbi* of cancerous disease, there was no compelling reason for Langenbeck not to suppose that cancer cells might spread from one human being to another, and even from a human being to an animal. Cancer had long been regarded as a possibly contagious (but not miasmatic) disease.[110] Langenbeck remarked that Jean Alibert, among others, had unsuccessfully attempted to "transfer carcinomas to men and animals by the injection of cancer ichor" and that he had repeated Alibert's experiment, again without success, using dogs and rabbits. But the reason for the failure of these experiments seemed clear. The cancer-molecules (*Krebsmolecuelen*) or cancer cells present in cancer ichor "would long since have lost their vitality."[111]

Accordingly, Langenbeck decided to introduce cancer cells from "freshly extirpated human carcinomas" into the circulation of animals —"little though it seemed likely to me that the body of an animal would be a soil suitable for their development." Several preliminary experiments on rabbits were fruitless. The animals died within twelve to twenty-four hours after the intravenous injection of cancer fluid, presumably—so Langenbeck concluded—owing to the obstruction of the pulmonary capillaries by particles in the injected fluid, since the rabbits died with evidence of respiratory distress. Then a successful experiment followed. Langenbeck withdrew eight ounces of arterial blood from a large dog, removed the fibrin by whipping, and added "one-half ounce of cancer-juice...fluid as thin cream and carefully cleared of tumor particles" obtained from a presumably malignant tumor occupying the freshly disarticulated humerus of a young man.[112] He then reinjected the mixture into the dog's femoral vein. Two months later the animal was killed. Langenbeck found several small nodules on the surfaces of both lungs and in the left middle lobe. Study of the nodules under the microscope left no doubt in Langenbeck's mind as to their carcinomatous nature. They consisted of fibers interspersed by closely packed large cells measuring about 1/100 of a line (roughly, 23 microns), together with smaller cells, some about the size of blood corpuscles and some only half that size. The same microscopic elements were visible in the original humeral tumor.[113]

Langenbeck was of the opinion that his autopsy and experimental findings furnished additional support for the views of Schleiden, Schwann, and Mueller: Schleiden had termed the plant-cell a "peculiar, small organism"; Schwann had drawn an analogy (functional and structural) between plant cells and animal cells; and Mueller had extended Schwann's analogy to include neoplastic as well as normal tissues. Contemporary botanists were well aware that plant cells (especially those of the simpler plants), singly or in small groups, were capable of independent life. But in higher animals the only cell capable of autonomous development seemed to be the fertilized egg, which customarily "metastasized" to the uterus, where it took root and flourished. Under pathological circumstances, however, other cells, particularly cancer cells, were capable of striking out in this manner. The cancer cell, like a detached plant-cell or an ovarian germ-cell, "must now appear as an organism endowed with life-force and developmental ability."[114]

Obviously it was a question of great importance whether individual cells from cancerous growths were identifiable under the microscope as "cancer cells" or not, and, if so, on the basis of what morphological criteria. Discussion of this topic began shortly after the publication of Mueller's monograph and has continued ever since. Gluge's paper of 1837 might be taken as the first in this series, but with the proviso that Gluge neither regarded his "globular bodies" as cells (in any sense) nor claimed that they were pathognomic of cancer.[115] A similar qualification applies to Mueller's earliest published statements on the microscopic structure of tumors. Mueller's presentation before the Berlin Academy of Sciences in 1836 contains no reference to cancer cells or globules, and the subsequent report in the *Archiv* (while it does mention certain globes and globules that are more or less characteristic of cancer) does not suggest that Mueller was already thinking along the lines of Schwannian cell theory—again, despite Mueller's implied claim to this effect in his monograph on tumors.[116]

The attempt to find a cell specific for cancerous growth can be regarded as a shift from the gross tissue level to the microscopic cellular level of the early efforts to define the features of abnormal, (heterologous or heteroplastic) in contrast to normal (homologous or homoplastic), tissues. Since Mueller was convinced that tumors, whether malignant or benign, contained no microscopic structural components not found in normal

embryonic or adult tissues, it is clear that the notion of a specifi
cell would have no appeal for him.[117] However, he did call atte
the frequent occurrence of tailed corpuscles (*Schwanzkoerpe*
certain malignant growths, in particular the so-called medullary carcinoma. Despite his disclaimer to the contrary, the tailed corpuscles were
taken by some impetuous microscopists to be pathognomic of cancer.[118]
But more careful microscopists directed their attention elsewhere.

The first and most unequivocal identification of a so-called cancer cell
came from the Danish pathologist Adolph Hannover in 1843. He
described it as highly variable in size, round or oval, its nucleus large
and sometimes multiple, its nucleoli large and peculiarly translucent (as
seen in unstained cell smears), and its surface finely granular. According
to Hannover, the cancer cell (*cellula cancrosa*), a "peculiar, heterologous
element," is the "true basis of cancerous degeneration." He also noted
that microscopic bodies resembling embryonic connective tissue cells
(presumably Mueller's tailed corpuscles) were often visible in cancers,
but he did not regard them as specific cancer cells.[119]

In an essay of 1843 entitled "Micropathological Observations on the
Nature of Contagion," P. F. Klencke made some interesting comments
with respect to the "foreign" character of cancer cells.[120] Klencke claimed
to have successfully repeated Langenbeck's transfer of cancer from a
human being to a dog, using human mammary cancer cells to generate
secondary pulmonary tumors. The experiment was essentially a transplantation procedure, of a kind long familiar to biologists. Nevertheless,
Klencke was uncertain whether the transplanted cells actually survived
and multiplied or merely furnished a blastema for the generation of new
cells. In principle, however, he agreed with Langenbeck that a cancer
cell was an "organism endowed with life-force and developmental
capacity" and capable, once formed from the cytoblastema, of taking root
anywhere in the body of a host organism. Such cells had become
"foreigners" within the very organism that had given them birth; their
commitment was primarily to a "foreign scheme of organic existence."
Hence they always acted in a manner "inimical to the normal conduct of
life"—not only in the host organism but wherever they might lodge.
Klencke generalized this hypothesis, suggesting that in cancer and in
many other diseases as well there arises within the afflicted individuals a
corresponding variety of deviant or "rebellious" (*abtruennige*) cells.[121]

Hannover's affirmative answer to the question of the anatomical
specificity of cancer cells was given support in 1845 by Hermann Lebert,
who argued that *all* tissue lesions contained cells having visible characteristics more or less specific for the kind of lesion involved. Cancer
globules (*globules cancéreuses*) were simply cells in which the "most striking
differences from every other species of cell" are manifest under the

microscope. The cancer cell, or rather its "cellular envelope," ranged in diameter from fifteen to 50 microns, and some of the larger cells were multinucleated. The nuclei themselves measured up to twenty microns in diameter and contained sharply defined, opaque nucleoli ranging from two to ten microns in diameter. Apparently wishing to distinguish normal tailed corpuscles from cancerous ones, Lebert described certain *corps fusiformes fibroplastiques*, present only in cancers and characterized by large nuclei and nucleoli.[122] Like Hannover, Lebert held that a cancer was a "heteromorphic production, without an analogue in the normal state of the organism." But he emphasized that only the cancer cell was heteromorphic; the connective tissue stroma comprised normal cells and other tissue elements. In Lebert's words: "The elements composing a cancer can be divided into elements peculiar to that morbid production and other elements found in a wide variety of morbid productions and even as a rule in the organism in the normal state."[123]

Julius Vogel, in his pioneering book on (Schwannian) cellular pathology referred to earlier, gave a detailed description of cells found in cancerous growths. Among the features he noted were variability of cell size (from six to over one hundred microns in diameter), large and sometimes multiple nuclei, and prominent nucleoli. Although Vogel spoke of "characteristic cancer cells," he was at pains to point out that there was no such thing as a "distinctive cancer cell." Despite the impossibility of deciding with absolute certainty whether a single cell was cancerous or not, when a large number of cells from a tumor were available the classification could be made with considerable confidence.[124]

In 1846 the morphologically specific cancer cell found two new defenders, one in France and the other in Germany. Charles Sédillot, a surgeon and a strong believer in the value of the microscope as a tool in cancer diagnosis, described his *cellule cancéreuse* rather imprecisely as a round or oval body up to ten times the size of a red blood cell.[125] The histopathological diagnostician in Sédillot's cases was Émile Kuess, who later devised and employed an instrument for obtaining punch biopsy specimens of tumors.[126] The new German defender of the thesis of the morphological specificity of cancer cells was Heinrich Meckel, who made the additional claim that cancer cells were the sole heterologous products of disease to be found in the body.[127] The opposite stance was taken by Virchow in one of his essays of 1847. Admitting the diagnostic value of certain distinctive microscopic features of cells found in cancers, particularly the overlarge nuclei, Virchow pointed out that such features could occasionally be misleading.[128] As for the other cells found in cancers, such as Mueller's tailed corpuscles, Robert Froriep's fiber-cells, and the cells composing small blood vessels, he derived them from the cancer blastemas but pointed out that they were not peculiar to cancerous growths alone.[129]

The question of the morphological specificity of cancer cells viewed singly, e.g., in smears prepared from cancer-juice, must be distinguished from the question of their morphological specificity when seen in large groups. Both questions became increasingly important for practical purposes in the decade following the publication of Mueller's monograph on the fine structure of tumors. The microscope rapidly became an instrument almost indispensable in the practical, surgical diagnosis of tumors—contrary to the prediction of Mueller himself, who had regarded the microscope as a tool useful only in research and valueless in the everyday diagnosis and treatment of tumors.[130] How contrary to his expectations matters had proceeded becomes evident from a reading of two outstanding monographs of the 1840s on the diagnosis of malignant tumors, Carl Bruch's *Die Diagnosis der boesartigen Geschwuelste* (Mainz, 1847) and John Hughes Bennett's *On Cancerous and Cancroid Growths* (Edinburgh, 1849). Bruch's monograph consists of a general discussion of the cancer problem followed by twenty-seven detailed case reports, complete with microscopic findings. Despite Bruch's apparent disillusionment with the chemical study of tumors—indicated by his statement that the microscopic anatomy of a tumor reveals more about its character than does its chemical constitution—he suggests that, if developed, techniques of microscopic histochemistry might be revealing. Cancer cells are neither specific nor heterologous; they somewhat resemble embryonal cells and do not differ in origin or development from normal cells, although they are prone to have multiple nuclei and large or multiple nucleoli. In spite of the individual cells' lack of specificity, cancers can usually be diagnosed with the aid of the microscope: although "there exists no elementary constituent of cancer that cannot possibly be found in some normal tissue...there exists no normal tissue that is composed of the sum of constituents met with in cancer."[131]

Bennett's monograph is even more impressive. It contains, in addition to a general discussion of the anatomy, physiology, pathology, diagnosis, and treatment of cancer, fifty-six well-documented case studies and a detailed description of the procedure to be employed in the examination of surgically removed tumors. Aside from the use of aniline dyes and the rotary microtome (which were introduced in the third quarter of the nineteenth century), Bennett's punctilious procedure could well pass muster today.[132] While he considered the microscope indispensable in the diagnosis of cancer, Bennett pointed out that it only became such when the microscopic anatomical evidence was assessed in conjunction with clinical evidence.[133] The chemical analysis of tumors had so far proved valueless in distinguishing tumors from one another or from normal tissues; what was needed, said Bennett, was a method that allowed for histochemical analysis at the microscopic level.[134] Bennett disagreed with Hannover and others who upheld the doctrine of the morphologically specific cancer cell, but he argued that the nonexistence of such a cell should not mislead anyone into believing that cancerous and normal tissues were not distinguishable under the microscope—a view that he erroneously attributed to both Mueller and Virchow.[135] However, he agreed that the "so-called cancer cell" often displayed certain distinctive features: it might present as a round, oval, oblong, caudate, spindle-shaped, heart-shaped, or otherwise contoured body varying in diameter from 0.01 to 0.10 millimeters; at least one and as many as nine nuclei were present, varying in size from one-sixth to four-fifths of the cell; the nuclei were provided with one or two nucleoli. But, when seen in isolation, such cells could not be distinguished from normal cells found in many epithelial tissues, especially when the latter cells were young and "plastic" or when they occurred free in exudates or other body fluids.[136]

Origin and Nature of Cancroids

Related to the dispute over the specificity of the cancer cell was another dispute that arose at about the same time in connection with the microscopic study of a long-recognized group of lesions of the skin and mucous membranes, some of which were characterized by a tendency to ulcerate, spread, and resist treatment. The most familiar was the *noli me tangere,* a papular and (later) ulcerative skin lesion whose name had served as a warning to generations of physicians. Lesions of this kind had usually been regarded as cancerous. However, even before the introduction of the microscope into histopathology, certain differences between superficial and deep-lying cancers had been recognized. Peyrilhe had suggested that a group of "cancerous ulcers" of the skin be distinguished from "true cancer."[137] Jean-Louis Alibert, in a treatise on skin diseases published a few years before the microscope transformed the study of pathological anatomy, classified a group of lesions as "cancerous dermatoses" and suggested the term *carcine,* to distinguish them from "cancer of the glands, and analogous alterations in the interior of the body." In this group he included *noli me tangere,* and *carcine verruqueuse,* the "sootwart."[138]

The two disputes overlapped to the extent that the distinction between true cancers and cancerlike lesions was made on the basis of the presence of specific cancer cells. Those who denied the existence of the cancer cell might still be inclined, however, to distinguish these lesions—then variously known as "pseudo-cancers," "cancroids," "epitheliomas," and "tumeurs épidermiques"—from so-called true cancers on the basis of histological structure, clinical behavior, or presumed origin, i.e., histogenesis. "Cancroids," "epitheliomas," and so on, were the first tumors to which—after the cell theory had become accepted in the 1840s—an origin from epithelial tissue was imputed.[139] The unitary epithelial origin of deep-lying cancers, on the other hand, seemed unlikely to most investigators at the same time, and not until the 1870s was it widely accepted. An understanding of the controversy over cancroids and similar lesions will help to show how this view of the histogenesis of carcinoma was possible and remained so even after the Schwannian belief in cell-forming blastemas had been discarded in favor of the postulate that all cells arise from preexisting cells. It should be understood that in terms of Schwann's theory a histogenetic inference did not necessarily imply a cytogenetic inference. In other words, the claim that cancroids were derived from epithelial *tissue* did not imply that the cells of cancroids necessarily arose from preexisting epithelial *cells*.

Perhaps the earliest statement of the problem occurs in Alexander Ecker's paper of 1844, which is chiefly concerned with lesions on the lower lip.[140] Ecker distinguished (1) an easily recognizable, harmless "wart-like formation," (2) "so-called cancer," and (3) "true cancer" (*wirklicher Krebs*). True cancer of the lip is a "carcinoma fibrosum," characterized by a microscopic fibrous stroma (*faserigem Stroma*) that contains cancer cells resembling those illustrated in Vogel's *Icones*.[141] Ecker's observations convinced him that "so-called cancer" of the lip was quite different in histological structure and origin from the "true cancer" with which it was frequently confused; the difference being that the former was composed of hypertrophied epidermis rather than of heterologous cancer tissue. Nevertheless, it was sometimes capable of deep extension into the underlying tissues and of recurrence after surgical excision. Since Ecker's criterion for distinguishing "so-called" from "true" cancer was not based on the presence or absence of cancer cells, it is histologic (and, to some extent, histogenetic) rather than cytologic in character. In contrast, Georges-François Mayor's later account of the microscopic findings in two similar lesions (one on the upper lip, one on the nose, both in older men) relies on a cytologic criterion.[142] The absence of specific cancer cells, *globules cancéreux*, persuaded Mayor that the two tumors should not be classified as cancers, even though both were invasive; they had been treated as cancers by the attending surgeons, but under the microscope Mayor found them to be composed of epidermal cells (*cellules épidermiques*).

The cytologic criterion was also used by Émile Kuess (working with the surgeon Charles Sédillot) at about the same time to distinguish pseudo-cancer from genuine cancer. Kuess described a *tumeur épidermique et cancéreuse* on the skin of the hand, with features of both "real" and "pseudo" cancer. He added that on other occasions as well he had "observed the presence of the epithelial cells in the heart of a reticular cancer." These findings led him to question whether there might be a "difference between cancers arising on the surface of the skin, from degeneration (*dégénérescence*) of the epithelium...and deep, vascular cancer, growing by endogenous generation of cells."[143]

Mayor, in a doctoral thesis published in 1846, revised his earlier assessment of the lesions in question after having become convinced that, regardless of their microscopic structure, they were clinically malignant. Abandoning the cytologic criterion, he stated that "the epidermal tumors commonly called *boutons de mauvaise nature, noli me tangere,* cancerous ulcer, or cancroid, cancers of the skin, are indeed true cancers, or, to speak more exactly, the cancerous affection may be the consequence of the development of an epidermal tumor.[144]

Lebert's views on the subject in 1845 (when his *Physiologie pathologique* was published) were determined by his firm belief in the existence of a specific cancer cell. Since cancroids did not contain such cells, as far as he was concerned they were not cancers. Like Ecker and Mayor, he attributed the origin of cancroids to epithelial tissue hypertrophy. In 1845 he had not yet seen cancroids give rise to tumor deposits in the regional lymph nodes.[145]

John Hughes Bennett's use of the term *cancroid* was highly idiosyncratic. For him it came to mean any tumor—not merely a tumor of epithelial character—that did not contain specific cancer cells. Thus he speaks of cartilaginous cancroid growths—"first described and separated from cancerous and osteosarcomatous tumors by Mueller under the name of enchondroma"—fatty and fibrous cancroid growths, and epidermal and epithelial cancroids. These tumors originate, grow, and decline in the same way as do the corresponding normal tissues, of which they are hypertrophied versions. It is sometimes apparent that "they, like all kinds of hypertrophies, originate in an increased exudation into a part, following a blow or injury; but at other times no apparent cause can be assigned."[146] Bennett's account of the origin, mode of increase, and character of cancer cells and cells in general, and of the relation between cancer cells and normal cells, is somewhat unclear. Although a firm believer in the existence of a specific cancer cell, he admits that the cells of cancroids, of normal adult epithelial and cartilaginous tissue, and of embryonal tissue in general may resemble cancer cells under the microscope. The question then arises whether specific cancer cells represent "only a modification of cells pre-existing in the body." Bennett's answer was that since cancer cells, like most cells, took origin from a formless blastema, presented the same microscopic appearance wherever they were found, and might be "actually seen to arise in tissues altogether separate from epithelium or cartilage," he doubted that the "true cancer cell" was ever "formed by the transformation of a previously existing one."

How then can true cancer cells be distinguished from morphologically similar cells found at times in cancroids, not to mention those in normal epithelial, cartilaginous, and embryonal tissues? Bennett replies that "a detection of their normal or anormal origin constitutes one of the distinctions between cancerous and cancroid growths."[147] In the place of an *observable* cytologic criterion for distinguishing between cancers and cancroids, he has substituted an *inferential* histogenetic or cytogenetic criterion, one that requires "a detection of their normal or anormal origin." While normal cells are never transformed into cancer cells, they may enter into the formation of cancroids owing to hypertrophy. New cells may then be added to the cancroid by the formation of cells in an appropriate blastema. Cancer cells, on the other hand, always arise primarily from a blastema, never by the transformation of preexisting cells. Once arisen, they may increase in number in two ways: by endocellular nuclear division or by endocellular formation. Bennett rejected the possibility, entertained by Kuess, that cancer cells were capable of "multiplying by division."[148]

Rudolph Virchow first addressed himself to the origin of cancroids in 1849,[149] and returned to the matter a year later in a paper on the histogenesis of a peculiar bone tumor composed of cells of epithelioid character.[150] In agreement with most investigators, Virchow held that cancroids began as hypertrophies of epidermal or epithelial tissue. But he argued that they become true cancroids only when they exceed the bounds of hypertrophy and spill over into the adjacent tissues in the form of "cavities and alveoli filled with cells of epidermoid character." According to Virchow, such alveoli could be distinguished from those found in true cancers, since they lacked the "new-formed layer of connective tissue which constitutes the walls of cancer alveoli." As for the epidermoid cells lining the alveoli of cancroids, Virchow admitted that they might well represent further extension and hypertrophy of the surface cells. But he was unwilling to derive *all* epidermoid cells in cancroids from epidermal tissue, for he had "seen an indisputable case in which the formation of a cancroid took place in a bone (the tibia) and only reached the exterior following the occurrence there of a fracture." Like other cancroids (as Virchow defined them), this tibial cancroid was composed of alveoli lined by "epidermoid cells."[151] This is probably the first report of that rare, and still controversial, tumor of the appendicular skeleton now usually referred to as an adamantinoma.[152] Virchow's chance encounter with it in 1850 not only influenced his view of the histogenesis of cancroid but also—long after he had abandoned the cell-blastema theory in favor of the view that all cells arise from preexisting cells —strengthened his conviction that epithelial cancers could originate from connective tissue.

Lebert dealt with the subject of cancroids again in his huge treatise

(1851) on cancerous and related diseases.[153] By that time he had become aware that cancroids were not as innocuous as he had first supposed. He now recognized that cancroids often recurred after surgical removal and that they might infiltrate into adjacent muscle and bone. Moreover, in the case of cancroids of the lip or penis, he observed that "epidermis may be carried by the neighboring lymphatics, and be transported to the nodes."[154] Nonetheless, Lebert remained convinced that cancroids and cancers differed in origin, microscopic structure, and clinical behavior. Cancroids—which he now called *tumeurs épidermiques* or *tumeur épithéliales*—were of epithelial (tissue) origin and were composed of cells of epithelial character, even though some of these cells might indeed resemble specific cancer cells. But only in cancroids, said Lebert, were to be found the peculiar *globes épidermiques* or *globes concentriques,* which at first sight resembled concentrically arranged fibers, but were in fact composed of concentrically arranged squamous epithelial cells. When a cancroid spread elsewhere these characteristic bodies were present in the locally invaded tissues and regional lymph nodes. Cancers, on the other hand, did not originate from epithelial tissue. Although they might contain a few cells resembling epithelial cells, they never contained *globes épidermiques.* Furthermore, cancer was a generalized disease with local manifestations, whereas cancroid was a local disease capable of limited spread.[155] Lebert admitted that there were difficulties in distinguishing the two diseases (he was of the opinion that perhaps one-fifth of the cases described as cancroids were in fact cancers). The difficulties were compounded when, as occasionally happened, a cancer and an epidermoid tumor simultaneously developed in the same location.[156]

Hannover, the original champion of the specific cancer cell in 1843 had not changed his allegiance when he published his 1852 monograph on epithelioma—"a peculiar tumor heretofore generally regarded as cancer."[157] Epitheliomas, i.e., cancroids, did not contain cancer cells and, unlike cancers, they arose from surface epithelium. In the course of their growth in the skin the Malpighian rete was somehow stimulated to "increased epithelial formation."[158] Epitheliomas, according to Hannover, arose only where pavement epithelium was normally present. Although the roots (*Wurzeln*) of certain epitheliomas might extend to involve underlying muscle and bone, and even reach out to the neighboring lymph nodes, the disease never became generalized. Nothing equivalent to the dissemination of cancer cells or cancer serum (*Krebssaft*) occurred. Remarkably, the cell that the cancroid cell most resembled was the *cancer* cell; hence, even with the microscope it was at times difficult to distinguish epithelioma from cancer.[159] Hannover's rejection of Virchow's claim that epithelial tumors could arise independently of epithelial tissue (as shown by tibial cancroid) is particularly interesting. It bears on the question of the fixity of cells and tissues under normal and pathological conditions, a question that continued to be debated throughout the nineteenth century. Hannover called Virchow's interpretation of the bone lesions in question "impossible."[160] "One tissue cannot be transformed into another," he says elsewhere, since this would contradict the "whole doctrine of development." For the same reason, he added, "an epithelial cell cannot become a cancer cell."[161]

4

CELL THEORY AND THE GENESIS
OF CELLS IN TUMORS, 1852-1900

BLASTEMA THEORY

Cytogenetic Uncertainty

Before Schwann, in the era of Bichatian tissue theory, the histogenetic question with respect to epitheliomas, cancroids, or *tumeurs épidermiques* could have been adequately (or at least unequivocally) answered with the assertion that they arose from normal epithelial tissue. However, Schwann's work destroyed the autonomy of the tissue concept. Tissues were now no more than structured aggregates of autonomous units —namely, cells—that had become variously transformed. Whether with respect to normal or abnormal embryonic or adult tissues, the question of histogenesis had become one of cytogenesis. But in Schwannian cell theory the autonomy of the cell was incomplete. Given the assumption that new cells arose partly from acellular blastemas, it was clearly impossible to trace adult tissue back to an embryonic precursor tissue. Similarly, if tumor cells arose *de novo* in pathological exudates, the statement that a given tumor originated in some one of the tissues of the body was equivocal, since the origin of the cells composing that tumor was not thereby accounted for.

The situation was even more unsatisfactory with respect to the origin of cancers. Although the resemblance of "cancer cells" to normal cells in epithelium or cartilage had been remarked from time to time, no one had suggested that cancers were derived from a precursor normal tissue, whether epithelium or cartilage. In retrospect the unsatisfactory character, as a working hypothesis, of the so-called free formation of cells from blastemas is evident, especially insofar as the search for the source of the "rebellious cells" (Klencke's felicitous phrase) constitutive of cancers was concerned. But if *all* cells arose from preexisting cells, it would be possible, in principle, to trace the cells composing all tumors, including cancers, back to the cells of one of the normal tissues, and then to look for the factors responsible for their conversion. It would also, of course, be possible to trace the cells of any normal adult tissue back to the cells of a

118

precursor tissue and eventually, through the succession of tissues in the embryo, back to the primal cell or zygote. The hazard to the autonomy of the cell, and certain other undesirable implications of the theory of free formation, now became evident. If cells arose *de novo* from what was generally agreed to be a proteinaceous substrate, i.e., the blastema, was this not equivalent to the spontaneous generation of life from lifeless matter, *generatio aequivoca?* And, as if aware of the undesirable implications of this notion, biologists—including Schwann, paradoxically enough —were attempting to dispose of it once and for all.[1]

Embryology

Today we might wonder why the data obtained from the studies of developing eggs and embryos with the improved microscopes of the 1830s did not at once obviate Schwann's hypothesis concerning the free formation of cells by revealing that the primal cell, or zygote, of all animals simply underwent cell division, without the participation of a hypothetical cell-forming blastema. Although the strongest objections to that hypothesis did in fact come from embryologists, the earliest observations on the developing egg were made before the cell theory as a whole could have been influenced by them in one way or another. The use of eggs containing large quantities of yolk as objects of microscopic observation, although convenient, suffered from the disadvantage that in the earliest stage of development the most obvious feature was the division of a fixed mass of yolk rather than the multiplication of new cell units. The drawings made in 1834 by von Baer accurately depict, to the eye of a modern biologist, the development of the batrachian egg from the zygote stage to the formation of embryonal germinal layers and membranes. Von Baer, of course, saw no such thing. Making no reference to cells as such, he described what occurred in the earliest stages as the cleavage (*Furchung*) of the yolk (*Dotter*).[2]

Schwann, discussing his own findings five years after von Baer made his drawings, does ask whether the "cleavage of the yolk described by Baer, Rusconi and others in the development of lower animals, e.g., in frog eggs, also depends on a cell-forming process, in which first two cells develop in the yolk, and then again two new cells in each of these, and so on." He asked, are the "globules of yolk-substance" actually "cells"? Although Schwann thought they were, he had to admit that definitive proof was lacking.[3] Even had he been able to produce conclusive proof, it would not have followed that the same rule held good for all later stages of embryonal development and for adult tissues, let alone pathological new-formations. The exudates seen by pathologists and physiologists in adult organisms, and regarded by them as blastemas, were real enough. The task of tracing the origin of the cells that subsequently appeared in these exudates was not so simple as it may seem today. Further, to the biologists of that time the temporal priority of the formless over the formed seemed almost self-evident.[4]

Nevertheless, the cell-blastema hypothesis was most vulnerable on the embryological side, especially with respect to the first stages of the development of the zygote. The step not taken by Theodor Schwann was taken by Karl Reichert. When Schwann's work became known in 1839, Reichert, an experienced embryologist, at once accepted and defended Schwann's "histogenetic" thesis, namely, the claim that cells and cells alone were the ultimate elements of animal tissues, from which all other structural elements were derived by transformation.[5] But Reichert did not accept Schwann's "cytogenetic" thesis, at least with respect to the new formation of cells in embryonic life. His own work had led him to conclude that from the beginning animal embryos were composed of cells and cells only; there was no trace of a "free intercellular substance" from which new cells could take origin.[6] Rudolf Koelliker, another well-known worker in the fields of microscopic embryology and histology, stated in 1844 that new cells were always derived from preexisting cells in the embryo.[7] But as late as 1851 Koelliker still held to a belief in the free formation of cells in *adult* organisms, especially under pathological circumstances.[8] And Reichert himself did not openly reject the free formation of cells under all circumstances until 1854.[9] The "cell-forming blastema" of nineteenth-century biology may be compared to the "luminiferous ether" of nineteenth-century physics. Both hypotheses reflected long-ingrained habits of thought; hence the readiness and tenacity with which they were accepted and held by most investigators in the absence of positive evidence to the contrary.[10]

Remak's Argument

Robert Remak, another of Johannes Mueller's outstanding pupils, seems to have been the first to dispense entirely with the hypothesis of free formation. Remak concluded that new cells arose only from preexisting cells on the basis of his embryological investigations.[11] The road then traveled by Remak to the generalized conclusion that *all* cells, embryonal and adult, normal and abnormal, arose from preexisting cells is set forth most clearly and succinctly in his paper of 1852, published in Mueller's *Archiv.*[12] Remak states that to him the extracellular origin of animal cells had always seemed "as unlikely as *generatio aequivoca."* Remak, like others, now saw the cleavage (*Furchung*) of the yolk as a process of continuing cell division in which the protoplasm (*Protoplasma*) of the egg-cell was divided up among the newly formed embryonal cells. There was no evidence whatsoever that the new cells arose from free nuclei or intercellular substance. As development proceeded, the embryonal cells separated off into the three germ layers: sensorial, motor, and trophic. Within these layers the continuing division of cells furnished the substance of the future tissues. Remak generalized his postulate (*Satz*) that "animal cells, like plant cells, have an *intracellular* origin only" in the following words:

> These findings are as closely related to pathology as they are to physiology. It can hardly be doubted now that pathological tissues constitute no more than variants of embryonal developmental types, and it is unlikely that they would have the privilege of the extracellular origin of cells. In this connection, the so-called "organization of plastic exudates" and the earliest stages in the formation of pathological tumors call for investigation. Supported by the confirmation of my long-standing doubts, I venture to express the surmise that pathological tissues no more take form from an extracellular cytoblastema than do normal tissues; they are, instead, derivatives or products of the organism's normal tissues.[13]

Remak's concern with the genesis of tumors was peripheral to his main interests (which lay in the field of embryogenesis), but it was strong enough to lead him to express the implied conclusion that tumors, like embryos, resulted solely from the successive division of a primal cell. This idea had already been expressed by Mueller, Walshe, and others, but not in combination with the postulate that all cells arose from preexisting cells. In the light of that postulate the old question whether tumors were truly new-formations or merely transformations or degenerations of preexisting tissues necessarily received a new answer. Remak was the first to give it. Writing on the subject of epithelial cancer in 1854, he stated that his own studies had confirmed his belief that in tumors, as in normal embryonic and adult tissues, new cells resulted only from progressive nuclear division (*fortschreitende, vom Kerne ausgehende Theilung*) followed by division of the whole cell, i.e., "multiplication by division" (*Vermehrung der Zellen durch Theilung*). No tumor, said Remak, not even a cancer, was, properly speaking, a "new-formation" (*Neubildung*) of pathological tissue from an amorphous blastema, as Virchow, Rokitansky, and others who built on the work of Schwann had supposed; a tumor was always the result of a "transformation of normal tissue" (*Umbildung normaler Gewebe*). Tumor cells, regardless of their atypicality, were ultimately derived from normal cells through nuclear and cell division.[14]

Remak and Cell Potency

Given Remak's assumptions, the cells of any tumor tissue are traceable to the cells of a precursor tissue, just as the cells of any adult tissue are traceable to those of an embryonic precursor. But to what particular precursor tissue? In other words, what are the limits of change imposed on normal tissues when they undergo transformation (*Umbildung*) into tumors? How much can a tumor cell deviate in character from its normal precursor cell? In the light of Remak's assumptions the general histogenesis and cytogenesis of tumors is clear enough, but the special histogenesis of particular tumors remains a problem. Remak's paper of 1854, however, contains a signpost pointing in the direction of future work on the histogenesis of particular tumors. With respect to Virchow's claim that the epidermal cells of cancroids could take form within the marrow of a bone (specifically, of the tibia) in the absence of any connection with the epidermis, Remak said that: "Since the penetration of epithelioma into bone has so often been observed, the derivation of aggregates of epidermal cells found within bones from similar detachments (*Ab-schnuerungen*) seems likely; these have perhaps taken place at an early developmental stage of the human embryo."[15] The importance of this remark is not that it anticipates (though it does) Julius Cohnheim's much later hypothesis of the origin of tumors from embryonic "rests" but that it introduces the problem of the developmental potency of cells and tissues into the field of tumor histogenesis. The reason for Remak's rejection of Virchow's claim that the epidermal cells of the tibial cancroid in question arise within the bone (independently of the overlying epidermis), and for the counterassertion that they arise from epidermal cells displaced during embryonic development, is his belief that the limits of tissue transformation (*Umbildung*) would have been exceeded. That is, the cells normally present within the marrow cavity of a bone are incapable of transformation into epidermal cells.

German Rejection of the Blastema Theory

The time-honored belief in the priority of the formless over the formed, shared by investigators from Aristotle's time through William Harvey's to John Hunter's, had rested on the observations of the naked eye. Hunter had extended the scope of its coverage from embryonic to adult tissue formation. Johannes Mueller had continued to accept it as he moved from the macroscopic to the microscopic dimension in the study of tumors. Schwann had made it part of his cell theory. But now it was being rejected in the very field of study where its strength had seemed greatest.

Remak was not alone. Other embryologists shared his conviction that a formless blastema played no role in the production of embryonal cells, that in the embryo all cells were derived from preexisting cells. And if the highly plastic substance of the embryo was incapable of the *de novo* formation of cells, it was hardly likely, as Remak pointed out, that the mature organism would somehow acquire this ability. A review of recent progress in microscopic anatomy by Reichert, published in Mueller's *Archiv* in 1854, reveals how far the tide of informed opinion in Germany had withdrawn from the assumption made by Mueller and Schwann. Reichert himself, who had never accepted the free formation of cells in the embryo, now called for a physiology and pathology likewise based on the tenet that new cells arise solely from preexisting cells.[16] Curiously enough, Schwann himself remained completely silent; the *Untersuchungen* of 1839 contain his final words on the subject.[17]

In 1854 Rudolf Virchow first expressed his misgivings as to the general validity of the blastema theory.[18] After calling attention to William Addison's claim that the new cells found in pathological exudates were actually migrant cells from the bloodstream, and to Remak's rejection of free cell formation under all circumstances, Virchow stated that there were four possible modes of cytogenesis: (1) by the division of pre-existing cells, (2) by budding (*Knospenbildung*), (3) by endogenous cell formation within "brood-spaces" (*Brutraeume*), and (4) by free formation where no other explanation seemed adequate, as in the case of patho-logical exudates and organizing thrombi. Under the heading of new-formation (*Neubildung*) Virchow included regeneration of lost tissue, scarring, diffuse hypertrophy and hyperplasia, partial hyperplasia, and heteroplasia. Partial, i.e., local, hyperplasia accounted for benign tumors (*gutartigen Geschwuelste*) of the thyroid, prostate, breast, uterus, and stomach, exostoses of bone, and lipomas. Heteroplasias involved the genesis of atypical cells and tissues, and under this heading Virchow placed local aggregates of pus corpuscles (*Eiterung*) in addition to "truly malignant tumors" (*die eigentlich boesartigen Geschwuelste*). The last named category included—in addition to "true cancer" (*der eigentliche Krebs*) and such tumors as cancroids, sarcoma, dermoid, and several others —"tubercle" (*Tuberkel*), that is the nodular proliferative lesion character-istic of tuberculosis. The common feature of new-formations, in this extended sense of the term, was (as Virchow saw it) the formation of new cells and tissues. But Virchow had by now largely discarded his belief in the genesis of cells and tissues from amorphous blastemas. "A great, indeed perhaps the predominating, part of new-formations is therefore to be derived from the progressive development of preexisting tissue components," he writes, after having enumerated the four possible modes of cytogenesis listed above.[19] It was in connection with the new formation known as *Tuberkel* that he first began to doubt the existence of a blastema.[20]

The four possible modes of cytogenesis described by Virchow in 1854 were all based on inadequate or misinterpreted microscopic evidence.[21] But the general abandonment of Schwann's belief in "spontaneous cell-generation"—as Henle called it in 1882—is best understood as the realization that empirical evidence of any role played by a cytoblastema in the cell-formation was entirely lacking, rather than as the consequence of anything approaching an accurate account of the actual mechanism of cell replication. According to Remak and Reichert, embryonal cells formed solely from preexisting cells; Remak then ventured to suggest that a cytoblastema likewise played no role in the adult organism. Those who had taken the cytoblastema on faith now reexamined their premises. The next step, taken by Virchow in 1855, was to assert that *omnis cellula a cellula*—all cells arise from cells.[22] Obviously, this postulate could never be verified fully; however, a single proved contradiction would suffice to falsify it. So also with the parallel postulate of spontaneous generation (*generatio aequivoca*).[23] The general assertions *omnis cellula a cellula* and *omne vivum ex ovo* are best understood as general denials of their contrary assertions. They pose a clear challenge to believers in the free formation of cells and the spontaneous generation of living organisms. Virchow now envisioned a "cellular pathology" (*Cellular-Pathologie* or *Cellularpathologie*)—a word apparently of his own coining—capable of reconciling the ancient and opposing claims of "humoral and solidary pathology" (*Humoral- und Solidarpathologie*).[24]

FOERSTER AND THE NEW CELLULAR PATHOLOGY

The first of the treatises on pathology to be written under the banner *omnis cellula a cellula* was August Foerster's *Handbuch*, the initial volume of which was published in 1855.[25] According to Foerster the new theory of the origin of cells, championed by Virchow, had by then found many adherents, among whom he counted himself. However, Foerster recognized that the available data were far from sufficient for a final conclusion as to the origin of new cells and was aware of all that this entailed in regard to the histogenesis of tumors.[26] Virchow himself did not put into print the necessary consequences of his new theoretical stance until several years later. Little more than a new interpretation of already available empirical evidence was involved, and, given a certain degree of intellectual intimacy between the two men, it is not surprising that the conclusions reached by Foerster in 1855 were essentially the same as those presented a few years later in Virchow's lectures on cellular pathology and in his three volume work on the pathology of tumors.

Foerster gives a vivid picture, drawn without *parti pris,* of developments in tumor theory since the introduction of microscopical and chemical data in the eighteen-thirties. The truth of the received dogma, he says, was not at first called into question. On the assumption that new-formations of all kinds arose from "plastic exudates," the new investigative tools had at first served only "to add histological and chemical detail to the already available gross-anatomical accounts of the course of develop-ment of new-formations." The cell theory, extrapolated from plants to animals by Schwann, had been integrated by Mueller into the old theory of the organization of pathological exudates and applied to the study of tumors. Then, continued Foerster, after years of effort to round out the "received theory" (*ueberlieferte Theorie*) and to secure it with new findings, the validity of the theory itself came under attack from two sides:

> In the first place, it soon became obvious that as far as most tumors were concerned no blastema whatsoever was demonstrable, and that all observa-tions made on blastemas were shaky and uncertain; further, it became clear that a certain number of tumors took form quite directly from normal tissues in consequence of hypertrophic growth and without any intercession on the part of a cell-forming blastema, e.g., fibroids, lipomas, vascular tumors and epidermoid cystic tumors. After it had been recognized that the formation of cells from a free blastema, heretofore assumed generally valid for both plants and animals, took place not at all or to a very limited degree, and that, instead, all cell formation took place by division of preexisting cells or endogenous cell production, the stimulus was given for revision of the theory in respect to pathological organization as well.[27]

Foerster also pointed out that new-formations that resulted from the organization of plastic exudates or blastemas in adult life were patho-logical analogues of embryonal new-formations, that is, of organs and tissues formed in the developing embryo.[28]

Like most pathologists, Foerster preferred a purely anatomical classifi-cation of tumors, unmixed with clinical criteria of malignancy or benignancy. He insisted, however, that the classifications should take account not only of the terminal structure (*fertigen Bau*) of a given tumor but also of the histogenetic course of development whereby the terminal structure was achieved. Attention to the total organization (*gesammte Organization*) was necessary to avoid the error of classifying a tumor solely in accordance with an outstanding histological or cytological feature of its terminal structure and thus overlooking the possibility that such features might have different developmental histories. Unfor-tunately, our knowledge of the developmental history of tumors was

extremely scanty.[29] In today's terms, Foerster was calling for a classification based on histogenetic rather than merely histological criteria. Two
tumors exhibiting the same histological structure may have entirely
different sites of origin and courses of development, hence they are best
classified separately. Although Foerster did not make the point, obviously
the chances of finding responsible causal factors are increased if tumors
are studied both where they begin and where they end.

    Excluding inflammatory and tuberculous new-formations as special
cases, Foerster drew up a provisional list of ten tumors (*Geschwuelste*)
properly so-called: (1) lipoma, consisting of fat tissue; (2) fibroid (*Fibroid*),
of connective tissue; (3) enchondroma, of cartilage; (4) osteoma, of bone
tissue; (5) angioma, of vessels; (6) adenoma (*Adenom*), of glandular tissue;
(7) cystic tumors, composed of one or more closed sacs; (8) papilloma,
composed of papillae; (9) sarcoma, consisting of elements of undeveloped
connective tissue; and (10) carcinoma, consisting of indifferent cells
growing without restraint (*indifferenten, schrankenlos wuchernden Zellen*).
The list began with tumors composed of tissues resembling those normally
found in the body and progressed to tumors deviating radically from the
normal; it began with the most benign and ended with the most malignant
tumors. Foerster states that the connective tissue, ubiquitously distributed
throughout the body, furnishes the matrix, or mother-substance, for the
majority of these tumors. The cells of the connective tissue, specifically
Virchow's connective tissue corpuscles (*Bindegewebskoerperchen*), are
capable, says Foerster, of yielding not only the nourishing stromal
framework of most tumors but also their specific cellular and histological
components; connective tissue cells serve as the starting point for all
varieties of new-formed cells (*den Ausgangspunkt fuer alle Arten neuge-
bildeter Zellen*). Thus the connective tissue "constitutes the matrix of all
fibroids, lipomas, enchondromas and osteomas, of many vascular tumors,
of all sarcomas and many carcinomas."[30]

    According to Foerster, then, the reservoir of indifferent connective
tissue corpuscles present throughout the body is not the sole histogenetic
source of tumors. Vascular tumors may arise from already existing small
blood vessels; adenomas of the breast, prostate, testis, skin, and mucous
membranes from the parenchymal cells constituting the glands in these
localities; tumors composed in whole or part of epithelial cells from the
epithelial tissues of skin and mucous membranes.[31] As used by Foerster,
adenoma refers only to the histogenesis and structure of the tumors so
designated. As for their clinical behavior, some are benign localized
tumors, whereas others, especially those occurring in the female breast,
may display the unrestrained cell growth that Foerster regards as the
hallmark of carcinoma.[32] Adenomatous tumors of the skin, which at times
resemble embryonic sebaceous or sweat glands, may take origin from

glandular epithelium or from the Malphighian rete. These tumors, too, may behave like cancers. Foerster states that he is unconvinced by the arguments of Hannover, Frerichs, and others in favor of the unitary origin of epithelial cancer of the skin from overgrowth of the epidermis. He considers true epithelial cancer of the skin (*eigentlichen Epithelial- krebs*) to be a tumor histogenetically independent of normal epithelium and glands, which originates in the cells of the connective tissue matrix.[33]

Origins of Epithelial Tumors

Foerster's category of papillomas—of new-formations composed of nipple- like protrusions of connective tissue with a covering layer of epithelial cells—includes a number of tumors having little in common except this one structural feature. A "simple" (*einfach*) papilloma amounts to a localized overgrowth of epithelium and connective tissue. The direction of growth is outward. In "destructive" (*destruierenden*) papillomas growth is inward, the underlying normal tissues (of the skin or mucous mem- branes) are damaged, and ulceration may result. In either case, the epithelium of the papilloma remains continuous with that of the adjacent normal skin or mucosa. In the third kind of papilloma, however, the epithelial and connective tissue cells grow in such a rapid and disorderly fashion that all continuity with the surface is lost. Detached clusters of cells appear in the depths of the invaded normal tissues, and the tumor is indistinguishable from a carcinoma. Foerster speaks of the third kind somewhat misleadingly as a "combination with carcinoma" (*Combination mit Carcinom*); he means no more than that they have secondarily developed into carcinomas, owing to unrestrained cell growth (*schranken- lose Zellenwucherung*).[34] A fourth kind of papillary tumor, differing histo- genetically from the third, but similar insofar as its final structure is concerned, is described by Foerster under the heading of primary cancer- formation (*primaere Krebsbildung*). Here the cells of the tumor, although they may resemble epithelial cells, do not arise from the hypertrophy and subsequent cancerous overgrowth of skin or mucous membranes; they arise instead from indifferent cells of the connective tissue reser- voir.[35] Thus histology yields to histogenesis in Foerster's classification of tumors.

Foerster's partial rejection of the category "epithelial cancer" (*Epi- thelialkrebs*) likewise reflects his belief in the primacy of histogenesis over histology in the classification of tumors. So-called epithelial cancers can take origin, he states, from three different sources. The "characteristic epitheliallike cells" of such tumors variously represent overgrowth of skin and mucosal epithelium, of glandular epithelium, and of deep-lying cells of the ubiquitous connective tissue reservoir. What they have in common is a tendency to grow destructively and without restraint.[36] *Carcinoma* and *cancer* (*Carcinoma, Krebs*), as used by Foerster, apply to a group of new-formations diverse in origin but alike in containing, as their essentially cancerous components, cells characterized by a lack of differentiation (*Indifferenz*) and a tendency to undergo limitless growth (*schrankenlose Wucherung*).[37] Presumably, cancers originating from undifferentiated connective tissue cells contain cells that never become differentiated, whereas cancers originating from surface or glandular epithelial cells contain cells that *de*-differentiate, i.e., lose whatever differential features they may possess.[38] According to Foerster, sarcomas arise solely from the undifferentiated cells of connective tissue. To the extent that they resemble the spindle-shaped cells found in mature connective tissues, the cells of sarcomas are more differentiated than those of cancers.[39]

VIRCHOW AND THE NEW CELLULAR PATHOLOGY

Neoplasms and Connective Tissue

Insofar as Foerster's histogenetic scheme rested on the postulate *omnis cellula a cellula,* his debt to Virchow was openly acknowledged. It is likely that his derivation of epithelial cancer from connective tissue also owed something to Virchow. In any event, Virchow's thoughts had been moving in that direction since his abandonment of the blastema theory. A crucial experiment of nature was the exceedingly rare tumor described by Virchow as a tibial cancroid. Enclosed within the thick, bony walls of the tibial cortex, this tumor appeared to be completely isolated from the overlying epidermis, the nearest source of epithelial tissue. If, as Virchow supposed in 1850, the tibial cancroid arose from a cell-forming blastema, the overlying epidermis could hardly have determined the direction of development; if, as he supposed in 1855, it arose from cells, these could only be those of the marrow connective tissues. In 1854 Remak suggested that it took origin from displaced embryonal epidermis; he had rejected the blastema theory but, for reasons discussed below, was unwilling to admit the transformation of connective tissue into epithelium. One could, of course, deny that the cells of a tibial cancroid were true epithelial cells—Hannover had done this in 1852.[40] Virchow, however, believed that they were, and he was unwilling to admit that Remak's embryologically based argument necessarily held good for pathological new-formations. But the paper in which Virchow proposed for the first time that epithelial tumors could originate in and from connective tissue dealt with another tumor, the "pearly tumor" (*tumeur perlée*) of Cruveilhier.[41] Virchow noted that the presence of epithelial cells in this tumor had first been described by Mueller. To Mueller's sixteen instances of the tumor in question, Virchow added five. The tumors, described by Virchow as *Perlgeschwuelste* ("pearly tumors"), were located in the meninges, ovary, and testis. Although none involved the skin or mucous membranes, they contained numerous "layered epidermal globes" (*geschichtete Epidermiskugeln*). These, said Virchow, were the *globes épidermiques* considered by Lebert and by Hannover to be characteristic features of tumors derived from epithelium. In his own opinion, however, their origin was threefold: some were derived from preexisting epidermal cells; others from glandular epithelial cells that had undergone epidermal transformation (*Umbildung*); and still others from connective tissue cells that had undergone epidermal transformation.[42] The connective tissue, says Virchow, is "the most important germinal source of heteroplastic new-formations, and the individual features of the various kinds of new-formations are revealed to be, for the most part, consequences of the relatively early differentiation of originally uniform tissue-germs (*Gewebekeime*)."[43] And, three years later, in the first edition of his twenty lectures on cellular pathology, Virchow states that "the vast majority of new-formations... arise from the connective tissue [*Bindegewebe*] and its equivalents.... One can therefore with a few *restrictions actually substitute the connective tissue and its equivalents for the earlier blastema and the later exudate, and for the original plastic-lymph of the older writers, as the common germinal stock* [*Keimstock*] *of the body.*"[44]

At this point a brief review of the concept of connective tissue, with particular reference to Virchow's own contributions to the subject, would be helpful. In the late eighteenth century the old belief that the connective tissue, or "cellular tissue" (*tela cellulosa, Zellgewebe, tissu cellulaire*), was composed of fibers and plates that intercepted "cellular" spaces had been rejected by such men as C. F. Wolff, Georg Prochaska, and Johann Blumenbach, who regarded the supposed fibers, plates, and "cells" as artifacts. Bichat, however, had followed von Haller in accepting their existence. In Germany, Bichat's doctrine of the tissues had been contested by Doellinger, Rudolphi, the younger Meckel, and others who believed that the so-called cellular tissue was actually, in the living state, an amorphous gel.[45] The controversy continued into the era of the microscope and the cell. According to Virchow, in his first edition of *Cellular Pathology* (1858), the situation was as follows. Some ten years earlier, Reichert had attempted to demonstrate that the fibers of connective tissue were optical artifacts resulting from the presence of folds in a more or less homogeneous and acellular matrix-substance that constituted the actual connective tissue or intercellular substance. Schwann, on the other hand, had claimed in 1839 that connective tissue in the embryo was composed of tailed, or caudate, corpuscles (*geschwaenzten Koerperchen*), i.e., of cells, corresponding to Lebert's "fibroplastic bodies," that underwent progressive splitting to yield the fibers of connective tissue; the nuclei of these cells remained behind, as such. Henle had proposed, in opposition to Schwann, that embryonic connective tissue was originally *acellular*, the nuclei and fibers later forming (independently of each other) from a blastema. Henle's view of the matter also conflicted with that of Reichert, who, although he denied even the existence of Schwann's tailed corpuscles, believed that the connective tissue was originally *cellular*, the boundary between cells and intercellular substance being obliterated later in life. Virchow's own studies on the microscopic constitution of connective tissue had led him to effect a synthesis of these conflicting accounts. Contrary to Reichert, he found that the tailed corpuscles or young connective tissue cells were present in adult as well as embryonic tissue and that the fibers characteristic of adult connective tissue were not optical artifacts; contrary to Schwann, such fibers were not the result of cell splitting but were formed in the originally more or less uniform intercellular substance (*Intercellularsubstanz*) of the connective tissue. Most important of all, insofar as his own theory of neoplastic histogenesis was concerned, Virchow held, contrary to the views of Reichert, Henle, and Schwann alike, that the structure of embryonic connective tissue was not essentially different from that of adult connective tissue. The essential cellular constituent of both was the "spindle-cell" (*Spindelzelle*) or connective tissue corpuscle (*Bindegewebskoerperchen*), first described as a tailed, or caudate, corpuscle by Schwann and Mueller.[46]

Objections to Remak's Derivation of Epithelial Cells

In 1858, in his book entitled *Cellular Pathology as Based upon Physiological and Pathological Histology*, Virchow stated that all tissues of the human body could be brought under three headings. In the first group were tissues composed solely of cells lying immediately adjacent to each other; these were cellular tissues in the modern sense (*in dem modernen Sinne Zellgewebe*). In the second group the constituent cells were separated by an intercellular substance (*Intercellularsubstanz*); this group of connective tissues (*Gewebe der Bindesubstanz*) included the "cellular tissue," i.e., the *tissu cellulaire, Zellgewebe*, or cellular texture of the older writers. The third group included tissues composed of cells that had undergone far-reaching structural transformations into muscle fibers, nerve fibers, blood vessels, and so on.[47] The layered mucosal surfaces, together with the epidermis, fell into the first group. Here the cells were constantly renewed from below. Curiously enough, in view of his theory of the histogenesis of skin cancer, Virchow held that the Malpighian rete was the starting point of most pathological processes involving the epidermis.[48] The epithelial glands were derived from epithelial surface layers in the course of embryonic development. One of Remak's greatest merits, according to Virchow, was the discovery that the outer and inner germ layers were the chief sources of these epithelial surface layers. The connective tissues had been regarded as more or less inert structural elements until Virchow's own investigations had shown that they, too, contained the germs (*Keime*) of new cells. Only then was he able to abandon Schwann's belief in the free formation of cells in blastemas. Having thus reached a new understanding of the nature of the connective tissues—namely, that they were, in the adult as in the embryo, composed of cells (in the modern sense of the term)—he was able to substitute the connective tissue for the recently discarded blastema in his theory of tumor genesis. It now appeared that the majority of tumors, and *all* cancers, took origin from undifferentiated connective tissue cells. The only exceptions to this rule were the relatively few pathological new-formations arising from epithelial tissues or from more highly organized structures, such as blood vessels.[49]

If, as Virchow stated in 1858, Remak had shown that glandular and surface epithelia in the adult organism were derived from the outer and inner germ layers of the embryo, why did Virchow propose that the majority of epithelial tumors arose from connective tissue? One reason already noted was his unwillingness to accept the unrestricted application to pathology of an embryologically based argument. Another reason seems to have been the recognition, indicated by his reference to the anomalous position of the gonadal apparatus in Remak's scheme of things, of an internal flaw in the argument itself, leaving aside the propriety of applying it under pathological circumstances. The argument, essentially, was that epithelia and derived epithelial structures were produced by the outer and inner germ layers, and connective tissues by the middle germ layer, in the normal course of embryonic development. But Remak had not shown that *all* secretory glands provided with epithelium-lined excretory ducts were so derived. Instead, much to his puzzlement, he had found that the primordial kidneys (*Urnieren*) and the ducts (*Urnierengaenge*), together with the male and female sexual apparatus (*Geschlechtswerkzeuge*), were derived from the middle germ layer.[50] And Virchow's own observations pointed toward the conclusion that the transformation of connective tissue into epithelial tumor cells was relatively commonplace in the course of neoplasia. It occurred in tumors arising in sites far removed from epithelial surfaces, such as the *Perlgeschwulst*. In the ovary, an organ derived, Remak thought, from the middle germ layer, so-called dermoid (*Dermoid*) tumors were found to contain typical epidermal tissue.[51]

Paradoxically, to a modern reader, the plausibility of Virchow's hypothesis that epithelial cancers arose from connective tissue was increased, rather than decreased, by the well-recognized phenomenon of metastasis. The problem of the histogenesis of secondary cancers had by no means been solved to the satisfaction of all concerned by Langenbeck in 1840.[52] His work had not proved that secondary growths resulted from the transfer of viable tumor cells to distant organs and tissues by way of the blood or lymph. On the basis of the same kind of evidence, it may be recalled, Langenbeck had claimed to have produced "secondary" tumors in the lungs of a dog by injecting cancer cells derived from a tumor in a man, evidence called into question by Virchow.[53] In the mid-nineteenth century—with the convincing demonstration that the spread of infectious diseases in the body was effected by the transfer of microbial cells still several decades in the future—the chemical, or zymotic, theory of metastasis was widely accepted. Championed by the great chemist Justus Liebig, the zymotic theory held that the spread of infectious diseases, whether from person to person or within the body of an afflicted individual, was brought about by "some morbific principle acting on the organism similar to a ferment."[54]

Virchow's advocacy of the central role of living cells in physiological and pathological processes did not prevent him from admitting the strength of the chemical point of view. Cancer cells might indeed serve to disseminate a primary tumor, he wrote in 1858, but it seemed "much more probable...that the conduction occurs by means of certain fluids, and that these fluids have the ability to generate an infection (*Ansteckung*) which disposes the individual parts to reproduce a mass of the same kind as that originally present." The often somewhat random spread of tumors in the human body influenced him in this direction. "Metastases of cancer," he noted, "very often do not correspond to those with which we have become acquainted in [the study of] embolism."[55] We owe to Virchow, incidentally, both the word and the concept "embolism."[56] It follows, then, that a ubiquitous source of undifferentiated cells, ready to respond so as to reproduce the inflammatory, tuberculous, or cancerous "tumor" appropriate to the zymotic stimulus, has to exist. This source Virchow finds in the connective tissue, the cells of which can undergo transformation variously into pus cells, tubercle cells, and the cells of cancerous tumors.

For Virchow, inflammatory, tuberculous, and cancerous tumors are histogenetically of identical origin. Pus formation (*Eiterbildung*) is the result of an increase in the size of connective tissue corpuscles or cells (*Bindegewebskoerperchen*), followed by nuclear and cell division. Toward the periphery a homologous new-formation (*Neubildung homologer Art*) composed of connective tissue becomes evident; in the center are closely packed aggregates of small cells, which later constitute round foci (*Heerde*) or diffuse infiltrates (*Infiltrationen*).[57] The genesis of tubercle—of what is still referred to as a "tuberculoma"—is explained by Virchow in the same way. The older medical writers, he says, designated small nodules (*Knoetchen*) in the tissues of the body by the term *Tuberkel;* they spoke of carcinomatous, scrofulous, and syphilitic tubercles. Laennec then gave the term a more limited and precise meaning. But by including the notion of diffuse "tuberculous infiltration" under the heading of tubercle, Laennec had moved away from the notion that a discrete nodular mass was an essential feature of the tuberculous process. The often cheesy or caseous consistency of tuberculous matter came to be accepted as the distinguishing feature of a tuberculous lesion. Virchow found that caseation occurred only at a later stage in the development of tubercles; in the beginning, tubercles were nodular aggregates of well-formed cells, contrary to the view of Lebert and Charles Robin in France that *corps tuberculeux* were solid, noncellular bodies. The hallmark of tuberculosis, said Virchow, was the cellular tubercle. A *Tuberkel* was, in fact, a cellular new-formation arising, like all new-formations, in consequence of some stimulus acting on the undifferentiated cells of the ubiquitous connective tissue so as to lead to their multiplication. Subsequently the mass of new cells underwent "caseous metamorphosis," a process that Virchow characterized as a kind of "transformation of inflammatory products."[58]

According to Virchow, the cells constitutive of new-formations, whether neoplastic, reparative, inflammatory, or tuberculous in character, are derived from preexisting cells, for the most part by simple division, although a few originate within intracellular "brood-spaces" (*Brutraeume*).[59] Since the great majority of new-formations arise from undifferentiated cells in the connective tissue (*Bindegewebskoerperchen*), their first rudiments, or *Anlagen,* are similar in appearance. In particular the divisions of nuclei and of cells are alike in all new-formations, regardless of whether they are destined to become benign or malignant in clinical behavior, heteroplastic or hyperplastic with respect to histological structure.[60] In tumors of this kind (including all varieties of cancer) there is an early state of apparently "absolute indifference" (*absoluten Indifferenz*), in which the dividing tumor cells resemble the "so-called formative-cells [*Bildungszellen*] of the embryo, which, too, quite resemble each other at first, regardless of whether an element of muscle, nerve or whatever will issue from them." Despite their similar appearance, Virchow thought it likely that there were as yet undiscerned differences (material rather than merely potential [*bloss Potentia*]) in these cells that governed their later transformations.[61]

The concept of heteroplasia was of course already available to Virchow; that of hyperplasia (*Hyperplasie*) was his own contribution. Heteroplastic new-formations, even those (such as cancer, tubercle, and suppuration [*Eiterbildung*]) that had no *tissue* prototype (*Vorbild*), had a *cell* prototype, namely, the undifferentiated cells of the connective tissue.[62] In the case of certain other heteroplastic new-formations a normal tissue prototype was evident, e.g., glandular, epithelial, or nerve tissue, but the tumor tissue was the result of cellular transformation (*Umwandlung,* later *Metaplasie*); cerebral substance or hair in ovarian tumors obviously had not sprung from preexisting tissues of the same kind. Hyperplasia, defined by Virchow as a numerical increase of cells resembling their parent cells, was of frequent occurrence in the body and accounted for a number of true tumors, such as lipomas arising in fat tissue and mature connective tissue tumors, but not for the more important ones. To call a tumor hyperplastic involves the histogenetic inference that it is *derived* from the tissue it resembles. Virchow did not deny that certain epidermal or epithelial tumors could arise in this way. But when a tumor of epithelial structure manifested itself in the lymph glands, in the depths of the body, even within a tubular bone, he saw no binding reason to suppose that it must have arisen from epithelium. Crucial to his decision here was his conviction that undifferentiated cells in the adult organism were capable of a wide range of transformations—where embryologists such as Remak tended instead to think of the progressive restriction, during development, of cell transformability—and his doubts of the feasibility of explaining the phenomenon of tumor metastasis by Langenbeck's hypothesis of viable tumor cell transfer.[63]

A final word remains to be said about Virchow's position with respect to the development of epithelial cancer from epithelial surfaces. Sometimes Virchow speaks as if he believed that cancroids arise from epithelium whereas "true cancers" arise from connective tissue, e.g., when he states that cancroid cannot be distinguished from "true" cancer (*vom eigentlichen Krebs*) on the basis of its epithelial elements, since they are present as well in "true" cancer.[64] Presumably, hyperplasia would overstep the bounds of normality under such circumstances and become cancerous. This view seems to have been shared by Foerster. Elsewhere Virchow appears to deny the possibility that cancers could so arise. He states, for example, that a papillary tumor of the skin or mucous membranes can only be called cancroid or carcinoma (here the terms are apparently synonymous) when cancerous changes are visible beneath the epithelial surface. Virchow was on guard against the misdiagnosis of superficial hyperplastic lesions as cancers. He mentions a penis that was amputated because of the presence of a syphilitic condyloma and states that some pathological anatomists consider any papillary or villous tumor a cancer when they find cancer cells (*Krebszellen*) in the covering epithelial layer, even in the absence of cancerous matter in the tissue beneath. While he has seen such tumors, he has "so far been unable to convince himself that cancer cells can arise on the free surfaces of skin and mucous membranes, that they simply arise from epithelium." On the contrary, a sharp distinction must be drawn between cases in which masses of cells, however abundant and peculiarly formed they may be, sit on an intact layer of ground-substance, and those in which the cells are formed within the parenchyma of the part itself.[65] With this statement Virchow seems to have completely ruled out the epithelial origin of carcinoma. Noninvasive epithelial carcinoma (the lesion today called carcinoma *in situ*) was of course ruled out as well, and Virchow's reluctance to make a diagnosis of cancer on the basis of superficial changes alone persisted, together with disbelief in morphologically identifiable cancer cells, into the 1880s, even after he had given up his theory of the connective tissue origin of all cancer.[66]

Virchow's Treatise on Tumors

Intended by Virchow to be his magnum opus on the subject of tumors, *Die krankhaften Geschwuelste* was published between 1863 and 1867.[67] This multivolume work can be dealt with briefly here, since it contains nothing new with respect to the histogenesis of tumors. In the course of its publication a large number of pathologists and surgeons abandoned the connective tissue theory of cancer histogenesis. Possibly due to a growing doubt on Virchow's part as to the general validity of that theory, the section of the work on epithelial cancer remained unpublished, if indeed it was ever written. In 1863, however, this doubt was yet unborn, and the first volume of the work, published in that year, contains some remarks that shed further light on the relationship between Virchow's understanding of the mechanism of metastasis in inflammatory and neoplastic disease, and the histogenesis of cancer. To repeat, he held that inflammatory tumors, tubercles, and true tumors (aside from those arising by direct hyperplasia, such as lipomas, fibromas, etc.) originated in response to some stimulus acting on the reservoir of undifferentiated cells in the ubiquitous connective tissue. These undifferentiated cells, in accordance with the nature of the unknown stimuli acting on them, are transformed into pus, tubercle, or tumor cells. When the anatomical lesions of inflammatory, tuberculous, syphilitic, or cancerous disease appear to spread throughout the body, i.e., to metastasize, what actually happens is that the appropriate stimulus, disseminated by the blood, lymph, or other body fluids, exerts its effect at a distant site and produces there the corresponding new-formation. Tumors do not constitute a sharply defined group of lesions, and no one can state what tumors truly are.[68] Although inflammatory tumors are customarily distinguished from true tumors, this is merely a matter of practical convenience. There is, in fact, no real basis for separating tumors from inflammatory swellings; an abscess is a tumor in the same sense as is a cancer. In practice, writes Virchow, only those lesions in connection with which the possibility of diagnostic error arises are classified as tumors. Thus abscesses, which as a rule are easily recognized, are excluded from that category. Likewise, a hydrocele of the testis is regarded as a tumor, but a collection of fluid in the pleural cavity is not.[69]

The more malignant (*boesartig*) a tumor, the more apt it is to spread throughout the body.[70] Not the spread of tumor cells, however, but the spread of the "harmful fluid," "juice" (*succus*), or "humor" that first provoked the primary growth is responsible for this phenomenon. The propagation is a consequence of the spread of the harmful agent by way of the blood, lymph, and other body fluids, "precisely as with the propagation of many inflammatory processes."[71] As we have seen, one of the reasons for Virchow's skepticism with regard to the role of tumor emboli in the dissemination of cancer was the frequency with which organs lying in the direct line of spread were skipped, the secondary or metastatic tumor manifesting itself at a more distant point. With some reservations, however, he accepted as valid observations on the presence of cancer cells in the blood and lymph made by other investigators, and he himself had seen indubitable tumor emboli in the pulmonary arteries.

Further evidence for the role of the "transport of morphological particles" in the spread of tumors was forthcoming in the case of peritoneal involvement. Here the findings at autopsy suggested that after a cancer, e.g., a gastric cancer, had spread to the peritoneal surfaces, clusters of tumor cells might drift down to the rectovesical or rectouterine pouch, where new tumor growths would then appear, just as if a seed (*Seminium*) had been sown and had then germinated. We are not to take this analogy literally, for, according to Virchow, the tumor cells function in such instances merely as the carriers of the hypothetical "harmful substance." Metastatic tumors, then, do not arise due to multiplication of the "seed" sown by the body fluids. The transmitted tumor cell is, rather, the carrier (*Traeger*) of a growth-stimulating, toxic substance that acts specifically on undifferentiated connective tissue cells elsewhere in the body to produce a secondary tumor of the same character as the primary. And, according to Virchow, the tumor cells are not only the carriers but also the producers (*Erzeuger*) of the harmful substance in question.[72] It is worth noting that in Virchow's scheme of things the idea that cells, normal or pathological, move of their own accord or are passively carried about the body via the fluids to grow or function at distant sites plays no role.[73] Of the germ theory of disease, which was to dominate medical thought in the last quarter of the nineteenth century, there is also no trace. In terms of the zymotic theory favored by physiological chemists in the mid-nineteenth century, Virchow conceives of the harmful causes of the spread of inflammatory, tuberculous, and neoplastic diseases not as invading, living agents but as, for the most part, self-generated substances.

MICHEL'S CRITICISM
OF VIRCHOW'S CONNECTIVE TISSUE THEORY

Early in 1855, before the publication of his two papers on the foundations of cellular pathology and the connective tissue origin of epithelial tumors referred to above, Virchow had sent a letter to the *Gazette Hebdomadaire* in Paris briefly setting forth the more important conclusions drawn in those papers. Cells, he informed his French audience, were always formed anew from preexisting cells by proliferation, never from amorphous blastemas by *génération spontanée.* Most tumors took their origin from embryonic cells of the connective tissue (*tissu cellulaire*). These undifferentiated cells persisted in the adult organism and furnished the "germ of most neoplasms, of malignant tumors in particular."[74]

Virchow's letter seems to have been the chief occasion of a long and thorough review by Eugène Michel of various aspects of medical microscopy, including the developments in cellular oncology since the appearance of Johannes Mueller's monograph on the subject.[75] Michel's comments on Virchow's letter to the *Gazette Hebdomadaire* are particularly interesting. He rejects both the connective tissue origin of cancer and the implicit postulate *omnis cellula a cellula.* Virchow claims that "every new production has for its point of departure preexisting cells," writes Michel, but for himself the *génération spontanée* of new cells from blastemas in accordance with Vogel's law of analogous formation is beyond doubt. He sees Virchow's denial of this mode of cell generation as responsible in part for his election of persisting, undifferentiated connective tissue cells as the source of origin of malignant neoplasms (*néoplasmes malins*), including carcinoma, cancroid, and sarcoma. According to Michel, Virchow's rejection of the epithelial origin of cancer is also based on the belief that a cancer only secondarily makes contact with the overlying epithelial or epidermal surface; he himself has observed, on the contrary, that epithelial tumors always originate on epithelial surfaces and sarcomatous or fibroplastic tumors in connective tissues.[76]

DECLINE OF VIRCHOW'S CONNECTIVE TISSUE THEORY

During the ten years between 1855 and 1865 the connective tissue theory of cancer histogenesis became, in Germany at least, the most commonly accepted textbook doctrine. Before entering into the reasons for its rapid decline thereafter, a brief recapitulation of certain key issues arising from the introduction of cell theory into the context of the problem will be helpful. We have seen that prior to 1855, before the belief that all cells were derived from preexisting cells began to win adherents, most pathologists held to the epithelial theory of cancer histogenesis, at least insofar as superficial cancers were concerned. But the theory did not at that time imply the genesis of epithelial cancer *cells* from preexisting normal epithelium. Rather, it implied that an acellular tumor "blastema" was somehow determined in respect of its cellular development by the presence of adjacent, preexisting, epithelial tissue. In the case of deeply-seated epithelial cancers, occurring where no normal epithelium was to be found, the theoretical situation was uncertain. The discovery of apparently primary epithelial tumors, cancerous or otherwise, in the meninges, the deep tissues of the neck, the ovary, and even in the marrow cavities of bones gave occasion for doubt. Where was the preexisting epithelial tissue that determined the development of tumors such as these? In the case of secondary cancers, this problem again presented itself. When a clearly metastatic cancer developed in a lymph node, under what influence did the new epithelial cancer cells develop? As far as secondary cancers were concerned, a ready solution to the problem followed from two assumptions; namely, that all cells arose from preexisting cells and that secondary cancers resulted from the multiplication of cells disseminated from primary growths. The first assumption had almost no adherents before 1855, and the second was slow in gaining them even thereafter.

The connective tissue theory, as formulated by Virchow and Foerster in 1855, differed from the old epithelial theory in two ways: not only did it derive epithelial cancer *tissue* from connective *tissue,* but it derived epithelial cancer *cells* from normal, undifferentiated connective tissue *cells.* When Virchow, in 1852, derived a tibial cancroid from marrow connective tissue he had not yet abandoned the blastema theory, hence he had not derived the epithelial cells of the cancroid from connective tissue cells. But when Remak, in 1854—with particular reference to Virchow's tibial cancroid—rejected the derivation of epithelial tumors from connective tissue, he at the same time abandoned the blastema theory. Hence Remak, in rejecting the derivation of epithelial cells from connective tissue cells, may be said to have rejected the connective-tissue theory even before it had been fully formulated by Virchow and Foerster.

Implicit in Remak's counterproposal that the tibial cancroid reported by Virchow (as well as other anomalously situated epithelial tumors) could well have developed from persisting, displaced embryonal epithelium were some conflicting assumptions. His embryologically based argument is without force unless he assumes that the laws of developmental history (*Entwickelungsgeschichte*) apply equally to both embryos and tumors. But he himself had found that the middle germ layer, the source of connective tissue, was also the source of epithelium indistinguishable from that derived from the outer and inner layers. His argument must then be shored up with the additional assumption that a middle germ layer derivative—namely connective tissue—cannot do in the adult what middle germ layer derivatives can do in the embryo.

Thiersch's Epithelial Theory

The signal for the abandonment of the connective tissue theory was given in 1865 by Carl Thiersch, who had been engaged since 1861 in histological studies of the genesis of cancers involving the skin and the mucous membranes.[77] Thiersch's monograph *Der Epithelkrebs, namentlich der Haut* was based on investigations of slightly over one hundred tissue specimens. Since neither the rotary microtome nor aniline dyes were then available, Thiersch cut the tissues, after fixation in alcohol or chromic acid, with a thin blade (*Messerblatt*) held under tension in a watchmaker's saw, and stained the sections in an ammoniacal solution of carmine. He then decolorized the tissue sections with absolute acetic acid, until the nuclei alone retained the dye.[78] Making use of serial sections, Thiersch tried to show that cancers of the skin, lips, and mouth arose in and from the epithelium and only later involved the underlying connective tissues; in no case, he claimed, did they arise in the connective tissues and subsequently spread to involve the overlying epidermis or mucosal epithelium.

Thiersch was aware that the histological evidence was in itself ambiguous. Even though he could demonstrate with serial sections that apparently isolated (in single sections) clusters of epithelial cancer cells were actually in continuity with overlying normal epithelium, proof that extension had occurred from epithelium to connective tissue, rather than the reverse, was lacking. The same doubt arose in connection with the so-called transitional cell forms (*Zwischenformen*) considered by Foerster and others to be intermediate between epithelial cells and connective tissue cells. Thiersch believed that such cells were transitional in outward appearance only, but he admitted that a sure conclusion could not be drawn from the histological findings alone; hence he resorted to the embryological argument implied by Remak ten years earlier.[79] "True" epithelium, stated Thiersch, was solely a product of the outer and inner germ layers. Connective tissue, a derivative of the middle germ layer, was incapable of yielding anything other than the so-called false epithelia of the vascular system, serous cavities, and synovial spaces. Still following Remak, Thiersch was forced to admit the existence of a "third epithelial group" in the genito-urinary apparatus, derived from the middle germ layer, but he passed over the troubling question raised thereby.[80]

As for the presence of epithelial cells in cancers arising in sites remote from normally occurring epithelium (including that of epithelial glands), such as the tibial cancroid described by Virchow, a transformation of connective tissue cells into epithelial cells seemed less likely than the abnormal segregation of epithelial cells during embryonic development. (Thiersch mentions, incidentally, that Remak's explanation was widely rejected as a too adventurous hypothesis [abenteuerliche Hypothese].)[81] Alternatively, epithelial cells from a surface layer or a gland might, during adult life, undergo cancerous degeneration (Degeneration) and then proceed to infect (inficiern) a distant organ or tissue before a lesion of any kind was apparent at the primary site. A secondary tumor would thus present as a primary tumor.[82] Thiersch mentions in this connection a case, described by Sir James Paget, of a chimney sweep whose inguinal nodes contained massive cancerous deposits, in the absence of any lesion on the scrotum.[83] Other cases in point—deep-seated cancers of the neck, without involvement of the overlying skin—had been described by Bernard Langenbeck.[84] What was the nature of the infectious agent responsible for the spread of epithelial cancer? The logical consequence of Thiersch's assumption that epithelial cancer arose only from epithelium was that it could be spread only by epithelial cancer cells. This is plain from his argument. He did not favor, he wrote, the generally accepted belief that cancer was spread by a "fluid or finely granular substance" carried in the blood or lymph. Such a substance might well be responsible for the nonspecific, metastatic inflammatory lesions commonly associated with cancer in the stage of ulceration. But how could a substance of this kind "bestow on cellular proliferation a specific histologic character"? On the other hand, if the infectious agent consisted of "nuclei, cells, or larger conglomerates" there would be no mystery involved, for it was well recognized that tissues transplanted from one site to another in the same organism often remained viable. In this way, Thiersch was led to favor what he called the transplantation hypothesis (Transplanations-hypothese) of the spread of cancer.[85]

An additional hypothesis put forward by Thiersch deserves comment here. He proposed that a disturbance of growth equilibrium (Stoerung des

Gleichgewichtes) is involved in the development of epithelial cancer. An epithelial cancer, Thiersch states, is made up of *two* cells or tissue components. The tumor proper consists of epithelial cancer cells, but these cells cannot continue to exist, much less grow and multiply, in the absence of a nourishing stroma composed of blood vessels and connective tissue. In certain benign tumors of organoid character—papillary tumors arising on epithelial surfaces and some tumors of epithelial glands—epithelial and stromal growth remain relatively within bounds. In epithelial cancers a disturbance of growth equilibrium of far more severe character becomes evident. Instead of maintaining their distance and offering each other mutual support (Thiersch does not tell us what the epithelium has to offer the stromal connective tissue in the way of support), they intermingle in total disorder and bring the whole structure down.[86]

To Thiersch the best available histological evidence was unable by itself to support the theory of the epithelial origin of cancer of the skin and the mucous membranes. The Remakian embryological argument, itself shaky, remained a necessary prop. It is interesting to wonder whether Thiersch's book would have been as effective had not Wilhelm His, shortly after its publication, proposed a revision of Remakian germ-layer theory, which—although discarded later—strengthened the embryological argument in favor of the epithelial origin of cancer at just the right time. His did this in a study of the development of the mammalian ovary, published in 1865.[87] According to His, the *outer* germ layer is the true source of the primordial kidney and its ducts, not the middle germ layer, as Remak had supposed. At a very early stage in embryonic development a fold of the outer layer became pinched off and included within the middle layer. Not only did it furnish the anlage for the primordial renal apparatus in the embryo, but part of that apparatus itself underwent a later transformation into the adult genito-urinary apparatus. All "true" epithelium was thus derived from the outer and inner germ layers. The class line separating epithelium from connective tissue was now complete. His pointed out that, in the light of his revision of germ-layer theory, the presence of hair, teeth, epidermis, and epithelial glands in dermoid tumors (*Dermoidgeschwuelste*) of the ovary was no longer a puzzle. In a footnote, His supports Thiersch's recently published work; by virtue of their middle germ layer origin, connective tissue cells cannot become epithelial cells.[88]

Billroth's Conversion

Thiersch's book made instant converts of some of his colleagues but left others partly, or not at all, convinced of the validity of the epithelial theory. Here the embryological argument rather than the histological evidence seems to have been the deciding factor. Theodor Billroth was one of the instant converts. In 1863, in his *General Surgical Pathology and Therapy in Fifty Lectures*, he had accepted without question the connective tissue theory as formulated by Virchow and Foerster.[89] In 1866, after the publication of Thiersch's book, he adopted, just as wholeheartedly, the epithelial theory.[90] His's work, in fact, made Billroth *paepstlicher als der Papst*, more dogmatic than Thiersch. Noting that His had repaired a serious flaw in the structure of Remakian embryology, a flaw that had "raised doubt as to its safety," Billroth claimed that the developmental potencies of cells were "determined by predestination," by "irrevocable laws of nature," once the germ layers had been formed. Hence a connective tissue cell could no more give birth to an epithelial cell than a dog to a frog (*wie ein Hund unfaehig ist, einem Frosch zu zeugen*).[91] In 1863 Billroth favored the chemical, zymotic, or infectious account of the spread of cancer.[92] In 1866 he was a "zealous proponent" of the transplantation theory of metastasis, or, as he preferred to call it, the embolic theory.[93] Since he had written the *Lectures*, Billroth stated, the doctrine of embolism, as formulated by Virchow, had undergone enormous development. Further, von Recklinghausen had shown that cells could "wander here and there" (*hin- und herwandern*) in the tissues. Formerly Billroth had thought of cells in general as "fluid-filled vesicles" more or less fixed in place. Now he saw them as capable of migrating elsewhere and continuing their lives as before (*anderswo als an dem ihnen urspruenglich angewiesenen Platze ihre Existenz fristen koennen*). Not only cancer metastasis but also the origin of primary epithelial cancers at sites where epithelium was normally not present might be explained in this way. Such primary tumors originated from aberrant epithelial germs (*aberrirte Keime*), as Remak had proposed, or perhaps from epithelial cells that had migrated from their sites of origin into the depths of the tissues and had, subsequently, become cancerous.[94]

Neoplasia and Inflammation Distinguished

The paper by Friedrich von Recklinghausen referred to by Billroth dealt only with the wandering movements of pus corpuscles and other inflammatory cells found in the connective tissues; it said nothing of similar movements by epithelial cells or cancer cells.[95] Billroth had, more or less justifiably, extrapolated from the findings of von Recklinghausen, and perhaps also from those of other investigators of the so-called ameboid movements of cells.[96] Von Recklinghausen's paper had certain other implications within the context of the tumor problem that demand comment here, even at the price of interrupting the account of the reception of Thiersch's book.

Virchow, it will be recalled, derived inflammatory, tuberculous, and noninflammatory, or true, tumors alike from the proliferation and differentiation of a reserve stock of undifferentiated cells in the connective tissues. But von Recklinghausen found no evidence that inflammatory cells originated in this manner; furthermore, he suggested that circulating white cells and pus corpuscles were not only similar in appearance (as Virchow and all others recognized) but were actually the *same* cells.[97] This suggestion called into question Virchow's theory of the genesis of inflammatory tumors, but von Recklinghausen, perhaps out of caution, carried the matter no further. In 1867 Julius Cohnheim, like von Recklinghausen a pupil of Virchow, extended the use of von Recklinghausen's technique for tagging cells with engulfed particulate dyes in order to follow their movements. After tagging white blood cells in this way, he inferred that similarly tagged pus corpuscles subsequently found at inflammatory sites had arrived there by way of the blood stream; at the same time he described in detail how untagged white cells made their way through the intact walls of small blood vessels.[98] Cohnheim, too, at first made no attempt to formulate a new theory of inflammation. In 1873, however, he discarded Virchow's theory in its entirety and defined inflammation as a "disease of small blood vessels." Partly due to the ideas of Simon Samuel, he had, in the interim, become convinced that the white blood cells, instead of actively making their way through intact capillary walls, were passively extruded through damaged walls at inflammatory sites. Their presence, as pus corpuscles, in inflammatory tumors was purely fortuitous.[99] (Only later, with the rise of the germ theory of disease, would they be assigned the task of engulfing bacterial invaders.) An inflammatory tumor, in the light of Cohnheim's theory, was always secondary; its characteristic cells came from elsewhere in the body, via the blood or lymph. Looking back, we see the concept of tumors and the tumor process, after having included within its scope for more than two thousand years tumors of both inflammatory and noninflammatory character, begin to undergo fission in the 1860s, eventually to yield the concepts of inflammation and neoplasia—disparate with respect to etiology, histogenesis, and physiopathological significance —that are familiar today.

French Conservatism

Before returning to the reception of Thiersch's work in Germany, it should be noted that in France neither the connective tissue theory of cancer genesis nor the Virchovian postulate *omnis cellula a cellula* was at first favorably received. Leading histologists, pathologists, and embryologists there, as in England, continued to espouse the theory of the free formation of cells in blastemas well into the 1870s.[100] Charles Robin, perhaps the most influential of these men, stated in 1865 that the "primary" cells of the embryo, i.e., those derived immediately from the fertilized egg cell, subsequently underwent "gradual liquefaction" to yield an amorphous blastema. The secondary "anatomical elements," including cells, constituting the embryo proper were then formed *de novo* from this blastema. Robin also held that the embryonic formative process repeated itself in the adult organism. The dissolution of adult cells and the subsequent regeneration of new cells from the resulting blastemas were, he stated, features of inflammatory and new-formative processes.[101]

In a series of papers that appeared in Robin's journal of anatomy and physiology in 1864 and 1865, André-Victor Cornil argued in favor of the origin of skin, breast, uterine cervical, and gastric cancer from epithelial *tissue* and rejected Virchow's contention that such tumors arose from undifferentiated connective tissue *cells*. In the first of these papers, Cornil brought forward the embryological argument: epithelial tissue and connective tissue were formed separately in the embryo and were not interconvertible thereafter, not even under pathological circumstances. As for the genesis of epithelial cells in epithelial cancers, Cornil accepted the "hypothesis of spontaneous generation, beginning with nucleated elements, then with pavemented...a genesis reproducing in the adult, under pathological circumstances, what takes place in the embryo under physiological circumstances."[102] What Cornil clearly had in mind was the dissolution of normal mucosal epithelial cells into a cancerous blastema from which the cancer cells were then formed *de novo*, by "spontaneous generation."

In a paper that appeared in 1865 after the publication of Thiersch's book, Cornil traced the origin of breast cancer to the "hypergenesis" (Robin's alternative to Virchow's *hyperplasia*) of terminal acinar epithelium. He expressed agreement with Thiersh (who had, of course, long since abandoned the blastema theory).[103] The point of difference is made clear in a paper by Louis Ranvier and André Cornil dealing with the extension of skin cancer to underlying bone. Cancers or cancroids (the terms are used interchangeably) of the skin develop at the expense of (*au dépens de*) the Malpighian layer or the epithelium of the dermal glands. Investigating a cancroid of the humerus, which had developed in association with an osteomyelitic sinus, they could find no histological evidence that the tumor had been "directly propagated from the epidermal tissue," as Thiersch would have supposed. Ranvier and Cornil believed, nevertheless, that the cancroid in question had its "primary origin in the glands and deeper layers of the skin."[104] In other words, they believed that it had reached the bone not in the form of cellular tissue but as a cancerous blastema.

The Debate in Germany

In Germany at this time the leading histologists, pathologists, and embryologists, whether or not they agreed with Thiersch's derivation of cancer from epithelium, subscribed almost without exception to the derivation of all cells from preexisting cells. The embryological argument in favor of the epithelial origin of cancer now called for the derivation of epithelial cancer cells from "true" epithelium alone, i.e., solely from epithelium of ectodermal (outer germ-layer) and endodermal (inner germ-layer) origin. The middle germ layer (mesoderm) and its derivatives in the adult organism were considered incapable, under any circumstances, of yielding "true" epithelium.[105] For the cell layers lining blood vessels, lymph vessels, and serous cavities, now regarded as "false" epithelia, His coined the term *endothelium*.[106]

Although lack of appropriate clinical material prevented Thiersch from demonstrating the epithelial origin of cancers of internal organs, this had been his original intent.[107] Others soon took up the work. The absence of established guidelines in the interpretation of histological evidence allowed histogenetic speculation to proceed rather freely. Oskar Wyss, for example, distinguished two histological varieties of prostatic cancer, one composed of glandlike structures resembling prostatic glands, the other of epitheliallike cell cords traversing the fibromuscular stroma of the prostate, independent of its glands. Ignoring the barrier between epithelium and connective tissue, Wyss drew from the histological evidence the histogenetic conclusion that the two varieties were of entirely different origin; the first arose from prostatic glandular epithelium, the second from stromal tissue of the prostate.[108] In 1866 Bernard Naunyn described clusters of proliferated bile-ducts adjacent to metastatic cancerous deposits in the liver and suggested that *primary* cancer of the liver took origin from bile-duct epithelium.[109] Naunyn rejected the connective tissue derivation of both primary and secondary (metastatic) cancers of the liver, at the same time maintaining that secondary cancers had *two* origins: they might arise "autochthonously," from native bile-duct epithelium cancerized by a zymotic, infectious agent coming from a primary cancer elsewhere in the body; or from actual cancer cells disseminated via the blood stream from the primary growth.[110] Naunyn's views may be contrasted with those of Carl Otto Weber, two years earlier.[111] Weber claimed that metastatic liver cancer resulted from the "catalytic effect of emboli" on undifferentiated connective tissue cells in that organ. The embolic material was, of course, not composed of cells; according to Weber metastatic cancers no more arose from the growth of transplanted cancer cells than did metastatic abscesses from transplanted pus corpuscles.[112]

Edwin Klebs, later to gain fame as a bacteriologist, expressed general agreement with Thiersch in 1867, as far as the genesis of *primary* cancers was concerned, in a paper that appeared in Virchow's *Archiv*. "There are," he wrote, "no two tissues so very different throughout in appearance and behavior during development, at least in the first stages of formation of the animal body, as epithelial and connective tissue."[113] This statement contains an escape clause. While Klebs agreed that cancers *primarily* originated in epithelial tissue, his histological findings convinced him that once a cancer had arisen it could grow and spread in two quite different ways: by proliferation, i.e., by division and multiplication of its own cells; and by infiltration. The histological evidence convinced Klebs that infiltration resulted not from the spread of cells derived from the original tumor but from the "transformation of other tissue elements into epithelial elements...as an epithelial infection." Cancroid epitheliomas (*cancroide Epitheliome*) spread by way of proliferation only, infectious epitheliomas (*infectioese Epitheliome*) by way of infiltration as well.[114] Klebs thought that the fixity of divisions between cell species, like those between animal species, had been exaggerated in the past. In his opinion the so-called embryological laws had limited sway, that is, they did not necessarily govern tissue development in the adult organism under pathological conditions.[115]

The histological appearances of infiltrative growth, Klebs stated, might conceivably be accounted for on the assumption that young cancer cells, not yet fully epithelial in character, wandered into the stroma (*in das Stroma eingewandert*). His reason for rejecting this view, and thus for postulating an infectious transformation of connective tissue cells into epithelial cells, is that "the stromal cells showing the closest resemblance to epithelium are found near the zones of most advanced epithelial proliferation," whereas the "small cell elements constituting the start of the new-formation in the connective tissue stroma" are *not* found within those same zones.[116] This piece of histological evidence, accurate enough in itself, was equally susceptible of the opposite interpretation. Furthermore, it is difficult to see how Klebs was able to reconcile in his own mind some of the conflicting statements in this paper. For example, he states that Thiersch has, "with logical precision," concluded that if epithelial cancers take origin only from epithelial cells, they must be disseminated (at least to parts of the body where epithelium is normally absent) in the form of epithelial cancer cells. But Klebs himself assumed that only primary epithelial cancers originated in this way; subsequently, they spread and metastasized by virtue of an infectious fluid capable of converting connective tissue cells into epithelial cancer cells.[117] Klebs gives no reason why the transformation is forbidden in the case of primary cancers and allowed in the case of secondaries.

The subsequent issue of Virchow's *Archiv* contained another response to Thiersch's work, a paper on lung cancer by Theodor Langhans, Virchow's successor at Wuerzburg.[118] After first having given a detailed account of Thiersch's views, Langhans remarked that the empirical evidence for the origin of cancer or cancroid from the epidermis presented by Thiersch was, for the most part, unconvincing. The argument really hinged on Thiersch's "attempt to apply an embryological 'law' in the sphere of pathological histology."[119] Langhans believed that the unknown agent responsible for the spread of malignant tumors was such that "cells of various kinds, connective tissue cells and epithelial cells, the nuclei of muscle-fibers, etc., could be infected [*inficirt*], stimulated to the production of cancer, cancroid or sarcoma cells [*Krebs- Cancroid- oder Sarcomzellen*]."[120] (The same agent was presumably responsible for the growth of the primary cancer; Langhans is silent on this point.) Langhans had at his disposal ten cases (one in a dog) of cancer involving the lung. All were "secondary in form," manifesting themselves as "nodules strewn throughout the lung."[121] None involved the bronchi. From our standpoint, as well as from Langhans', these were metastatic tumors. Langhans divided them into two groups, cancer and cancroid. The latter group he subdivided into squamous cell cancroid (*Plattenepithelialcancroid*) and cylinder cell cancroid (*Cylinderzellencancroid*). The basis of Langhans' classification was entirely histological; he did not infer from the resemblance of cancroid cells to epithelial cells that they had arisen from epithelial cells. On the contrary, it seemed to him that epithelial cells of one and the same tumor might have a dual origin, the epithelium and the connective tissue. He argued (in keeping with his notion of the way in which tumors spread) that the occurrence of entirely isolated clusters of epitheliallike tumor cells in the pleura spoke for their derivation from pleural connective tissue cells, regardless of the source of similar cells in foci of tumors lying deep in the lung.

Briefly recounting the history of what he called the genetic principle in tumor theory, Langhans pointed out that the designation *homeoplastic* (or *homologous*) had originally meant that a tumor contained histological elements resembling those of normal tissues; in contrast, *heteroplastic* (or *heterologous*) tumors did not. Virchow had then given the terms a different meaning: a tumor was homologous or heterologous to the degree that it resembled or differed from the tissues *at its site of origin*. For Virchow the distinction was of practical as well as theoretical importance, since he believed that homologous tumors were usually benign and heterologous tumors usually malignant. The practical value of the distinction, continued Langhans, had been called into doubt by Thiersch's derivation of skin cancroid, an "outspokenly malignant" tumor, from the epidermis rather than from the connective tissue, thus shifting it from the category of heterologous to that of homologous tumors. Langhans denied that there was any valid basis, theoretical or practical, for so classifying tumors. From the practical standpoint, a high degree of cellularity was a more reliable sign of malignancy in a tumor than the heterologous character of its cells. And the theoretical basis of the distinction was invalid if (as he supposed) tumor cells and tissues of similar appearance could be, in one and the same tumor, of different genetic origin.[122]

LIMITS OF CELL SPECIFICITY

A larger question lay behind the debate over the histogenesis of epithelial cancer. Not only the interconvertibility of epithelial and connective tissue cells but also the limits of cell specificity in general was at issue. Were cell species as fixed and immutable, in the adult organism at least, as animal species? Did Billroth's quaintly phrased statement that a connective tissue cell could no more sire an epithelial cell than a dog could a frog apply to all species of cells? Or, as Virchow and others supposed, was there not a reservoir of undifferentiated cells in the connective tissues, and were not even differentiated cells capable, to some degree, of transcending the limits of cell specificity?

The generalized thesis of cell specificity was stated in 1865 by Ludwig Buhl, in an account of two recurring tumors composed of striated muscle fibers.[123] Buhl pointed out that Zenker, in a study a year earlier of regenerative changes in the body musculature of typhoid fever patients, had derived the new muscle fibers from intrafascicular connective tissue. Buhl claimed that the process of new-formation of muscle fibers began instead with the transverse division of muscle — not sarcolemmal — nuclei. As the fibers grew longer, the nuclei of the resulting arrays moved apart. Longitudinal division of these nuclei and subsequent splitting of the fibers completed the growth process. Unwilling to accept the received notion of connective tissue cells as the undifferentiated source of all kinds of cells, given the proper conditions, Buhl tendered an alternative scientific hypothesis (*wissenschaftliche Hypothese*); namely, "that in the adult a specific tissue element cannot be formed anew other than from a preexisting tissue of the same specific character, already laid down in the embryo by spontaneous generation, so to speak."[124] Anticipating a phrase that would be coined two decades later, Virchow's *omnis cellula a cellula*

became *omnis cellula a cellula ejusdem naturae.* That Buhl cited August
Weismann (as well as Lebert, Remak, and Koelliker) in support of his
account of the mode of origin of new muscle fibers is worth noting, for
Weismann later based the idea of cell specificity on his theory of
determinants (*Determinanten*). According to this theory, the sum total of
determinants, or specifying particles (*bestimmenden Theilchen*), was present
in the germ plasm only; in the course of cell division during embryonic
development, they were parceled out as needed.[125]

Buhl himself recognized that the empirical evidence had no binding
force. In 1867 Carl Otto Weber not only disputed Buhl's findings,
claiming that the development of smooth muscle fibers from connective
tissue and of striated from smooth fibers was clearly evident, but argued
that it was precisely the study of muscle regeneration and tumor formation that threatened the "new gospel of cell specificity," and he supported
the received view that new cells developed from a reservoir of undifferentiated cells. In the case at issue, said Weber, the young cells destined
to become muscle cells certainly possessed no *visible* distinguishing
features. "The elements arising in consequence of a simple, traumatic
irritation," he continued, "or of a specific (cancerous, sarcomatous, suppurative) irritation can assume the type of the mother tissue . . . but they
can also turn into pus corpuscles, sarcoma cells, epithelial cells, and pale,
large nucleated epithelioid cancer cells; indeed single cells can strike out
in different directions at the same time." This "cardinal question" should
be approached from all sides, according to Weber, and chemical reagents
were needed by means of which epithelial cells could be distinguished
from connective tissue cells, and connective tissue from nerve tissue.[126]
He failed to realize that such reagents could help ascertain only what a
cell (or a cell line, where successive divisions were involved) had become
—that is, what it had differentiated into, and not what it had been. This
or any other means of positively identifying the various cell types would,
of course, solve the problem of tumor histogenesis for an investigator
who accepted Buhl's hypothesis. But that hypothesis was based on the
very doctrine of cell specificity that Weber rejected.

Waldeyer's First Paper

In a long and closely reasoned paper, published in Virchow's *Archiv* near
the end of 1867, Wilhelm Waldeyer summed up the evidence and arguments in favor of a purely epithelial origin of epithelial cancer, whether
external or internal, primary or metastatic.[127] Waldeyer's presentation of
his own histological evidence garnered in favor of this view was admirably
clear. But such evidence was inherently ambiguous. The strength of his

argument lay, rather, in his demonstration that further histogenetic assumptions were not needed to account for the histological findings and that germ-layer theory and the associated doctrine of cell specificity argued against the propriety of making these assumptions. Since the epithelial theory as formulated by Waldeyer was destined to become textbook dogma within the next few decades and to remain so down to the present time, Waldeyer's paper is worth considering in detail, the more so because it contains a wealth of acute histopathological observations.

Waldeyer put the question at issue as follows: Do carcinomas arise solely from connective tissue cells—Virchow's "common generative source of all pathological new-formations"—solely from epithelial cells in the organ primarily involved, or from both?[128] Reviewing the recent spate of papers on the histogenesis of tumors, Waldeyer pointed to a babel of voices—some claiming that epithelial cancer cells could develop from muscle corpuscles, others that both carcinomas and sarcomas arose variously from epithelium and connective tissue; some deriving metastatic cancers from transplanted tumor cells, others from pathologically stimulated cells in secondarily involved organs (epithelial cells, connective tissue cells, or both); some attributing the local extension of cancer to the mobility of cancer cells, others to the spread of an infectious agent capable of transforming normal connective tissue cells into cancer cells.[129] The critical question of the relationship between the cells of a tumor proper and the cells of its supporting stroma remained unsettled.[130]

Waldeyer presented a detailed account of his own histological studies of scirrhous cancer of the breast—the cancer (*Krebs*), scirrhus, or carcinoma *kat' exochēn*, as he says. Aside from mentioning the use of carmine as a nuclear stain, he had little to say of his technical procedures. He employed large sections, where possible, and implied that they were thinner than those ordinarily used by histopathologists. Methodologically, his interpretative procedure was the usual one of attempting to reconstruct temporal sequences from spatial arrangements—a procedure obviously open to objection but enforced by the nature of the data, on the one hand, and of the questions asked, on the other.

His conclusions, in brief, were as follows. The earliest state of a breast cancer is marked by the proliferation of epithelial cells in breast acini. The epithelial proliferation is always accompanied by an "intralobular" or "periacinar" proliferation of small connective tissue cells, the "constant companion[s] of acinar epithelial cell proliferation." Only the presence at this stage of complete glandular lobules indicates that epithelial proliferation occurs first. As epithelial growth proceeds, the acini become filled with atypical epithelial cells. Next, these cells break through the basal membranes of the acini and spread irregularly in the surrounding connective tissue—not in the small-cell intralobular connective tissue already mentioned, but in the ordinary, fibrous, interlobular connective tissue that, at this stage, lies between widely separated acinar formations. There is no evidence of a transition from connective tissue cells to epithelial cells; wherever the dividing line between the two appears blurred, the examination of very fine sections (*sehr feine Schnitte*) suffices to establish its existence. The distinction between intralobular and interlobular connective tissue growth is a special case of the accompanying connective tissue proliferation (*begleitende Bindegewebswucherung*) and introductory connective tissue proliferation (*einleitende Bindegewebswucherung*) generally characteristic of carcinomas.

Depending on the relative rates of epithelial and connective tissue proliferation, a breast cancer has more or less connective tissue stroma. A so-called medullary carcinoma is, although composed almost exclusively of epithelial cancer cells, not essentially different from a scirrhous carcinoma, in which cancer cells are at times so rare that they must be searched out. The difference lies only in the amount of stromal connective tissue present; between these two extremes lie tumors composed of varying proportions of stromal and epithelial tissue. Further, the stromal connective tissue presents itself in a variety of forms: fibrous, fatty, myxomatous, vascular, cartilaginous, and even sarcomatous (*sarkomatoese*). The essential element of carcinoma is the epithelial cancer cell, which is somehow able to generate its own supporting stroma. Only in this sense is the "infectious theory" of cancer valid. Wherever they arrive and manage to survive, cancer cells, "these tiny living organisms," are capable, like all foreign bodies—in particular, entozoal embryos and vegetable parasite-germs (*pflanzliche Parasitenkeime*)—that have wandered into the tissues, of stimulating the growth of the surrounding connective tissue.[131]

Always the paradigm for malignant growths, carcinoma of the breast appropriately received more attention in Waldeyer's paper than any other tumor. The histological sequences of carcinoma of the stomach, according to Waldeyer perhaps the most common of all malignant tumors, were also given in some detail. Using large sections, Waldeyer attempted to trace the destructive spread of cancerous mucosal glands through the *muscularis mucosae* into the loose submucosal tissues and the muscular wall of the stomach, pointing out that continuity between the cancerous epithelium in the mucosa and that in the wall was always demonstrable (this, of course, is what Thiersch had shown in cancer of the skin). Likewise for carcinoma of the uterus: all primary epithelial cancers of that organ could be traced to an origin in epithelium.[132]

The spread of cancer could thus be adequately explained without recourse to the old hypothesis of "infectious" transformation of connective tissue, for which there was no positive evidence. Local spread of carci-

noma took place in consequence of the migration, or wandering-in
(*Einwanderung*), of epithelial cancer cells. Distant spread was the result of
embolization, "embolic masses of cancer cells in the branches of the
portal vein" being a prominent accompaniment of carcinoma of the
stomach.[133] In summary, Waldeyer states: "I consider carcinoma to be,
essentially, an epithelial new-formation, and I believe that it arises as a
primary tumor only where true [*aecht*] epithelial formations are present.
Secondary carcinoma can arise only from the direct propagation of
epithelial cells, or by way of embolic transmission through the blood and
lymph vessels, since cancer cells [*Krebszellen*], insofar as they are brought
to a suitable site, are, like entozoal germs [*Entozoenkeime*], capable of
further reproducing themselves."[134]

Waldeyer, like other pathologists before him, was insistent that the
notion of malignancy (*Boesartigkeit*) ought not to be reified; malignancy
was no ontological something (*ontologisches Etwas*) inherent in cancers.
Rather, "a cancer is malignant because it is an atypical epithelial tumor."
The varying degrees of clinical malignancy exhibited by different tumors
reflect the atypical character and behavior of their constituent cells. A
scale extends from the most malignant to the most benign of epithelial
tumors. Warts, cutaneous horns, trichomas, naevi pilosi, epithelial cysts,
and adenomas of the breast and stomach are mentioned by Waldeyer as
instances of relatively benign tumors. While carcinomas must be distinguished from such tumors, the mere term *carcinoma* ought not to
conjure up a spectre (*Popanz*) before which the physician is helpless.
Further, the belief that anatomical indices alone suffice for the prediction
of the clinical behavior of a given tumor should be abandoned; the
relative malignancy or benignancy of a tumor depends on its structure,
its site of origin, and the general condition of the patient.[135]

Additional support for the assumption that carcinomas developed
from epithelial cells in the tissues or organs where they primarily arose
came from the similar character of changes met with in corresponding
normal and cancerous cells. "In every organ," Waldeyer states, "the carcinomatous bodies predominantly go through the same metamorphoses as
those most frequently seen in epithelial cells under normal circumstances
at the same sites." But the evidence for this generalization was scanty:
Waldeyer could adduce only the familiar cornified "globes épidermiques"
of Lebert, as seen in skin cancer, and the fatty changes frequently present
in epithelial cells of breast cancers. He admitted that "keratoid bodies"
were sometimes found in deep-seated primary cancers of the medullary
variety and that "fatty degeneration" was rather common in cancer cells
generally. With reference to Weber's call for a reagent to distinguish
epithelial from connective tissue cells, however, Waldeyer commented
that cornification (*kornige Umwandlung*) was itself a cellular chemical

transformation found only in epithelial cells, whether normal or cancerous; it never occurred in connective tissue cells or tumors derived
therefrom.[136]

Waldeyer admits that if only *one* proved case of a primary carcinoma
originating at a site where derivatives of neither of the "two epithelial
germ layers" were normally present could be adduced, his argument
would collapse. But, although a variety of supposedly primary carcinomas
arising in tissues derived from the middle germ layer—lymph nodes,
spleen, bloodvessels, peritoneum, and bone—had been reported by
competent observers, he could not find a single unimpeachable case.
Very fine sections of such tumors reveal them to be composed of round
and spindle-shaped connective tissue cells, sometimes in formations that
mimic epithelial alveoli; these tumors are in reality sarcomas, that is
"true connective tissue tumors." Unlike carcinoma cells, sarcoma cells
have a tendency to secrete an intercellular substance, traces of which are
often visible and thus furnish the histopathologist with still another
criterion for distinguishing epithelial from connective tissue tumors.
The other so-called primary cancers of tissues and organs derived from
the middle germ layer are actually secondary cancers and therefore of
purely epithelial origin. For the rare and still doubtful cases of truly
primary cancers in those organs and tissues, Waldeyer suggests two
possible explanations: they arise from epithelial germs (*verirrte Keime*)
displaced in the course of embryonic development or from epithelial
cells that have been included in scar tissue and have then undergone
abnormal growth. Waldeyer called attention to Cornil's report (discussed
above) of an epithelial cancer that had arisen in an osteomyelitic sinus;
oddly, he had nothing to say of Virchow's report—the original stimulus
of Remak's *verirrte Keime* hypothesis—of a cancroid of the tibia. Waldeyer
recognized that the proposed explanations were ad hoc in character; in
order to settle "this difficult question"—whether epithelial cells could
ever be derived from connective tissue cells—a host of carefully made
observations, beyond the power of any one person to accomplish, would
be necessary.[137]

Waldeyer's paper implicitly contains the following propositions:
(1) the sole source of the original epithelial cancer cells constituting a
given carcinoma is normal epithelium, i.e., the various derivatives of the
two epithelial germ layers; (2) the transformation of normal epithelium
into cancerous epithelium does not involve cell dissolution (the rule
omnis cellula a cellula remains valid here); (3) multiplying by cell division,
the original epithelial cancer cells generate all additional cancer cells of
a given carcinoma (to the extent that the local transformation of normal
into cancerous epithelium no longer takes place); (4) the movement,
active or passive, of cancer cells into the adjacent tissues is the sole

mechanism of local spread; (5) distant spread, or metastasis, likewise results solely from the transport of cancer cells, via the blood, lymph, or other body fluids, to sites far removed from the primary tumor, where the cells grow and multiply as before; (6) neither local nor distant transformation of connective tissue cells into epithelial cancer cells ever takes place; (7) the multiplication of cancer cells incites or is accompanied by two forms of connective tissue proliferation: a small-cell accompanying (*begleitende*), and a more fibro-cellular introductory (*enleitende*) proliferation, the latter constituting the newly formed stroma of the tumor; (8) the connective stroma of some carcinomas, e.g., carcinoma of the breast, presents itself in a wide variety of forms (fibrous, fatty, cartilaginous, and so on).

Although Waldeyer's chief concern was with the histogenesis of carcinoma, his paper contains indications of a generalized thesis. Sarcomas, he states, are true connective tissue growths (the above propositions apply, *mutatis mutandis,* to sarcomas as well as to carcinomas). It may also be assumed without hesitation that, according to Waldeyer, benign epithelial tumors (trichomas, adenomas, etc.) and benign connective tissue tumors arise from corresponding normal cell types—taking into account, of course, the rather protean character of connective tissue.

Finally, it should be noted that Waldeyer had nothing to say of the cause of the transformation of normal cells into tumor cells; nor did he offer an explanation why cells so transformed, in particular the atypical cells of carcinomas, behave more or less as if they were hostile foreigners in the commonwealth of the body—invading near and distant tissues, stirring up the growth of connective tissue, and proliferating, like "entozoal embryos" or "vegetable parasite-germs," almost without restraint.

Histogenetic Inference: Tibial Adamantinoma

Since Waldeyer's account of the genesis and mode of spread of carcinoma is essentially the account that is found in all textbooks of oncology and pathology in use today, the story is essentially complete, and what follows is largely in the nature of an epilogue. One might suppose that Waldeyer's thesis, whose tentative character he recognized, was subsequently verified by direct observation rather than inference, as one tumor after another was traced to its origin in normal cells of the same type and general arrangement. But nothing of the sort took place; nor could it have, given the limitations inherent in the histological procedures that were the mainstay of tumor studies in both laboratory and clinic. What did happen was that the assumptions so clearly articulated and skillfully employed by Waldeyer in 1867 continued to suffice, as the nineteenth century wore on, to more or less satisfactorily explain all additional histological data garnered by students of the tumor problem. Histological techniques, with the introduction of the rotary microtome and aniline cell and tissue stains, became increasingly refined in the 1870s and 1880s, and apochromatic objectives and substage condensers sharpened the microscopic image.[138] The perfection of these techniques was a powerful stimulant to convert pathologists into histopathologists and to stunt the growth of other procedures in the study of tumors. As Virchow pointed out in 1898, pathologists were becoming captive interpreters of static images, "readers" of glass slides.[139] Meanwhile, no decisive evidence in favor of any of the alternatives to Waldeyer's set of assumptions appeared: those hypotheses gradually lost credibility, because they were unnecessary rather than because they were refuted by further observation.

No matter what refinements were introduced into the study of the primary object of visual analysis — then, as now, a slice of tumor tissue, growing ever thinner — available to the microscopist, tumor histogenesis was still interpretative, whereas tumor histology was descriptive. To pass from the observed histological data to the histogenesis of a given tumor required an inference. In some tumors — in cancer of the skin, for example — the very earliest stages of tumor genesis at times seemed to present themselves directly to the observer. But this, too, was deceptive. Leaving aside the near certainty that the initial step in the transformation of a normal cell into a cancer cell is not visible under the light microscope, it was still necessary for histopathologists to infer temporal developmental sequences from statit spatial arrangements. And in most instances tumors became available for microscopic study only after they were well past their initial states of development and growth.

Before bringing this story to a close, I want to give a brief account of the long succession of attempts to ascertain the histogenesis of a particular kind of tumor, thereby showing that the procedure for ascribing histogenetic origins to clinically available tumors has, with all its inherent uncertainty and the resulting wide differences in opinion, remained unchanged in principle for the last one hundred years.

The kind of tumor in question, first described and designated by Virchow in 1850 as a primary cancroid of bone and today known variously as adamantinoma, ameloblastoma, pseudoameloblastoma, synovial sarcoma, and malignant angioblastoma of the appendicular skeleton, is exceedingly rare. Fewer than one hundred instances have been reported since 1900.[140] Compensating for the infrequency and consequent lack of clinical importance of this unusual tumor is its great theoretical interest. Since 1850 the tibial cancroid has occupied a pivotal position with respect to the perennial question of the derivation of epithelial tumors from connective tissue. Virchow, as we have seen, first derived the tumor from an acellular blastema; then, after postulating *omnis cellula a cellula,* from undifferentiated connective tissue cells. Remak, unwilling to admit the transformation of connective tissue into epithelium in the light of his germ-layer doctrine, had derived it instead from aberrant embryonal epithelium. Accepting Remak's hypothesis, Thiersch added another: the tumor cells might originate deep in the epidermis overlying the tibia and make their way into the bone before reaching the skin surface.

Returning to the topic in 1872, Waldeyer called attention to the paucity of reports of primary carcinoma of bone since the appearance of Thiersch's book seven years earlier. Before that time, said Waldeyer, such cases had been reported, admittedly rarely, by competent observers. He himself had never seen a carcinoma arising other than in association with preexistent epithelium, and even if it were true (as some of the opponents of the exclusively epithelial origin of carcinoma asserted) that tumors in all respects similar to carcinomas could arise from endothelium, Waldeyer was of the opinion that those tumors should be designated by a term other than *carcinoma* to distinguish them histogenetically from the vastly larger class of true carcinomas arising from epithelium.[141]

In 1882 Richard Volkmann affirmed the existence of primary carcinoma of bone as a rare disease. He described two varieties of primary "cancroid" of bone—squamous cell and cylindrical cell—and asserted that they occurred most frequently in the mandible. The next most frequent site was the tibia. Volkmann thought it possible that some or all of the tibial cancroids actually arose from the overlying epidermis, in the absence of a visible lesion of the skin.[142] Even before Volkmann's article on the subject, certain centrally placed epithelial tumors of the jaw were being derived by investigators in France and Germany from rests of the dental enamel organ. Among the names applied to these tumors were *epithelioma adamantinum* and *adamantinoma.* By the first decade of the twentieth century, case reports of adamantinoma of the jaw were relatively common in European and American medical literature.[143] Since the enamel organ and its residues were real structures, the inference that the tumors in question arose from epithelial rests was, while still an inference, on firmer ground than was the case of similar tumors in the tibia. In 1900 Otto Hildebrand suggested that Volkmann's cancroids of bone (presumably those in the appendicular skeleton) were in fact angiosarcomas or endotheliomas. Hildebrand also reevaluated a supposedly primary carcinoma of bone discussed by Karl Sudhoff in 1875. It was clear from Sudhoff's descriptions, said Hildebrand, that the tumor in question was an angiosarcoma (*Angiosarkom*) or an endothelioma (*Endotheliom*).[144]

In 1900 Carola Maier again called attention to the subject of primary epithelial cancer of bone.[145] Noting Ernst Ziegler's categorical denial, in 1892, that such tumors could occur, she remarked that the universal acceptance accorded to Thiersch's and Waldeyer's thesis of the exclusively epithelial origin of carcinomas lent extraordinary interest to those rare instances in which primary carcinomas appeared to have originated in tissues of nonepithelial (germ layer) derivation. In the past, said Maier, before a sharp histogenetic line of distinction had been drawn between sarcomas and carcinomas and before the present level of technical skill had been reached, it was no doubt true that sarcomas had erroneously been taken for carcinomas. Overlooking a real primary tumor elsewhere in the body had been another pitfall. In a survey of reports during the preceding twenty-five years or so, she had found at best only one or two convincing cases of primary carcinoma of bone.[146]

Maier then reported a case of apparently primary carcinoma of bone from her own experience. The patient was a twenty-year-old woman with a centrally located tumor of the ulna. The overlying skin was uninvolved. A diagnosis of myelogenous sarcoma had been made from a roentgenogram. One year before the appearance of the tumor the woman had injured her arm while sailing. The immediate result was a hematoma, but no further sequelae were apparent. Under the microscope the tumor proved to be a "squamous cell carcinoma, a typical cancer of the skin with cornification." Three years after amputation the patient was alive and well, without evidence of a primary tumor elsewhere. The possibility that the tumor might have arisen from connective tissue or endothelium was not one that Maier recognized. In her opinion it could have arisen only from ectopic epithelium, whether displaced in embryonal life as a germ (*Keim*) or, in adult life, from the overlying epidermis in consequence of trauma. She opted for the latter, proposing that the trauma sustained in the boating accident had displaced epidermal cells through a fissured ulnar cortex into the medulla.[147]

In 1913 Bernhard Fischer extended the term *adamantinoma*, by then in general use for the tumor of the jaw supposedly derived from rests of the enamel organ, to include the similar tumor of the appendicular skeleton.[148] Since it was textbook doctrine that primary epithelial cancer of bone did not exist, said Fischer, tumors apparently of this character had been reported under various other names. Frequently they had been termed *endotheliomas*, in part because they often contained mucoid matter intermixed with cylindromatous aggregates of epitheliallike cells. He himself, however, regarded endothelioma as a diagnosis of despair (*Verlegenheitsdiagnose*). Fischer was struck by the resemblance of a tumor of this character from his own experience (a tumor of the tibia, involving subperiosteal and cortical bone) to the adamantinoma of the jaw. In both tumors there was a similar disposition of mucoid matter and epithelial cells. He concluded that the tibial tumor was to be explained by means of the doctrine of displaced embryonal germs (*die Lehre von der versprengten embryonalen Keimen*). But, short of a fetus biting its leg at the time the enamel organ was being laid down, such a distant displacement was out of the question. In order to account for this peculiar ectopic tumor (and for ectopic tissue generally, e.g., pancreatic tissue in a Meckel's diverticulum), Fischer proposed a modification of the accepted doctrine: it was not a specific embryonal epithelial germ that was deposited in such instances, but an epithelial germ whose cells had not lost all their original potency for further development. In the case in question, adjacent dermal epithelium had been displaced into the bone from the overlying skin at a stage of embryonal development in which the epithelial cells had not yet lost the potency for developing into enamel organ tissue.[149]

Commenting on Fischer's hypothesis in 1930, C. S. Richter remarked that, while it could hardly be disproved, no one had yet demonstrated the actual presence in normal bone of the required nests of displaced embryonal epithelial cells. Richter regarded the resemblance of Fischer's tumor to adamantinoma of the jaw as purely fortuitous. In his own instance of the tibial tumor Richter, too, found an abundance of mucoid or myxomatoid material present in addition to epitheliallike cells, but he took this to mean that the tumor was an analogue of the mixed salivary gland tumor. "Theoretically," stated Richter, "we must assume that primary epithelial tumors of bone cannot occur." He preferred to call his tumor an endothelioma, with the implication that it was a pseudoepithelial tumor of nonepithelial origin.[150] Still another reassessment of the controversial tumor was offered in 1936, when Brunner, one of Uehlinger's pupils at Zurich, suggested that Fischer's tumor was really of synovial origin. Arnold Lauche, who was Fischer's successor to the chair of pathological anatomy at Frankfurt, followed up this suggestion in 1947. After reviewing Fischer's case material, Lauche decided that the tumor in question resembled synovial membrane rather than enamel organ tissue. He included Fisher's case, along with nineteen additional tumors involving bursae or joint capsules, in a list of "synovialomas," "synovial endothelio-fibromas," and "synovial sarcomas."[151]

Seven years later, two papers dealing with adamantinoma of the appendicular skeleton appeared in the same issue of the *Journal of Pathology and Bacteriology*. The first, by J. Douglas Hicks, reviewed the literature on the subject. Hicks pointed out that in at least six of fourteen recorded tumors squamous epithelium and keratinized epithelial cell nests had been found. Unwilling, on the basis of the available evidence, to accept an origin from developmentally displaced embryonal epithelium or from traumatically displaced adult epithelium, Hicks argued that the tumors were derived from synovial connective tissue and that the presence of keratinized squamous epithelium was the result—the sanctity of the germ layers not withstanding—of squamous metaplasia. His view, he reminded his readers, meant a return to the old concept that these tumors were derived "from an endothelial source—on the understanding the synovium is 'endothelium.'" Hicks presented a new case and reevaluated the tissues from an earlier one.[152]

In the second paper H. Lederer and A. J. Sinclair described a tibial tumor, which they termed a "malignant synovioma," in an eleven-year-old girl. After reviewing the descriptions and photomicrographs of other such cases, reported in the literature as adamantinomas of the appendicular skeleton, they concluded that the tumors were all of synovial origin; hence, the term *adamantinoma* should be discarded.[153] Neither Hicks nor Lederer and Sinclair appear to have known of the papers of Brunner and Lauche on this subject. Hicks cited Richter's words, "Theoretisch muessen wir annehmen, dass primaere Epithelgeschwuelste des Knochens nicht vorkommen koennen," as an epigraph, but did not include in his bibliography the paper (see note 150) from which the words were taken.

Fischer's tumor was once again reappraised, in 1957, by Changus, Speed, and Stewart. They reviewed twenty-five case reports and added eight cases of their own. In six of their tumors, alkaline phosphatase positive cells were present. On the basis of this and "sufficient presumptive evidence . . . obtained from the routine hematoxylin-and-eosin-stained sections," they decided that the tumors, including Fischer's, were all of angioblastic origin, hence "malignant angioblastomas." Changus, Speed, and Stewart added that Lauche's earlier reappraisal of Fischer's tumor as a synovial sarcoma was open to objection on clinical and pathological grounds.[154] F. Gloor, however, replied in 1963 that such tumors of bone were of mesenchymal and probably synovial origin after all and argued that synovial cells, too, contained alkaline phosphatase.[155] In 1968 Albores Saavedra, Díaz Gutiérrez, and Altamirano Dimas, using the electron microscope, described tonofibrils and desmosomes in the cells of a tibial adamantinoma. They concluded that the tumor cells were genuinely epithelial in nature, if not in origin.[156] Their work was independently confirmed by Juan Rosai two years later. Rosai stated that under the light microscope his tumor (a tibial tumor in a thirty-seven-year-old man with no history of preceding trauma) had in places "an epidermoid appearance, with whorling suggestive of pearl formations." His electron micrographs clearly show that the tumor cells contained dense bundles of microfilaments—presumably tonofibrils—and desmosomes, characteristic of epithelial cells.[157]

Leaving aside the possibility that adamantinomas of the appendicular skeleton constitute a group of histogenetically unrelated tumors, does a demonstration, however definitive, that the epitheliallike cells of the tumor are truly epithelial establish its histogenesis? Apparently Rosai thought so. Whether the tumor represents a "basal cell carcinoma, a squamous cell carcinoma, a sweat gland carcinoma, or a true amelo-blastoma" are histogenetic questions that cannot yet be decided, but he believes that his findings "establish with reasonable confidence that the present case of tibial adamantinoma is of epithelial derivation."[158] Harlan Spjut et al. also argued that the findings of Albores Saavedra and Rosai, if confirmed, would rule out a derivation from endothelial, angioblastic, or synovial cells, leaving only two histogenetic possibilities: "(1) congeni-tal cell rests; such cell rests, however, have not been identified in or around the tibia; (2) trauma with possible implantation of basal cells of the epidermis deep into the subcutaneous tissues."[159] Such traumatic implants, however, have not been identified in or around the tibia, either. Spjut's conclusion that one of the two "possible" explanations of the histogenesis of the so-called adamantinoma must be valid is precisely the conclusion reached seventy years earlier by Carola Maier, and in both instances the implicit premise was *omnis cellula a cellula ejusdem naturae.* The theoretical grounds for assuming that mesodermally derived cells, mesenchymal cells, or connective tissue cells, or their progeny can under no circumstances become transformed into true epithelial cells, complete with tonofibrils and desmosomes, are even less certain today than they were seventy or one hundred ten years ago. Such transformations, and others of the same or greater degree, may indeed be rare, or may not occur at all, but this is an empirical matter rather than one to be dealt with on an a priori basis.

The above excursus into the attempts of successive generations of histopathologists to fathom the histogenesis of a particular kind of tumor, the so-called adamatinoma of the appendicular skeleton, with depth-lines spun from histological data aimed to show how little change has occurred since Waldeyer's time with respect to the technical means available for ascertaining the histogenesis of clinical (as opposed to experi-mental) tumors and the premises underlying data interpretation. It is true that immunological and genetic techniques currently in laboratory use in the study of tumors make possible the accurate tracing of cell lines. These techniques may prove applicable to the study of clinically available tumor material, or the results of their application in the laboratory may call into question the assumptions made in the interpretation of clinical material. In any case, this is a matter for future investigators to study and is beyond the scope of the present book.

A second purpose of the above excursus is to offer some justification for the decision not to proceed further with a detailed account of the successive attempts of histopathologists during the past century to deal with the histogenesis of the enormous variety of tumors recognized in clinical practice. It is true that such attempts, based on increasingly refined histological data and at times carried out in full awareness of the inferential character of the interpretative procedure and its various pitfalls, are often both of great intrinsic interest and useful in the identification and classification of tumors, insofar as they lead to finer histological and histochemical discriminations. But, too often, the same questions are endlessly debated; the names of tumors change, change again, and sometimes repeat themselves as different inferences are drawn from essentially the same data. Admittedly, adamantinoma of the appendicular skeleton is, like all tumors of bone, a hard case. Even concerning the skin, however, where circumstances would seem most favorable for detecting the initiating cells of tumors, tumor names—all intended, more or less, to carry histogenetic information—have continued to proliferate. W. G. MacCallum's witty comment to the effect that histogenetic classifications of tumors are little more than "tissue[s] of assumptions" is worth quoting here in full:

> If, now, we speak of a fibrous tumor as a fibroma, a fatty tumor as a lipoma, and cartilaginous or bony tumors as chondromata or osteomata, it is rather because their tissues closely resemble fibrous, fatty, cartilaginous, or bony tissue, than that we can actually trace their origin to these tissues. Our classification is, therefore, rather a tissue of assumptions than one formed on a true histogenetic basis. Probably it is true that an epithelioma *is* definitely derived from the epithelium in which it began, and a fibroma from preëxistent connective tissue. It would be difficult to conceive of any other explanation, but the absolute proof is not at hand. Classification is at best unsatisfactory on a histogenetic basis, since so often we cannot make a good guess at the tissue which the tumor most resembles, or the point from which it actually sprang.[160]

Lest it be supposed that MacCallum's remarks have since been outdistanced, Leslie Foulds' comments in 1969 on the same subject are worth repeating: "Identification of the parent cells of a tumor, as attempted in histogenetic classifications, is not the only problem in early neoplastic development. The point of origin is often inferred, more or less plausibly, but it is scarcely ever seen, and the validity of inferences about histogenesis is rarely subjected to crucial tests."[161]

The topic was given its most acute analyses by A. von Albertini in 1955 and again in 1956. He, too, concluded that it was "in general not possible to set forth the precise lineage of a tumor cell." The common belief that we can do so, observes von Albertini, rests on the "assumption that the demonstration of a specific cell type in a tumor justifies the derivation of that cell from a corresponding normal cell."[162]

Waldeyer's Second Paper

A few remarks from the concluding half of Waldeyer's paper, published in 1872, on the histogenesis of carcinoma were cited above in connection with the problem posed by the development of apparently primary carcinomas at sites where epithelium is normally not present. Amounting to about one hundred pages in Virchow's *Archiv*, the second half of Waldeyer's paper reviewed published work in the field of tumor histo-genesis since 1867, rehearsed old and presented some new arguments and evidence favoring the exclusively epithelial origin of carcinomas, and refuted the counterarguments of a decreasing number of whole-hearted opponents of that theory, as well as of those who accepted it only in part. Waldeyer's conclusions were now supported by observations of an additional two hundred or more tumors.[163] The second half of his paper contains a wealth of acute reasoning and empirical histological observations. (The two halves were considerably longer than the whole of Thiersch's book.) Waldeyer's work—brilliantly argued, convincingly documented, and clearly stating that the generalized thesis of the exclusively epithelial origin of carcinoma was not susceptible of positive proof but must rest on circumstantial evidence, theoretical embryological considerations, and its superior ability to account for the observational data—constitutes a landmark in the field of tumor studies even more impressive than Thiersch's.

Among the textbook writers who had come to accept, to one extent or another, the epithelial theory of cancer genesis, Waldeyer lists Theodor Billroth, Edwin Klebs, Georg Rindfleisch, Ernst Neumann, Georg Luecke, Ernst Wagner, and Rudolf Maier. A host of investigators had demon-strated the epithelial origin of particular carcinomas, but many of them remained, Waldeyer points out, eclectic in their views. In France, Robin, Cornil, and others had argued for the derivation of carcinomas from epithelial *tissue,* although they differed with Waldeyer (and German investigators generally) in regard to the mode of origin of the epithelial *cells* of carcinomas. Virchow remained a proponent of the connective-tissue theory of cancer genesis. Aside from his followers, there were other whole-hearted opponents of the epithelial theory, such as Karl Koester, "who derive[d] all carcinomas from lymph vascular endothelium," and August Classen, who held that cancer cells were emigrated ameboid blood cells (*ausgewanderte amoeboide Blutzellen*). Further, the eclectics

Rindfleisch, Neumann, and Klebs variously derived carcinomas from "preexistent epithelial cells...connective tissue corpuscles, colorless blood corpuscles, and lymph vascular endothelium."[164]

Since all the cells of a given organism are directly derived from a fertilized egg cell, continued Waldeyer, it was obvious that epithelial, connective tissue, muscle, and nerve cells were, in some sense, all potentially present in that primal cell. There was, therefore, nothing a priori absurd in the notion that epithelial cells in an adult organism could arise from endothelial or connective tissue cells. It was simply a matter of embryological fact that this transformation did *not* occur after the germ layers had made their appearance. From that time on "not a single genetic intermixture of the various cell forms and cell types takes place." Still unshaken by a single, confirmed observation to the contrary, this "fundamental proposition of our modern histology" is, says Waldeyer, the foundation on which the "whole doctrine of the epithelial development of carcinoma rests." Waldeyer carried the doctrine of cell specificity to the extreme by claiming that even the various *types* of epithelial cells breed true. Whether under normal or abnormal circumstances, one "never sees squamous epithelium making its appearance where cylindrical cell epithelium is the typical form, and vice-versa," evidence to this effect so far brought forward by other investigators notwithstanding.[165]

Waldeyer (who after 1872 devoted himself to studies in comparative anatomy, embryology, and cytology) pointed out that embryology was a rapidly developing science; therefore, its applicability to the study of tumors, as well as to other aspects of pathology, required continual reassessment. Remak's derivation of urogenital epithelium from the mesoderm had been disputed by His, who—to Billroth's great satisfaction—derived it from a pinched-off portion of the outer germ layer, but Waldeyer's studies of the development of the ovary had shown that the matter was far from settled. And His had since come out with a radical revision of germ-layer doctrine, according to which the archiblast (*Archiblast*)—the sole derivative of the fertilized egg cell—was supposed to deliver all tissues of the body, other than blood, bloodvessels, and connective tissue. These three were supposed by His to be derived from the parablast (*Parablast*), which was constituted by the white yolk (*weisser Dotter*); they were, therefore, genetically distinct from all archiblastic tissues. Waldeyer regarded this thesis as unproved; subsequently, he reinterpreted the data on which it was based in such a way as to bring them into the mainstream of embryological thought.[166] Although he believed that "true" epithelial cells derived from the ectoderm, endoderm, and possibly, the mesoderm (i.e., urogenital epithelium) were as genetically distinct from one another as connective tissue cells were from epithelial cells, Waldeyer saw no reason to subdivide carcinomas into separate classes derived from each of the three germ layers. Although justified in theory it would be quite without practical value, for all carcinomas had a similar structural arrangement, characterized by the presence of closely packed epithelial cells lying in a supporting stroma of vascularized connective tissue. In contrast to the cells of sarcomas, the epithelial cells of carcinomas were not separated by an intercellular substance of their own making, nor did they ever form the linings of blood or lymph vessels.[167]

Waldeyer thought it odd that certain investigators denied to epithelial cells what they readily granted to connective tissue cells, namely, the capability of reproducing by division, budding, or endogenous cell formation. As evidence for the ability of epithelial tumor cells to do so, Waldeyer pointed to the presence of multinucleated tumor cells and to cells with constricted nuclei suggestive of imminent division. He had, he said, attempted directly to observe—so far without success—the possible processes of cell division in carcinoma cells, using a heated stage and freshly extirpated tissues.[168] Waldeyer added that it was well known that Virchow and his numerous partisans had insisted on deriving the cells of all inflammatory masses and most tumors, carcinomas and sarcomas alike, from fixed connective tissue cells. Recently, however, the "unsure empirical foundations" of Virchow's theory had been exposed by "the recognition of the Waller-Cohnheim doctrine of emigration,"[169] and it was now "almost comical to see a great horde of investigators, obviously blinded by this new and significant achievement, striving to derive from the emigrated colorless blood corpuscles not only muscles, nerves, connective tissues, and epithelia of the normal body, but of each and every pathological new-formation as well." Thus they fell from one extreme to the other.[170]

In recognizing and clearly stating the inferential character of all accounts of tumor histogenesis, including his own, and in marshaling the circumstantial evidence in favor of the exclusively epithelial origin of carcinomas, Waldeyer is at his best. What, he asked, was the justification for Virchow's supposition that the connective tissues were the source of most tumors, or the supposition of others, after the work of Cohnheim, that emigrated blood cells were the source of new-formations of all kinds? Why had no one suggested that fibrous tissue tumors had an epithelial origin, rather than the other way around? The fact is that "no one has actually seen how a fibroma of the skin arises, how the elements of the preexistent connective tissue or, if you will, the wandering cells, go about transforming themselves into the constituents of one or another kind of fibroma." One simply concludes that a given fibroma arises from connective tissue on the basis of the observed fact that similarly structured elementary components are present both in the skin and in the fibroma in question. A conclusion drawn in this way, by inferring the histogenesis of a tumor from its histological structure, was, in Waldeyer's opinion, justified. The right to do so, he says, "indisputably holds for all other tissues, and I ask no further right in support of my view of the epithelial origin of carcinoma." (Waldeyer's "right" is obviously a corollary of the doctrine of the specificity of cells and tissues.)

Moreover, in the study of some two hundred epithelial tumors he had found that they always arose in association with preexistent normal epithelium, whereas he had seen no evidence that they arose from the epithelial cells of blood and lymph vessels or by way of *generatio aequivoca.* His conclusion is nonetheless inferential; with reference to Koester's claim that carcinomas develop from the endothelium of lymph vessels, Waldeyer says: "No one, admittedly, has heard the grass grow, and likewise no one has as yet seen an undoubted cancer cell take form before his own eyes from an epithelial cell, an endothelial cell of the lymphatic vessels, or a fixed connective tissue cell. The demand for strict proof will be met only when we succeed in experimentally growing cancers at will on transparent media. Until then we must be content to draw conclusions from dead images regarding the possible life-processes that have determined them."[171]

Waldeyer points out that the epithelial theory of the histogenesis of carcinomas (although, like all histogenetic theories, based on inference) is consonant with the findings of embryology and better able than alternative theories to account for the observed data of oncology. It does not require, as does the connective tissue theory, the additional assumption that connective tissue cells can be transformed into epithelial cells. And Koester's inference that carcinomas arise from endothelial cells (which are already somewhat epithelial in character) conflicts with the observed data. Why do carcinomas of the skin and mucous membranes, asks Waldeyer, make their first appearance in the epithelium? Why do carcinomas arise only in epithelial tissues and organs, whereas lymph vessels are as ubiquitous in serous membranes, the diaphragm, and so on as they are in those organs? Why have no indisputably positive instances of carcinomas arising primarily in the spleen, lymph glands, muscles, and bones been reported? Why do we find squamous cell nests in carcinomas of the skin, cylindrical epithelial cells in carcinomas of the gut, and cells resembling those of the convoluted tubules in carcinomas of the kidney? Why does a squamous cell carcinoma metastatic to the liver yield a secondary growth of squamous cell character, and a cylindrical cell carcinoma of the stomach a secondary of cylindrical cell character? All these findings are readily explained by the assumption that the epithelial cells of carcinomas arise from corresponding normal epithelial cells and thereafter, in accordance with the doctrine of cell specificity, breed true. No additional assumptions are needed.[172]

The so-called infectious theory of carcinomas—supported, in part, by Virchow—had a number of variants. Waldeyer regarded this theory as quite shaky and constantly in need of the support of subsidiary assumptions. Rudolf Maier, for example, "took refuge in a completely unsupported hypothesis"; namely, that the cells of carcinomas might indeed first arise from epithelial cells but that the disease process was not really under way until an "epithelial infection" had generated (possibly from the epithelial cells) an infectious agent capable of transforming neighboring connective tissue cells, endothelial cells, or wandering cells into epithelial cancer cells.[173] Another proponent of the infectious theory, Wilhelm Mueller, held that both epithelioma and carcinoma were infectious diseases, but caused by different viruses. In Mueller's own words: "The virus at the basis of carcinoma is, however, essentially different from that calling forth epithelioma formation, in that it, like the virus of syphilis, is characterized by a specific relationship to the cellular elements of the connective tissue of the body, whereas the virus whose effect has in train the formation of epithelioma possesses a specific relationship to the epithelial components of the body."[174]

In order to explain the histological character of metastatic carcinomas, Waldeyer says that the adherent of the infectious theory must have recourse to an additional hypothesis, such as: "The character of the epithelium at the point of origin determines the form of all developing cancer cells, which then retain their once inherited character in all metastases." But the infectious theory itself is mostly hypothesis, according to Waldeyer. What kind of agent is this infecting virus, he asks, and where does it come from? Why is it so lacking in contagiousness that a carcinoma can be handled with impunity? How is the virus able to change the form of the cell that it infects? Does the theory not "smuggle the hardly banned specific cells [of cancer] back into tumor doctrine"? And further, with the advance of histological technique, the so-called transitional forms between cancer cells and connective tissue cells or wandering cells have been revealed as illusory.[175]

In retrospect, the infectious theory of cancer genesis, together with attempts on the part of certain investigators to derive carcinoma cells from emigrated "wandering cells," may appear as no more than a way station on the road toward the differentiation of inflammatory and neoplastic diseases. There were, however, some findings of genuine histological interest involved in the matter. In 1870 August Classen interpreted the clusters of small round cells seen adjacent to carcinomas (termed *begleitende Bindegewebswucherung* by Waldeyer in 1867) as inflammatory wandering cells undergoing transformation into tumor cells.[176] Writing in 1872, Waldeyer emphasized the essentially inflammatory character of both *einleitende* and *begleitende* changes in the connective tissues associated with carcinoma. "On the border between a carcinoma and adjacent healthy tissue," he wrote, "one always meets with changes in the interstitial connective tissue, which appear now as more acute, now as more chronic inflammatory processes." And he concluded that "if any kind of tumor exhibits relationships to inflammatory processes in respect to its etiology or earliest manner of development...it is carcinoma." Further, a primary carcinoma usually differs from its metastases in this respect: while the primary is apt to be diffusely infiltrative in its growth, and associated with considerable inflammatory reaction, the secondaries usually present as well-circumscribed masses with little evidence of a surrounding inflammatory reaction.[177]

For Waldeyer, then, a carcinoma is, histologically and histogenetically, an atypical epithelial tumor, just as a sarcoma is, histologically and histogenetically, an atypical connective tissue tumor. Both are characterized by "unrestrained new-formation"—of epithelial cells in the former and of connective tissue cells in the latter. In most instances these tumors are readily distinguishable under the microscope; there are a few exceptions, notably Billroth's alveolar sarcoma and his own plexiform angiosarcoma. These tumors mimic carcinomas. Waldeyer had become interested in some peculiar, darkly granulated cells with numerous fine processes more or less attached to the adventitia of small blood vessels. The cells were most evident in bats, mice, and rats, but were also seen in human beings. Waldeyer's terms for these cells were *perithelium* (*Perithel*) and *perithelial cells* (*Perithelzellen*). Peculiar connective tissue tumors, particularly the so-called plexiform angiosarcoma, in the brain, lymph glands, testes, and serous membranes perhaps arose from these cells. In the brain, an organ that is a "touchstone for the doctrine of the epithelial origin of carcinoma," he had never seen a carcinoma; one that he had formerly taken to be such he now regarded as a plexiform angiosarcoma mimicking a carcinoma.[178]

Inflammation and Neoplasia: New Developments

Despite the newly recognized association of inflammatory changes with those of beginning carcinomatous neoplasia, and the attempts of certain investigators to promulgate the so-called infectious theory of carcinoma, the line of distinction between inflammatory and noninflammatory tumors—otherwise expressed, the line between inflammatory and neoplastic processes—received additional emphasis during the decade following the publication of the second part of Waldeyer's paper. The line was first drawn on a physiopathological basis. Cohnheim's slighting reference, in 1873, to Klebs's work on gunshot wounds as the product of a bacteria-happy (*bacterienfroh*) age is revealing. Speculation was rife, but the evidence scanty. Cohnheim added that to him the role of causal agent of inflammation assigned by some workers to micro-organisms seemed unlikely.[179]

Progress in the field of bacteriology was such that by 1877, when the first edition of Cohnheim's *Lectures on General Pathology* appeared, he had changed his mind. He devotes ten pages to a discussion of bacteria as causal agents of inflammation in traumatic and infectious diseases, remarking to his readers: "You see that I am truly not inclined to underestimate the significance of schizomycetes for traumatic inflammation." At the same time he was unconvinced that one could "comprehend the whole of traumatic infection as the effect of bacteria."[180] Evidence continued to accumulate. Richard Koch, who had described the role of the anthrax bacillus in 1876, in 1877 made public his technique for staining dry smears of bacteria with aniline dyes (simultaneous with the publication of Paul Ehrlich's similar procedure for staining blood cells). Koch's monograph on the etiology of wound infections was published in 1878; he described the use of solid (gelatin) media for the isolation of pure cultures of micro-organisms in 1881; and in 1882 he identified, cultured, and stained the tubercle bacillus—the etiological agent responsible for perhaps the most striking of the "inflammatory tumors."[181]

To the physiopathological distinction between inflammation and neoplasia an etiological distinction was now being added. For, aside from the continued fruitlessness of the search for tumor or cancer "viruses," the contagiousness and ready transmissibility of inflammatory diseases was in striking contrast to their absence in neoplastic diseases. A third distinction, based on the physiopathological significance, or lack of it, of the two processes, gained additional credence in the 1880s with the advent of the so-called biological theory of inflammation, promulgated (although it had already made itself felt) by Ilya Metchnikov.

For centuries there had been an argument as to whether inflammation was a disease or a defensive reaction against disease.[182] Virchow, in 1854, had stated that the teleological interpretation of the inflammatory process was exaggerated, but at the same time by no means entirely off the mark.[183] Cohnheim's interpretation of the inflammatory process as no more than the result of a lesion in the capillary vascular system entailed, it would seem, the withdrawal of its teleological significance. Cohnheim at first paid little attention to the matter. Rejecting (in 1877) the notion that muscle, nerve, and epithelial cells were derived from white cells in inflammatory exudates, he proposed that they gave rise to the fibrous tissue of scars and the callus of bone fractures; in some instances this was beneficial to the organism and in others it was not.[184] In the second edition of his *Vorlesungen* (1882) Cohnheim repeated these statements, but added to them (on grounds that are not made clear) the claim that inflammation was a "reaction" and a "remarkable adaptation" on the part of the organism to harmful agents. What this reaction consisted in, and the nature of the harmful agents, was left unstated.[185] Metchnikov's explanation of the reaction (first put forward in 1883) was that the function of the inflammatory process was to bring phagocytes, the colorless corpuscles of the blood, into contact with invading harmful agents, including micro-organisms, which they would then ingest and destroy. His own work along this line had been with water fleas, larval starfish, and other lower forms of life until, stimulated by the *Vorlesungen* but dissatisfied with Cohnheim's theory of inflammation, he moved into the field of human pathology—encouraged, incidentally, by Rudolf Virchow. Metchnikov's first article written for a medical audience appeared in Virchow's *Archiv* in 1884, and in 1885 Virchow himself dealt favorably with the biological theory of inflammation in an article entitled "The Battle of Cells and Bacteria."[186] An inflammatory tumor, or, more accurately, the inflammatory process of which it was an incidental manifestation, could thus be interpreted as an adaptive response of the organism to invading agents of disease. Inflammation, in other words, made sense within the context of the physiological economy of the body. True tumors—excluding, of course not only inflammatory masses but also local hypertrophy or hyperplasia occurring in response to some obvious physiological demand—did not. On the contrary, such tumors were useless at best and lethally destructive at worst. Writers of textbooks, among them Cohnheim, first began to call attention to this third distinguishing feature of true (*echte*) tumors in the second half of the nineteenth century.[187]

Cohnheim's Cell Rests

In the field of oncology, Cohnheim is best remembered today as the proponent of the theory that tumors arise from embryonal cell rests. As a histogenetic theory this was by no means new; as far as cellular pathology in Virchow's sense was concerned, it had been put forward by Remak in 1854 to account for the epithelial character of a primary tumor (Virchow's cancroid) arising in the bone marrow. But in Cohnheim's hands the theory, aside from being generalized to account for the origin of *all* tumors, acquired etiological overtones; it was now offered in explanation of the *growth* as well as the cellular makeup of tumors.

In Cohnheim's first paper on the subject, published in Virchow's *Archiv* in 1875, the new aspect of the theory is not evident. The paper reports a case of bilateral kidney tumors in a five-year-old girl. The larger of the tumors was 25 cm in greatest dimension. Cohnheim, who expected that the tumor would reveal itself under the microscope to be an ordinary sarcoma, was surprised to see, at first, "nothing but the most beautiful cross-striated muscle fibers." In addition he found vascular, fibrous, and fatty connective tissue, together with foci of "sarcoma" made up of small round cells about the size of white blood corpuscles. The tumor was thus, said Cohnheim, the "striated muscle sarcoma," or *myosarcoma strio-cellulare,* described by Virchow in his book on tumors under the heading of "teratoma." However, according to Cohnheim, striated muscle fibers had not heretofore been found in renal tumors. Cohnheim's tentative explanation of their presence was Remakian in both substance and phraseology. In consequence of a developmental error, germ-cells of future striated muscle fibers had been segregated from the primitive vertebral plate, where they were normally present, and included in the urogenital rudiment (*Anlage*). The cells resulting from this faulty inclusion (*fehlerhaft Abschnuerung*) persisted and became the source of the striated muscle in the renal tumor. This hypothesis, remarked Cohnheim, was more attractive than the assumption that any of the normally present renal constituents were capable of yielding striated muscle. As for the small round cells of the tumor, it was an open question whether they were the germ-cells in question or merely intramuscular connective tissue cells.[188]

Cohnheim's idea that the growth as well as the structure of tumors might be accounted for on the assumption of an origin from embryonal cells is set forth in the first edition (1877) of his *Vorlesungen.* After dealing with regeneration, hypertrophy, and infectious tumors (*Infectionsge-schwuelste*) in a separate chapter, he introduces the subject of true (*echte*) tumors with some remarks on the growth process in general. The sudden growth of the genitalia at puberty and of the uterus during pregnancy cannot, he states, be explained as the result of work hypertrophy, the way in which we account for localized growth of skeletal muscle or, when the outlets of the bladder and stomach are obstructed, of smooth muscle. We must assume, on the contrary, that the cells of those organs are, from their earliest existence as embryonal rudiments, predisposed to undergo partial growth, the remainder of the body remaining relatively unaffected. The repeated growth of the uterus represents the "most extraordinarily pregnant example of growth dependent on the original germ-rudiment but is nevertheless exceptional; only because it is grounded in the type of our organization do we not call it abnormal." Likewise, the growth of congenital malformations, ectopic organs and tissue, and the phenomenon of local gigantism are to be explained in terms of an abnormality of the embryonal rudiment (*Abnormitaet der embryonalen Anlage*). This far-from-mystical conception (*mystischer Begriff*) that among the causes of excess growth we must include a predisposition of the embryonal rudiment of an organ or tissue should be broadened, Cohnheim was now proposing, to cover the entire field of true tumors, i.e., those tumors that are not the result of physiological or pathological hypertrophy (the pregnant uterus, "splenic tumor," etc.) and do not fall into the class of retention tumors (*Retentionsgeschwuelste*) or infectious tumors.[189]

The etiology of tumors, says Cohnheim, is a dark chapter, if there ever was one, in the science of pathology. Age, sex, social position, and so forth—each has its place, but as no more than a predisposing cause. Trauma and local irritation of a chemical or mechanical nature are much spoken of as direct causes. Aside from the lack of correlation between trauma and neoplasia, however, both experiment and experience show us that "through trauma of various kinds certain products of hypertrophy and inflammation, but no *true tumors*, arise." The evidence for the infectious origin of true tumors is likewise slight. In contrast to the so-called infectious tumors (*Infectionsgeschwuelste*), there is not a single confirmed case of the transfer of a true tumor from one person to another: "Never has a surgeon been 'infected' while operating on a tumor; never has a man acquired a cancroid of the penis from the uterine cancer of his wife." Nor has the transfer of tumors from one animal to another ever been successfully carried out. As for harmful aliments and the emotional and nervous disturbances so emphasized in the older literature in connection with the origin of tumors, Cohnheim is unable to see that they can influence local growth except by disturbing the circulation. There remains, then, the idea of an embryonal rudiment (*embryonale Anlage*) as the necessary starting point of a tumor. This explanation, he points out, had already been used by Georg Luecke to account for teratomas, but that is no reason why it should not be held valid for all other tumors, Virchow's histioid and organoid tumors included.[190]

The simplest hypothesis was the supposition that at an early stage of embryonal development more cells than necessary for the part involved were produced. As development proceeded a "quantum of cells" remained behind unused, perhaps only of very small dimensions but—because of the embryonal nature of the cells—of great reproductive capability. In support of the hypothesis that tumors arise from residual embryonal rudiments, Cohnheim adduced the occurrence of congenital tumors, ectopic tissues, and the parallel case of congenital malformations. But the real value of the hypothesis, as Cohnheim saw it, was that it accounted for both the growth *and* the structure of neoplasms. "Our hypothesis," he writes, "makes it understandable that *each and every tissue* can occur in tumors, and indeed just as well in tissues in which elements are continually produced throughout the whole of life, such as epithelial and connective tissues, as in tissues which only add substance physiologically under the influence of specific stimuli, such as muscle and gland tissue, and also finally, tissues which after a certain period of life no longer bring forth new elements at all, such as the central nervous system." And, at the same time, the hypothesized embryonal rudiment has, from the beginning, the "capability of abundant cell production. . .because of its embryonal nature." His "etiological interpretation of the tumor concept," wrote Cohnheim, went to the "heart of the matter," for etiology, rather than morphology or chemical constitution, was the ultimate distinguishing point in oncology, as in all pathology.[191] A final comment: In Cohnheim's opinion, the hypothesis did not stand or fall on the empirical evidence for the actual existence of residual embryonal cells in adult organs and tissues. On the contrary, he writes that "it is quite conceivable that the cell groups representing the rudiment of the future tumor are, with our technical means, quite impossible to distinguish from the physiological elements of a part. . .how can one look at a group of epithelial cells, cells of lymph glands or cells of the bone marrow and determine whether they are left over from embryonal development or not?"[192]

Cohnheim's belief that embryonal tissues, as opposed to tissues in the adult, were peculiarly capable of growth seems to have been based on nothing more than the relatively rapid growth manifest in embryonic life. This thesis, however, received some experimental support in 1877, when Friedrich Wilhelm Zahn, a former pupil of von Recklinghausen, read a paper on the fate of tissue implants at the Fifth International Congress of Medical Sciences in Geneva.[193] After describing previous work by investigators who had transplanted bits of tissue from one animal to another of the same or a different species, making use of the body cavities, subcutaneous tissues, and the anterior chamber of the eye as implant sites, Zahn stated that his experimental results had been successful only when he used fetal tissues, cartilage in particular; adult tissues were resorbed. Further, he had a successful outcome in one animal out of three when he implanted a fragment of a maxillary enchondroma (from an old woman) into the anterior chamber of the rabbit eye. After eighty days the fragment had increased in size, and the cartilage cells showed evidence of proliferation. Embryonal tissues, he concluded were "more closely related to neoplasms than to normal adult tissues." Zahn thought that his experiments proved the relevance of Virchow's doctrine of the genesis of certain tumors.[194]

Investigating the mechanism of tumor metastasis, Cohnheim and Maas, in 1877, had injected bits of periosteal tissue into the jugular veins of animals (dogs, rabbits, and chickens), their aim being to ascertain whether tissue removed from its site of origin would grow and proliferate within blood vessels of the lung.[195] Curiously enough, in view of Cohnheim's theory of tumors, the thought of using embryonal tissues evidently did not occur to them. In 1881, stimulated by the work of Zahn, G. Leopold reported on experiments carried out in Cohnheim's Institute at Leipzig over a period of two years.[196] According to Leopold, Zahn was the first person to employ embryonal tissues as implants. In following up Zahn's work, Leopold asked whether the growth of the implanted tissue depended on the age of the embryo from which it was derived. Carrying out the operations with strict antiseptic precautions, Leopold implanted tissues from 2½, 4, 6 and 8 cm rabbit embryos into the anterior ocular chambers, peritoneal cavities, and subcutaneous tissues of sixty-one adult rabbits, using cartilage, bone, skin, and even whole extremities as implants. The report deals chiefly with the fate of cartilage in the anterior ocular chamber.[197] Adult cartilage implants failed to grow. Leopold obtained his best results with cartilage derived from the youngest embryos. An implant measuring less than 1 mm in diameter, taken from a 2½ cm embryo, reached 8 mm in greatest dimension after about six months. Leopold did not hesitate to claim that he had experimentally produced "true" tumors, namely, enchondromas. The admissibility of Cohnheim's hypothesis that tumors developed from embryonal rudiments had, said Leopold, now received experimental confirmation.[198] In the second edition of the *Vorlesungen* (1882), Cohnheim likewise claimed no more than that the admissibility (*Statthaftigkeit*) of his hypothesis had been shown by Leopold's experiments.[199]

Cohnheim's attempt to give etiological as well as morphological significance to the old hypothesis that aberrant germs (*verirrte Keime*) are the starting point of tumor growth was seriously flawed. By his own admission, the hypothesized embryonal cell rudiments were identifiable only where they differed, in consequence of embryonal displacement, from the surrounding adult tissues. Furthermore, even admitting the proneness of embryonal cells to undergo rapid growth, the hypothesis offered no satisfactory explanation of why they underwent rapid growth at one time rather than another.[200] The net result was that potential verification of the hypothesis existed only in the case of tumors differing in morphological character from the tissues in which they arose. Hence, insofar as the hypothesis proved viable at all, it was viable in its morphological rather than in its etiological sense. It survives today as a histogenetic, that is, a morphological, hypothesis of the origin of teratomas from "aberrant germ cells."[201]

Virchow: Neoplasia and Metaplasia

In contrast to those who held, as Billroth did, that cell species were as incapable of interconversion as were animal species, Virchow continued to lay emphasis on the plasticity of cells and tissues under pathological circumstances. In the fourth edition (1871) of the *Cellularpathologie*, he stated that he had always emphasized the histogenetic identity of cancroid and true cancer (*Carcinom*) and had held that if one was essentially a hyperplastic new-formation, so was the other. The view that carcinoma was an epithelial proliferation had come to be widely accepted, added Virchow, but rather than deny the existence of primary carcinomas in sites where epithelium was not normally present, or derive them from lymphatic vessels, he preferred to regard connective tissue as the source of cancer—"to hold with the primary heteroplasia [*Heteroplasie*] of all cancer."[202] He also coined a new term, *metaplasia* (*Metaplasie*), to designate the transformation, or metamorphosis, of one kind of tissue into another. Virchow did not, at this time, use the term with special reference to pathological tissue processes, including the development of tumors; as we have seen, he referred to the transformation of undifferentiated connective tissue into epithelial cancer as *heteroplasia*, a term that antedated cellular pathology and the cell theory itself.[203]

In 1880 Virchow argued against the morphologists (*Morphologen*) who seemed to wish to reduce the whole of pathology to embryology. "I will never admit," he stated, "that the word 'embryonal' adds anything essential to the pathology of the adult." Not even the limits of metaplastic change in the adult were prescribed in embryonal development. Bursae, for example, were not present in the embryo; they arose in the adult from connective tissue and came to be "lined by epithelial or, if you will, endothelial cells." It was sheer "embryological mysticism" to deny that epithelium could ever arise from connective tissue.[204]

This reproach of "embryological mysticism" was directed less against Cohnheim than against Franz Boll and Carl Hasse. The former held that the argument over the relative merits of the epithelial versus the connective tissue theory of cancer was meaningless, since cancers actually arise from a germinal vascular tissue (*Gefaesskeimgewebe*) representing a reversion to the embryonal state; the latter (who believed he was extending Cohnheim's theory) held that *all* tissues of the adult contain embryonal cells capable of yielding tumors.[205] Hasse's amplification of Cohnheim's theory appeared to Virchow as a *reductio ad absurdum:* in effect it simply defined all cells capable of growth as embryonal cells. Boll's "germinal vascular tissue," the matrix of all tumors, was like his own "indifferent granulation tissue," according to Virchow, the difference being that it was labeled embryonal. The only proper sense in which a tissue in the adult organism could be called embryonal was, said Virchow, with reference to tissues that had persisted in their embryonal form; for example, bones were originally laid down in cartilage, therefore persisting remnants of cartilage in the shaft of a bone could be termed embryonal. With reference to Cohnheim's theory of tumor genesis, Virchow remarked that he himself had coined the term *teratoma* in part because such tumors appeared to have an embryonal origin. Cohnheim was unable to see why Luecke's account of the histogenesis of teratomas should not be extended to all tumors; he, on the other hand, was unable to see why it should be. How, asked Virchow, would Cohnheim account for an amputation neuroma? By assuming the presence of an embryonal rudiment as needed? Virchow's paper contains much else of great interest, the consideration of which would take us too far afield.[206]

Virchow returned to the topic once again, in 1884, in an address entitled "On Metaplasia."[207] Here he extended the sphere of meaning assigned to the term *metaplasia. Hypertrophy,* he reminded his auditors, referred, strictly speaking, to an increase in cell size; *hyperplasia* (his own term), to an increase in cell number. *Metaplasia* referred not only to a "plastic process" in which a new tissue took form from a precursor tissue of different character, but also to the production of new tissue elements, that is, it had some features of hyperplasia. Further, the metaplastic process corresponds to some degree to the "differentiation" of the embryologists and the "transformism" of the Darwinists. In the adult organism metaplasia occurred in both physiological and pathological circumstances. It also played a role in the histogenesis of tumors. A myoma of the uterus, said Virchow, could be regarded as the result of hyperplasia; a myxoma of the uterus, on the other hand, resulted from secondary metaplasia. The limits of metaplasia in the adult organism had not been defined. The transformation of cylindrical cell epithelium into squamous cell epithelium was generally admitted, but the majority opinion categorically denied the possibility that connective tissue could be transformed into epithelium, or vice-versa. Virchow himself, however, was "still convinced that tumors of epithelial structure can arise by metaplasia from connective tissues." A final decision on this matter was premature, but it should be made on the basis of observation, not theory. He concluded with the following comment on germ-layer theory: "Now I shall not give decisive value to the fact that precisely this aspect of embryology has not yet been explained to everyone's satisfaction, and that each new embryological finding brings to light for itself another formula. But I cannot admit that embryology, especially in its histological aspect, is decisive for pathology. Here everything depends on experience."[208]

Virchow's concept of metaplasia was not formulated precisely enough to allow for a clear distinction between the direct transformation of one cell into another (say, of a columnar epithelial cell into a squamous cell) and the transformation involving one or more divisions or replications of the original cell, in the course of which the new cell type would appear. In the main, he seems to have envisioned the latter as the more common path of metaplasia. In the case of the "indifferent" cells of the connective tissue, supposed by Virchow to be the common source of tumors, this is plain enough, since he states that new formations of widely different kinds—even as different as cancer and tubercle—are hardly distinguishable in the earliest stages of their growth. However this may be, the point on which Virchow most strongly insisted was that the limits of cell transformability, insofar as the genesis of tumors was concerned, ought to be derived from oncological experience rather than prescribed by embryological theory. He was thus the first in the long series of pathologists who have declared their independence from overrestrictive interpretations of the histogenetic significance of the germ layers, and of embryologists who have protested against the undue generalization of germ-layer theory, whether in pathology or within the broader confines of comparative anatomy.[209]

Bard: Specificity of Cellular Elements

A year after the appearance of Virchow's essay on metaplasia, Louis Bard, professor of pathological anatomy at Lyons, restated the doctrine of absolute cell specificity in relation to the histogenesis of tumors.[210] Granting that the derivation of all cells from preexisting cells, as set forth by Remak and Virchow, was now almost universally accepted, Bard rejected Virchow's "notion of an undifferentiated tissue, capable of almost unlimited metaplasia," i.e., the connective tissue, in favor of the "notion of *the absolute specificity of differentiated anatomical elements.*" His notion of cell specificity, said Bard, was at once more general and more restrictive than Remak's "specificity of the three embryonal layers": more general in that it did not assign each layer an absolute monopoly of certain cells and tissues; more restrictive in the sense that the specificity of cells was still more rigorously conceived, since a germ layer is itself a "complex organ which may, and does in fact, contain specific elements of very different character, as in the case of the ectoderm, which gives birth to the cells of the covering epithelium and cells of the central nervous system."

By the "specificity of cellular elements," Bard means that "the various cell types constitute so many families, genera and species, which, like the families, genera and species of animals, may well be traced through an ancestral series to a common stock, but which have pursued their collateral courses of evolution and have become incapable of undergoing transformation into each other." This means, according to Bard, that all tumors arise from normal cells of the same type as those composing the tumor. The specificity of tumor tissue, like that of normal tissue, "pertains to the cell itself, considered as the primordial element, rather than to the overall structure of the tissue, which is no more than a secondary production." Since tumors arise from anatomical elements like themselves, nothing is easier, says Bard, than to account for the presence of neoplasms similar in structure to the tissues in which they first appear. In the relatively few instances where this is not true, Cohnheim's theory may be invoked. As for mixed, or composite, tumors, we must suppose that they have originated from a "bouquet cellulaire"—that two or more cell types have undergone neoplastic growth.[211] In 1886 Bard deplored the recourse taken by certain pathologists to "differentiations," "adaptations," "metaplasias," "dedifferentiations" (*retours des éléments nobles à l'état indifferent*), and "redifferentiations" in their attempts to unravel the threads of tumor histogenesis. They appear to believe, says Bard, that "everything is in everything, and everything can come from something else." He holds, on the contrary, that Virchow's aphorism *omnis cellula e cellula* must yield to *omnis cellula e cellula ejusdem naturae*, insofar as reference is made to fully developed cells in adult organisms.[212]

For the most part, Bard was saying no more than what Thiersch, Waldeyer, and others had said; the analogy between cell species and animal species, which in Bard's hands gains phylogenetic overtones, originated with Billroth. But by this time ideas of the way in which cell potentialities might be progressively restricted in the course of embryonic development were beginning to be formulated more clearly and to be given an observational base. The notion of a genetic substance of definable chemical character, present as a whole in the fertilized ovum and subsequently distributed to diverging series of descendant cells, was being considered in the light of the precise splitting and equal distribution of the threadlike components of the nucleus recently discerned in dividing cells.

In 1879 Walther Flemming summed up his work and that of other, chiefly German, investigators on the indirect, or *mitotic* (as Flemming termed it), division of cells in a monograph so definitive that little could be added to it until the middle of the present century.[213] Bard was aware of these developments. In his second paper he distinguished two quite different modes of cell proliferation. In the first, which he terms *multiplication*, the resulting cells are like their parent cells in all respects; in the second, termed *dédoublement* ("division"), the "original elements of several different specific cells" contained in parent cells are sorted out and passed on to their progeny. In the fertilized ovum, of course, *all* "original elements" are represented. The process of *dédoublement* occurs throughout embryonic development, as the elements of specific cells are progressively segregated and come to express themselves openly. It is, said Bard, somewhat comparable to a "chemical analysis that separates two or more bodies closely united in a single composite body and, in so doing, returns to each one of them its special properties, which had remained immanent in the composite body, and had not, in this temporary state of fusion, lost any of their respective qualities." The fertilized ovum is thus the source of two distinct series of cells: one, proceeding along the path of *dédoublement*, yields the cells of the embryo proper; the other, by way of *multiplication*, yields the future egg and sperm cells.[214]

MOLECULAR BIOLOGY FORESHADOWED

Similar ideas had been taken much further in Germany. In 1880 Moritz Nussbaum presented evidence to show that in a number of lower animals the primordial germ-cells or sex cells originated outside the embryo proper and only later, by means of wandering ameboid movements (*Einwanderung*), reached the middle germ-layer rudiment in which most embryologists thought they took origin.[215] The belief that primordial germ-cells, guarding as they did the entire inheritance of the species, were entirely distinct from the somatic cells that went on to differentiate into the specialized cells of the adult organism, now arose. Connected with it was August Weismann's belief in the continuity of the germ-plasm (*Keimplasma*), of which the germ-cells were the carriers as well as the transmitters, and his claim that cell determinants, or specifying particles (*bestimmenden Theilchen*), present as a whole in the germ-plasm, were separated out in the course of embryonic development to yield the specific cell types found in the adult organism.[216]

Diametrically opposed to Weismann's views were those of Albert Koelliker; in 1886, *sine ira et studio*, as he says, he reviewed the evidence in favor of his contentions that no sharp distinction between germ-cells and somatic cells existed and that the structure of the "idioplasm" in the fertilized ovum passed over unchanged to the nuclei of all somatic cells engaged in the formation of the embryo.[217] Koelliker and Weismann, as well as other biologists who engaged in this controversy during the closing years of the nineteenth century, were strongly influenced by Carl Wilhelm Naegeli's hypothetical concept of the idioplasm, with which Naegeli hoped to account for cell function, embryonic development, and the phenomena of heredity on a common molecular basis.[218] Naegeli proposed that the idioplasm, which he conceived to be a self-reproducing substance of proteinaceous nature arranged in linear strands consisting of differently arrayed "crystalline molecular groups or micelles," present as a whole in the fertilized egg cell, was distributed as a whole to each one of the innumerable descendants of that cell constituting the adult organism. The multiple spatial configurations possible in such a structure determine, according to Naegeli, the total activities of all cells. In his words, "the form, size, and arrangement of the idioplasmic micelles yield innumerable combinations of effective powers and, thereby, also innumerable chemical and formative processes in living substance, which bring about just so many differences in growth, inner organization, external form, and function." Naegeli suggested that the nuclear threads that became visible during mitotic division of cells might represent the actual cords of idioplasm.[219] Koelliker, who agreed with Naegeli that the idioplasm was fully present in every adult cell, made the further suggestion that it consisted of "nuclein," the nucleoprotein isolated from leucocytes and fish sperm by Friedrich Miescher in the 1870s.[220] But this false dawn of the era of molecular biology antedated the event itself by seventy years.

During the nineteenth century the life sciences, in particular those with which we have been concerned in our study of the problem of tumor genesis—histology, cytology, embryology, pathology, and to a limited extent, bacteriology and biochemistry—moved ahead at an extraordinarily rapid pace. An enormous distance lies between the conceptual worlds of, say, Bichat at the beginning of the nineteenth century and Naegeli near its close. The forward movement of these sciences was undeniably much slower during the first half of the twentieth century, whether in consequence of purely internal reasons or, as seems more likely, owing to the occurrence of wars and political persecutions on a new and unprecedented scale. As for progress in the understanding of the histogenesis and cytogenesis of tumors, its pace during the same period might be characterized as glacial. Only within the past decade or so have investigators begun to move beyond the charmed circle of techniques, ideas, and observations already current by the end of the nineteenth century.

NOTES

INTRODUCTION

1. L. J. Rather, "Systematic Medical Treatises from the Ninth to the Nineteenth Century: The Unchanging Scope and Structure of Academic Medicine in the West," *Clio Medica* 11 (1976): 289-305.

1

1. Roy L. Moodie, *Paleopathology.*
2. Marc A. Ruffer, *Studies in the Paleopathology of Egypt.* For a recent review of human paleopathology see Emiliano Aguirre, "Paleopatología y medicina prehistórica," *Historia Universal de la Medicina*, 1: 7-31.
3. Jacob Wolff, *Die Lehre von der Krebskrankheit,* 1: 4-5.
4. A. D. Godley, trans. *Herodotus, with an English Translation by A. D. Godley,* 2: 163-65.
5. Émile Littré, *Oeuvres complètes d'Hippocrate,* 8: 99; see also 7: 347 and 8: 339.
6. Ibid., 5: 259, 461.
7. Ibid., 8: 282.
8. Ibid., 9: 33.
9. Ibid., 5: 701.
10. Ibid., 4: 573.
11. Cf. Wolff, *Die Lehre von der Krebskrankheit,* for the use of the term *cancer* by Cato the Elder (234-149 B.C.) and by Celsus.
12. Cf. L. J. Rather, "Disturbance of function (*functio laesa*)," *Bull. N.Y. Acad. Med.* 47 (1971): 303-22; also "Galen on Inflammation: The True Story," in *The Healing Hand,* by Guido Majno, p. 413. The "true story" is that Virchow "first spelled out the *functio laesa* as a fifth sign" in the *Cellularpathologie* and that Galen had nothing to do with it. But what Virchow actually said (*Cellularpathologie*, p. 347) was that "all newer schools are at least in agreement that to the four characteristic symptoms *functio laesa* must be added"; the idea, if not the phrase, was already current in 1858. As early as 1852 and 1854, Virchow had included disturbance of function (*Funktionstoerung*) among the features of inflammation. In 1838 James Macartney had made a remark along similar lines, the ultimate source of which is clearly a passage in one of Galen's most widely read works, the *Ars medica,* wherein it is stated that local affections (not inflammation alone) are characterized by "swelling, pain, disturbance of functions, and difference of excretions" (*tumore, dolore, functionum offensione et excrementorum differentia*). Galen adds that function can be disturbed in three ways (*trifariam autem functio laeditur*). It would thus seem that the fifth sign does, in a sense, go back to Galen; the step from *functio laeditur* to *functio laesa* is not great. Nonetheless it remains true that Galen did not add anything to the four cardinal signs of Celsus and that *functio laeditur* refers to *any* local affection. Apparently it was Nicholas Tendeloo who first linked Galen to Celsus in 1919, and implied that the Latin tag *functio laesa* came from the writings of the former (cf. Rather, "Disturbance of Function").
13. Caelius Aurelianus, *On Acute Diseases and on Chronic Diseases.*
14. Cf. L. J. Rather, "Two Questions on Humoral Theory," *Medical History,* 15 (1971): 396-98, for a rationalization of the interchange of *dynameis* between water and air.

15. Cf. Raymond Klibansky, Erwin Panofsky, and Fritz Saxl, *Saturn and Melancholy*, esp. pp. 3-15.

16. Erich Schoener, "Das Viererschema in der antiken Humoralpathologie," *Sudhoff's Arch. Gesch. Med. Wiss.*, suppl. 4.

17. Rather, "Two Questions on Humoral Theory," p. 398.

18. Galen, *Opera omnia*, 15: iv.

19. Ibid., vol. 11. For a translation of *Ad Glauconem de medendi methodo libri II* see Charles Daremberg, *Oeuvres anatomiques, physiologiques, et médicales de Galen*, vol. 2. In keeping with the psychosomatic orientation of Greek humoral theory, melancholy humor, i.e., black bile and its variants, has connections with cancer on one side and emotional melancholy on the other. The history of Western medicine might possibly include an unbroken chain of attempts by physicians to assign to emotional disturbance an etiological role in the development of cancer. Such attempts would have been in keeping with the traditional etiological doctrine of the six nonnaturals (Galen's six nonnecessary conserving causes of health and disease), the sixth of which includes all emotional disturbances (cf. L. J. Rather, "The 'Six Things Non-Natural,'" *Clio Medica* 3 (1968): 337-47. However, the earliest reference to cancer in this connection, with which I am acquainted, occurs in the writings of Johannes Pechlin, a seventeenth-century physician. "I have seen," he writes, "an affection which was formerly a benign sort of tumor (*quodque nuper benignus erat tumor*) in women's breasts turn into a carcinoma when changed for the worse by fear or sorrow. Indeed, I have never seen a cancer of the breast so thoroughly removed, even after extirpation, that would not, in consequence of fear and sorrow, rather suddenly once again slowly recrudesce and, after long difficulties, at length put an end to life. Truly, nothing so much weakens the ferments and increases the sharpness of acid as a constant struggle with sorrows; for the volatile spirits, and rulers of the mixtures of juices and fluids, perish and are carried away due to that emotion; whence, all being fixed, viscous and acrid, they usually bring on manifest putridity, and, with putridity, death." J. N. Pechlin, *Observationum physico-medicarum libri tres*, p. 447.

Some sixty years later Gerard van Swieten, commenting on Hermann Boerhaave's inclusion of sad and bilious emotions (*affectus animi tristes et biliosi*) among the contributory causes of scirrhus and cancer, remarks that an atrabiliary temperament following on sorrowful emotions is well suited to the production of such ailments (*cum atrabiliaria temperies, tristes illos animi affectus sequens, illis malis producendis apta sit*) (Gerard van Swieten, *Commentaria*, pp. 876, 877). About one hundred years later Sir Astley Cooper stated that "anxiety of mind, tending to the presence of slow fever and suppressed secretions are the predisposing causes of the complaint. A person, the prey of disappointment from reduced circumstances, and struggling against poverty, when her prospects begin to brighten, finds a malignant tumor in her breast; costive state of bowels, a dry skin, a paucity of other secretions have attended this anxious state of mind, and laid the foundation of that destruction which awaits her" (*Principles and Practice of Surgery*, 1: 335).

20. Galen, *Opera omnia*, 14: 786.

21. Ibid. vol. 18, bk. 1, 60, 61.

22. Ibid., 11: 141, 142. Cf. Rudolph E. Siegel, *Galen's System*, pp. 285-87.

23. Galen, *Opera omnia*, 7: 702-32. The most readily available translation of the essay on preternatural tumors has heretofore been Paul Richter's *Ueber die krankhaften Geschwuelste*, in vol. 21 of *Klassiker der Medizin* (Leipzig, 1913). A translation is now available in English, cf. Jeremiah Reedy, "Galen on Cancer and Related Diseases," *Clio Medica* 10 (1975): 227-38.

24. Paul Richter, "Ueber die Entwicklung des aristotelischen Begriffes der Tumores praeter naturam," *Monats. prak. Derm.* 44 (1907): 65-70. Richter derives the notion of preternatural tumor from Aristotle's statement (*Problemata* IV, 13; wrongly given in his paper as XIV, 13) that many things growing on the body are preternatural and thus alien to the body; they are to be removed or cast out by the physician.

25. Jean Fernel, *Universa medicina*, lib. 7, *De externis corporis affectibus*, cap. 1, pp. 644, 645. These lesions are of course not always to be identified with their modern counterparts of the same name.

26. Cf. Rather, "Disturbance of function," p. 321, on the almost universal neglect of the technical medical term *inflammatio* until the end of the sixteenth century.

27. Fernel, *Universa medicina*, cap. 2, pp. 646, 647; cap. 3, pp. 648-51.

28. *Gabrielis Falloppii Opera omnia*.

29. Ibid., 1: 618-82; 2: 256-324.

30. Ibid., 2: 256.

31. Ibid., 2: 256, 257. "Non-natural" in this context means preternatural or contranatural; it has nothing to do with the meaning of "non-natural" in the medical phrase "six things non-natural (*sex res non-naturales*) current at the time. Cf. Rather, "The 'Six Things Non-Natural.'"

32. Ibid., 2: 261.

33. Ibid., pp. 262, 263.

34. Ibid., p. 262.

35. Ibid., p. 262.

36. Ibid., p. 262. The term *kakoëthes*, translated by Littré as *malignité*, is used in the Hippocratic writings, but not in connection with tumors (cf. Littré, *Oeuvres d'Hippocrate*). Celsus, however, uses the term in his brief discussion of cancer and claims that he is following the Greek physicians in doing so. The first stage of the disease, he says, is called *cacoethes* by the Greeks. It develops into *carcinoma*, then into an ulcus and lastly into a *thymium* (presumably, a wartlike growth). Only the *cacoethes* is to be removed; the other stages are irritated by treatment of any kind. Cf. Celsus, *De medicina*, trans. W. G. Spencer, 2: 128-31; 3: 589-92.

37. For discussions of these matters in a different context cf. L. J. Rather, "Pathology at Mid-Century," in *Medicine in Seventeenth-Century England*, ed. Allen G. Debus, pp. 71-112; also L. J. Rather, "Some Aspects of the Theory and Therapy of Inflammation," in *Proceedings of the 23rd Congress of the History of Medicine*, 1: 8-12.

38. Hippocrates (Littré, *Oeuvres d'Hippocrate*, 9: 110). "rhidzōsis phlebōn hēpar, rhidzozi artēriōn kardiē. Ek touteōn apoplanatai es panta haima kai pneuma, kai thermasiē dia toutōn phoita."

39. The best study of pre-Harveian theories is John C. Dalton's *Doctrines of the Circulation*, which includes passages from the older literature, in both the original and in translation; cf. pp. 19-36 and 229-46.

40. Cf. Dalton, *Doctrines*, vol. 3, passim.

41. Galen in Kuehn, ed., *Opera*, vol. 3, passim.

42. Ibid., vol. 11, passim. Galen comments that in the course of a fluxion vascular blockage may occur in consequence of excess quantity (*plēthos*) or viscidity (*pachos*) of the fluxed humors, which become impacted in the small blood vessels (*emphrachthe . . .en mikrois angeiois*). This notion outlived the Galenical "circulation." Donald Fleming has traced the erroneous notion that Galen described an ebb and flow of blood from the right ventricle to page twelve of Sir Michael Foster's *Lectures on the History of Physiology during the Sixteenth, Seventeenth, and Eighteenth Centuries*. Combined with an earlier error (that the fuliginous wastes were discharged on the *right* side of the heart) made by Heinrich Haeser and perpetuated by Julius Pagel, this notion appeared in Charles Singer's *A Short History of Science to the Nineteenth Century*, pp. 91-92. Cf. Donald Fleming, "Galen on the Motions of the Blood in the Heart and Lungs," *Isis* 46 (1955): 14-21.

43. See J. H. Randall, Jr., *The School of Padua and the Emergence of Modern Science*. Harvey's essay on scientific method is available in the reprinted edition of Robert Willis's translation (first published in London, 1847, by the Sydenham Society) of his complete works (*Sources of Science*, no. 13 [New York and London: Johnson Reprint, 1965], pp. 154-67).

44. Cf. Dalton, *Doctrines;* also Charles D. O'Malley, *Michael Servetus.*

45. The best study of Harvey's work on circulation is John G. Curtis's *Harvey's Views on the Use of the Circulation of the Blood.*

46. Cf., for example, F. R. Jevon, "Harvey's Quantitative Method," *Bull. His. Med.* 36 (1962): 462-7; E. V. Ferrario, F. N. C. Poynter, and K. J. Franklin, "William Harvey's Debate with Caspar Hofmann on the Circulation of the Blood," *J. Hist. Med. Allied Sci.* 15 (1960): 7-21.

47. Jean Riolan, "De motu circulatorio sanguinis in corde," in *Joannis Riolani filii. . .opera anatomica,* pp. 537-603.

48. Ibid., p. 549.

49. Ibid., p. 590.

50. Gregor Horst, *Gregorii Horstii, senioris. . .operum medicorum. . .cura Gregorii Horstii junioris,* 1: 80. In describing the circulation, Horst says that the right and the left ventricles attract (rather than receive) blood from the liver and the lungs respectively, i.e., he is still committed to a Galenical attractive force rather than to a Harveian mechanical *vis a tergo.* See 1: 439 for Horst's remarks on the subject of inflammation.

51. It would be a mistake, however, to suppose that Harvey regarded the heart as no more than a mechanical pump. On the contrary, he believed that it "concocted" and "perfected" the contained blood, that the expansion of the heart in diastole was due to "effervescence" of the contained blood in consequence of the "innate heat" of the latter, and that the heart was the actual (not merely the metaphorical) seat of the emotions (see L. J. Rather, "Old and New Views of the Emotions and Bodily Changes," *Clio Medica* 1 [1965]: 1-25).

52. See L. J. Rather, *Addison and the White Corpuscles,* for an account of some of the developments in the theory of inflammation.

53. Walter Pagel, *Paracelsus,* pp. 20, 21.

54. Ibid., pp. 130, 131. The notion of an antithesis between the classical Greek emphasis on the concrete physiological disturbance operative in the ill individual, and the modern emphasis on 'abstract disease entities in which ill individuals "participate," was given wide currency by Henry Sigerist. Its source was an essay by Owsei Temkin, "Die Krankheitsauffassung von Hippokrates und Sydenham in ihren Epidemien," *Arch. Gesch. Med. Wiss.* (Sudhoff's) 20 No. 4 (1928): 327-52. See Rather, "Towards a Philosophical Study of the Idea of Disease," in *The Historical Development of Physiological Thought,* ed. C. M. Brooks and P. F. Cranefield, wherein the notion of the disease species is traced to Plato (*Timaeus,* 89), and Owsei Temkin, "The Scientific Approach to Disease," in *Scientific Change: Symposium on the History of Science,* ed. A. C. Crombie, wherein the same notion is found in the writings of the Greek Empiricists.

55. Ibid., pp. 133, 134. A few additional references to cancer may be found in Pagel's work. Paracelsus calls cancer the *morbus arsenicalis:* a cancer in the human microcosm corresponds to an arsenical deposit in the macrocosm (p. 146). Echoing Dioscorides, Paracelsus says that crabs can be used against cancer (pp. 147, 149).

56. Levinus Lemnius, *The Touchstone of the Complexions,* pp. 86, 87. (Spelling and punctuation have been modernized.) Lemnius's description of drawn blood is moderately accurate: melancholy is the red cell mass; choler (yellow bile), the serum; and phlegm, the inconstantly present "buffy coat" of later writers. For early-nineteenth-century studies of the buffy coat with the microscope, see Rather, *Addison and the White Corpuscles,* ch. 1, passim.

57. Jean Baptiste van Helmont, *Ortus medicinae,* p. 790. Paracelsus himself did not escape the lash of van Helmont's tongue; he is called a great idiot, and even a blasphemer, for supposing that the spleen and kidneys are dispensable (p. 800).

58. Ibid., p. 791. The changes could be seen, of course, but were, according to van Helmont, indicative of the decomposition of blood. He argues that blood must be studied while it is moving within the vessels and contains "spirits and life." Van Helmont continued

that the school physicians, in accounting for the changes of color observed in superficial bruises or contusions, contend that the blood escaping from damaged vessels is transformed successively into black bile and yellow bile (incidentally, not far from the present-day concept of its transformation into bile pigments); they ask us to believe that the different colors represent humors that were always present in the blood. But that line of reasoning would require us to hypothesize innumerable humors to account for the many changes observable in the blood. Van Helmont concludes that blood is a simple substance whose changes do not reflect the preexistence of the Galenic humors, but rather demonstrate "the effects and operations of the Archeus or seminal spirit" (ibid., passim).

59. See Walter Pagel, *J. B. van Helmont;* also his "The Religious and Philosophical Aspects of van Helmont's Science and Medicine," *Suppl. Bull. Hist. Med.,* no. 2 (1944).

60. *Ortus medicinae,* p. 129. With a little hindsight, the conclusion of this statement could be that cancer, unlike many other diseases, requires no external "seed," but provides its own from within.

61. For additional remarks on this line of thought, which was unbroken by the advent of modern chemistry at the end of the eighteenth century and evident in the "zymotic" theory of disease championed by Justus Liebig in the 1840s, see L. J. Rather, "Medicine in Seventeenth-Century England."

62. Daniel Sennert, "De chymicorum cum Aristotelicis et Galenicis consensu et dissensu," in *Danielis Sennerti...operum in sex tomos divisorum...editio, Tomus primus,* pp. 180-284; cf. p. 231.

63. Daniel Sennert, *Practicae medicae liber quintus,* 1: 1-195; cf. pp. 105, 106.

64. Horst, *Institutiones medicae,* 1: 434.

65. Ibid., p. 439.

66. See Rather, "Medicine in Seventeenth-Century England," for illustrations.

67. William Harvey, *Opera omnia,* p. 105.

68. Marcello Malpighi, *Opera omnia,* pp. 328, 329. The question of the existence of discrete, membranous, capillary walls was still under debate in the 1840s. Cf. Rather, *Addison and the White Corpuscles,* pp. 59-69.

69. Gasparo Aselli (Asellius), *De lactibus.* The three other "necessary vessels" referred to in the title of this work are nerves, arteries, and veins.

70. Wilhelm His, "Ueber die Entdeckung des Lymphsystems," *Z. Anat. Entwickelungsgeschichte,* 1 (1876): 129-143. His states that according to the testimony of Galen the lymph vessels had been known to Herophilus and Erasistratus, but that Galen did not subscribe to their findings. For a good history of the subject see István Rusznyák, Milhály Földi, György Szabo, *Lymphatics and the Lymph Circulation,* pp. 2-28.

71. His, *Entdeckung.* The passage from Bartholin is cited in the original; it antedates Malpighi's description of the capillaries and combines Harveian "percolation" with Galenic "anastomoses."

72. Cf. Castelli's *Lexicon medicum Graeco-Latinum,* p. 694.

73. Cf. "Antonius Nuck," in *Biographisches Lexikon der hervorragenden Aerzte aller Zeiten und Voelker* 4: 389.

74. For a discussion of the opposing views of Stahl and Hoffmann cf. L. J. Rather "Georg Ernst Stahl y Friedrich Hoffmann," *Historia Universal de la Medicina,* vol. 4.

75. Georg Ernst Stahl, *Theoria medica vera,* ed. Johann Ludwig Choulant, 1: 252, 253. (The first edition of Stahl's work was published in 1708.) The lymph corpuscles referred to by Stahl should not be identified with present-day lymphocytes; they were small particles of variable size, destined to be incorporated into the solid parts. But there may well be a series of links connecting Stahl's notion with the early-nineteenth-century belief that tissues are nourished by "globules," or "corpuscles," which pass from the blood to become intercalated in tissues (cf. Rather, *Addison and the White Corpuscles,* pp. 7, 8, 82-89).

76. Stahl, *Theoria medica vera,* 2: 297.

77. Ibid., 3: 256, 257.

78. Ibid., 3: 304, 306.

79. In the words of the English translator of his *Fundamenta chymiae*, Stahl was "one of the greatest masters in all parts of chemistry that Europe ever produced" (Peter Shaw, *Philosophical Principles of Universal Chemistry*, p. vii). Nevertheless Stahl believed that the physician should not concern himself with the details of chemistry while engaged in the task of working out *medical* theory. Chemistry, even more than anatomy, was foreign to that task (*alienor est ab illa spe boni atque solidi usus ad medicam theoriam, chymia*). According to Stahl, those among the physicians who called themselves chemists had many unsupported hypotheses regarding the roles of acids, alkalis, and ferments in disease—e.g., "ophthalmic acid," "pleuritic acid," "nephritic acid," "hysteric acid." (*Theoria medica vera*, pp. 67-71). G. W. Leibniz took issue with Stahl's apparent rejection of anatomy and chemistry, and a private polemical interchange ensued, which was made public in 1720. See L. J. Rather and J. B. Frerichs, "The Leibniz-Stahl Controversy I. Leibniz' Opening Objections to the *Theoria medica vera,*" and "The Leibniz-Stahl Controversy II. Stahl's Survey of the Principal Points of Doubt," *Clio Medica* 3 (1968): 21-40, and 5 (1970): 53-67.

80. Stahl, *Theoria medica vera*, 3: 291, 302, 303.

81. A phrase more often associated with John Hunter. Cf. Rather, "Some Aspects of the Theory and Therapy of Inflammation," and "G. E. Stahl's Psychological Physiology," *Bull. Hist. Med.* 35 (1961): 37-49.

82. Friedrich Hoffmann, *Fundamenta medicinae*, p. 96.

83. Hermann Boerhaave, *Opera omnia*, pp. 197-205, passim. See note 19 for his remarks on emotional melancholy in relation to cancer.

84. Pagel, "The Religious and Philosophical Aspects of van Helmont's Science and Medicine," pp. 16, 18.

85. Walter Pagel, "The Prime Matter of Paracelsus," *Ambix* 9 (1961): 117-35.

86. See Gershom Scholem, *Sabbatai Sevi*, pp. 37-66, for the Lurianic doctrine of the *tiqqun*. For the influence of Kabbalism on European scientific thought see L. J. Rather, "Alchemistry, the Kabbala, the Analogy of the 'Creative Word' and the Origins of Molecular Biology," *Episteme* 6 (1972): 83-103. The notion of seeds of disease continued to play a significant role in eighteenth-century medical thought. Near the end of the eighteenth century Jerome Gaub worked out a threefold classification of the *seminia morborum:* (1) general, natural seeds of disease; (2) specific, natural seeds of disease; and (3) preternatural seeds of disease (*seminia morborum, quae praeter naturam sunt*). For Gaub, a seed of disease is any material disposition of the human body rendering it liable to disease (Jerome Gaub, *Institutiones pathologiae medicinalis*, 2d ed., pp. 235-42); not an external agent but an internal disposition renders the body unequal to the effects of some external agent. The phrase *seminia morborum* is translated in the German edition of Gaub's book as *praedisponierenden Ursachen* ("predisposing causes") or *Krankheitsanlagen* ("disease-primordia" or "disease-anlagen") (*Anfangsgruende der medicinischen Krankheitslehre*, pp. 248-58). The first of Gaub's three classes of seeds includes the inherent liability of the human body to disease and injury under the circumstances of everyday life. It also includes the fixed laws of commerce between mind and body (*mutui denique mentem inter et corpus commercii leges statae, nec pro lubitu variandae*). The second class includes the influence of age, sex, temperament, and so on in the production of disease. Of interest is Gaub's account of "idiosyncrasy" (*idiosynkrasis*), a condition in which certain individuals are harmed by agencies that thousands of others bear with impunity. Gaub's third class includes hereditary diatheses, which, "like seeds lie hidden, often for years, in the absence of sensible defect or lesion of functions" (*functionum laesione*).

87. Claude-Deshaies Gendron, *Recherches sur la nature et la guérison des cancers.*

88. Gendron's book is not listed in Pauly's *Bibliographie des sciences médicales*, Engelmann's *Bibliotheca medico-chirurgica et anatomico-physiologica*, Ersch's *Literature der Medizin*, Choulant's *Bibliotheca medico-historica*, or Garrison and Morton's *Medical Bibliography;* it is mentioned in

passing in Wolff's *Die Lehre von der Krebskrankheit* (p. 67). Garrison and Morton state that François Le Dran, in his "Mémoire avec un précis de plusieurs observations sur le cancer," *Mém. Acad. Roy. Chirur.* (Paris) 7 (1757): 224-310, first discarded the humoral theory of the disease (*Medical Bibliography*, p. 28). That statement is doubly incorrect, for Le Dran did not discard the humoral (lymph) theory; nor, had he done so, would he have been the first.

89. Gendron, *Recherches*, pp. 6-9.

90. Ibid., pp. 43-46.

91. Ibid., pp. 49, 50.

92. Ibid., pp. 52, 53. Gendron adds that it is superfluous to invoke a "corrosive acid" to explain the pain of advanced cancer; the pain can more adequately be explained as the result of pressure on "nerve fillets" that have undergone "metamorphosis in addition to extension" (p. 54).

93. Ibid., pp. 92, 93.

94. Ibid., pp. 94.

95. Ibid., pp. 81, 82.

96. Ibid., pp. 82-87.

97. Jean Astruc, *Traité des tumeurs et des ulcères;* Bernard Peyrilhe, *Dissertatio academica de cancro.* A Latin translation of Astruc's treatise, *Tractatus de tumoribus et ulceribus ex Gallico sermone versus,* was published in Venice in 1766 (available in the Kofoed collection, University of California at Berkeley).

98. Astruc, *Tractatus,* 1: 1, 2.

99. Ibid., pp. 3, 4.

100. Ibid., pp. 4, 5.

101. Ibid., 2: 5.

102. Ibid., pp. 4, 5.

103. Ibid., pp. 25, 26.

104. Ibid., pp. 29, 30.

105. Bernard Peyrilhe, *A Dissertation on Cancerous Diseases.*

106. Peyrilhe, *Dissertation,* pp. 10, 11. He adds that grief is among the many causes of "inspissating the lymph" and thus bringing about a cancerous change.

107. Ibid., pp. 14-16, 51.

108. Ibid., pp. 56, 57.

109. Hunter's *Lectures on the Principles of Surgery,* which were delivered in 1786 and 1787, were not published until 1835, long after his death. *A Treatise on the Blood, Inflammation, and Gun-Shot Wounds* was published one year posthumously. These two works contain the sum of his views on cancer and on tumors generally. I have used James F. Palmer's *The Works of John Hunter, F.R.S.*

110. Wolff, *Die Lehre von der Krebskrankheit,* 1: 80-82. Wolff finds essential differences between the Hunterian and what he calls (for reasons not entirely clear) the Cartesian lymph theories. *Cartesian lymph* is an inactive substance present in the vessels, subservient to physical laws alone, and "accumulating in consequence of obstruction and extravasation rather than of secretion": *Hunterian lymph* "derives from the blood, is exuded from the vessels, and organizes itself in accordance with biological laws." Wolff continues that with respect to tumors, the "essential advance lying in this theory is Hunter's demonstration that *tumors arise through the activity of the organism itself, that they are comparable to normal tissues, that they live, grow and are nourished by the organism."*

111. Hunter did not use the term *fibrin.* This term was in use by 1800, however, as shown by a citation in the *Oxford English Dictionary* taken from the *Philosophical Transactions* of that year (90: 375), which reads, "The substance called fibrin by the chemists." The *Oxford English Dictionary* defines *fibrin* as *coagulable lymph.*

112. Cf. *Addison and the White Corpuscles,* and L. J. Rather, "Some Relations between Eighteenth-Century Fiber Theory and Nineteenth-Century Cell Theory," *Clio Medica* 4

(1969): 191-202.

113. *Works of John Hunter,* 1: 233.

114. Ibid., p. 251.

115. Others had been the Alexander Monros (*secundus* and *tertius*), Watson (probably Henry W.), and Albrecht von Haller; cf. Drewry Ottley's *The Life of John Hunter,* in *Works,* 1: 18.

116. Ibid., 3: 2. Annotating this passage, Palmer states that Hunter's coagulating lymph has more recently been called *gluten, fibre of the blood,* and *fibrin,* the latter being the "term now most frequently adopted, from its being in some degree expressive of the fibrous or half-organized texture which this substance exhibits." Present day terminology distinguishes circulating *fibrinogen* from its derivative, *fibrin.*

117. Cf. Kenneth D. Keele, *William Harvey,* pp. 196, 197.

118. John Hunter, *Works,* 1: 229-31. "That the blood has life," he writes, "is an opinion I have stated for above thirty years, and taught it for near twenty of that time, in my lectures; it does not, therefore, come out at present as a new doctrine, but has had time to meet with considerable opposition, and also acquire its advocates" (3: 104). Palmer cites a long passage from Harvey's *De generatione* in which the doctrine of the life of the blood is stated and referred back to the Bible and to Aristotle, but he adds that Hunter's work gave it a "solid basis" (3: 104, 105).

119. Ibid., 2:242.

120. Ibid., 1: 293; 3: 296. Hunter does not mention Stahl in his writings, but his debt is apparent. Stahl had spoken of salutary inflammation, *inflammatio salutaris* (see n. 81). His successor in the chair of medicine at Halle also called inflammation a salutary act or operation (*actus salutarius*) (Michael Alberti, *Introductio in medicinam universam,* pp. 257, 258). Despite important points of resemblance, however, the ideas of Stahl and Hunter differ in an important respect: Stahl's "salutary act" is the overcoming of a vascular block, whereas Hunter's is a reparative process.

121. John Hunter, *Works,* 3: 296, 297. Hunter's statement that inflammation may (in an unspecified fashion) be capable of altering a diseased mode of action—presumably a mode of action due to the specific principle of the disease in question—foreshadows the nineteenth-century interpretation of inflammation as a defensive process.

122. Ibid., 1: 566.

123. Ibid., pp. 568, 571.

124. Ibid., pp. 571, 572. Among the hydatids described by Hunter are: (1) hydatids in sheep liver; (2) multiple hydatids of the kidneys; (3) hydatids of the lungs, brain, and thyroid gland. Also described are cystic ovarian tumors containing "fatty, cuticular and hairy" matter (ibid., 1: 572-74). A modern pathologist would regard only the last as true tumors: the liver hydatids result from parasitic flukeworm disease, and the multiple hydatids of the kidney from "polycystic disease"; the nature of the other hydatids described by Hunter is more or less indeterminate.

125. Ibid., 1: 618, 630. The fungoid growths in question constitute a "specific well marked disease." Unlike cancer, they occur in all parts of the body and seldom, if ever, involve the neighboring lymph glands. They may be present in solid or cystic form, and Hunter has seen them in the antrum, tibia, eye, testicle, penis, rectum, and sole of the foot (*ibid.,* 1: 630). Some of these features, particularly the lack of involvement of the neighboring lymphatic structures, suggest to a modern reader that the tumors in question were malignant tumors of connective tissue character, i.e., sarcomas (in the modern sense of the term). Palmer (writing in 1835) equated them with his category of fungus haematodes, or medullary disease, and remarked that Hunter had "classed together several diseases which modern pathologists have very properly separated." Fungus haematodes, says Palmer, usually occurs before the age of forty, cancer usually after that age (ibid., 1: 622).

126. Ibid., 1: 309, 619-22, 627, 628. Elsewhere Hunter states that axillary glands draining

a cancerous breast may enlarge without becoming cancerous. "The glands in the axilla will often inflame and subside again, which they would not do if they were affected with cancer" (ibid., 1: 329). Hunter's differential diagnosis of cancerous and scrofulous tumors is worth noting. "If cancer," he says, "it will vary its appearance by becoming less circumscribed, not having so determined an outline, from the cellular membrane around becoming diseased; the skin will be less moveable, the nipple more or less retracted, and the lymphatic glands going to the axilla will swell. But in scrofula there will be no surrounding disease, no affection of the nipple or axillary glands, no adhesion, even though the tumour be large" (ibid., 1: 618, 619).

2

1. Albrecht von Haller, *Bibliotheca anatomica,* 1: 1-4. We have little knowledge of the prehistory of anatomical science. From a study of the extensive anatomical knowledge and vocabulary of the Aleuts and contiguous Eskimo tribes at the time they made contact with Europeans, William Laughlin infers that precise and extensive anatomical knowledge was acquired, largely for practical purposes, i.e., hunting, toolmaking, clothes-making, very early in the evolutionary development of the human being. "The organization of the mammalian body," he writes, "provides a basis for intellectual organization, and anatomical analogies and reasoning are found in all cultures" ("Acquisition of Anatomical Knowledge by Ancient Man," in *Social Life of Early Man,* ed. Sherwood L. Washburn.)

2. A. E. Taylor, *A Commentary on Plato's Timaeus,* pp. 590, 591.

3. Aristotle, *Historia animalium,* trans. D'Arcy Wentworth Thompson, 520b.

4. *Galen on the Natural Faculties,* trans. A. J. Brock, pp. 152, 153, 328, 329. Brock remarks that the elementary fibers of Erasistratus and Galen are more or less the structural and functional equivalents of the cells of modern biology.

5. Rudolph E. Siegel, *Galen's System of Physiology and Medicine,* p. 234.

6. Aristotle, *Historia animalium,* cf. footnote to 486a.

7. Aristotle, *Parts of Animals,* trans. A. L. Peck, pp. 28, 29.

8. Aristotle, *De partibus animalium,* trans. William Ogle, 647b, 1-10; cf. Peck, p. 117.

9. Leonhard Fuchs, *Institutiones medicinae,* pp. 140-43.

10. Gabriele Falloppio, "De partibus similaribus," in *Opera omnia,* 2: 96-156.

11. Bartholomaeus Perdulcis, *Universa medicina,* pp. 19, 20, 38.

12. Robert Burton, *The Anatomy of Melancholy,* pp. 94-98.

13. Andreas Vesalius, *De humani corporis fabrica,* p. 512.

14. C. D. O'Malley, *Andreas Vesalius,* pp. 138, 166.

15. Moritz Roth, *Andreas Vesalius bruxellensis.*

16. Nehemiah Grew, *The Anatomy of Plants,* see pp. 120, 121.

17. Robert Hooke, *Micrographia,* p. 138.

18. See Rather, *Addison and the White Corpuscles,* ch. 1/2 text and notes for a full discussion of this point.

19. Fielding H. Garrison, *An Introduction to the History of Medicine,* p. 255.

20. Albrecht von Haller, *First Lines of Physiology* and *Primae lineae physiologiae.* The word translated as "cell" in the English edition is *spatiola,* i.e., "little space." (*Primae,* p. 3).

21. François Marie Arouet de Voltaire, "La Pucelle" (chant. 21), Another revealing instance of eighteenth-century usage occurs in the writings of Joseph Addison: ". . . nay, we find in the most solid bodies, as in marble itself, innumerable cells and cavities that are crowded with such imperceptible inhabitants, as are too little for the naked eye to discover" (Addison, *Works,* vol. 4).

22. Philippe Pinel, *Nosographie philosophique,* 1: xix, 2: 130-240.

23. François-Xavier Bichat, *Treatise of the Membranes*, pp. xii, xiii, 23.

24. Ibid., p. 5 (numbering is the same in English and French editions).

25. Ibid., p. 21.

26. Ibid., p. 96.

27. Ibid., pp. 170-73.

28. Ibid., pp. 238-42.

29. Ibid., pp. 40-42.

30. François-Xavier Bichat, *General Anatomy Applied to Physiology and Medicine.*

31. *Dictionnaire des sciences médicales*, 1821 ed., s.v. "tissu" by Jean-Baptiste Montfalcon.

32. Bichat, *Anatomie générale.*

33. Bichat, *General Anatomy*, 1: vi, vii.

34. Montfalcon, s.v. "tissu."

35. Burkard Eble, *Versuch einer pragmatischen Geschichte der Anatomie und Physiologie, 1800-1825*, pp. 20, 21. Rudolphi's monograph on the tissues was entitled *Programma de solidorum corporis humani partibus similaribus. Tela carnea* is a typographical error for *tela cornea* (epidermis, nails, hair, etc.); cf. Rudolphi's *Grundriss der Physiologie*, 1: 71.

36. Eble, *Versuch*, pp. 173, 174.

37. Bichat, *Anatomie générale*, 1: 12.

38. Eble, *Versuch*, p. 72, 73. He cites Théophile Bordeu's *Recherches sur le tissu muqueux* and C. F. Wolf's [*sic*] *De tela quam dicunt cellulosa*, stating that Bichat "followed the older mode" of depicting the cellular tissue.

39. J. B. Lamarck, *Histoire naturelle des animaux sans vertèbres*, 1: 337-43.

40. Hippolyte Royer-Collard, "Considerations générales sur les lois d'organisme dans l'état de santé et dans l'état de maladie," *Bull. Soc. Anat. de Paris* 3 (1828): 135-50.

41. Johannes Mueller, *Handbuch der Physiologie*, 1: 410. Mueller was Rudolphi's pupil.

42. Bichat, *General Anatomy*, 1: 148.

43. Ibid., p. 158.

44. Ibid., p. 159.

45. Ibid., pp. 160-62.

46. *Anatomie pathologique.* A contemporary account calls the book a mere publisher's gamble and claims that Béclard did not come to Paris until six years after Bichat's death (*Dictionnaire historique de la médecine ancienne et moderne*, 1: 396).

47. Cf. Matthew Baillie, *The Morbid Anatomy of Some of the Most Important Parts of the Body.* Baillie's chapters are "Diseased Appearances of the Liver," "Diseased Appearances of the Heart," etc., whereas Bichat's are "Diseases of the Cellular Tissue," "Diseases of the Serous System," etc.

48. Jean Cruveilhier, "Essai sur l'anatomie pathologique en général."

49. Guillaume Dupuytren, *Bulletin de l'École de Médecine* 2 (1805): 13-24.

50. S.v. "Anatomie pathologique" by René Laennec, *Dictionnaire.*

51. Ibid., passim; for Laennec's use of the term *scirrhus* as a synonym of *cancer*, see *Dictionnaire*, s.v. "Encéphaloïdes," p. 165.

52. Laennec, s.v. "Anatomie pathologique."

53. Ibid., p. 47. See in this connection L. J. Rather, "An Early Nineteenth-Century View of Functional vs. Organic Disease," *A.M.A. Arch. Int. Med.* 108 (1961): 502-6.

54. Laennec, s.v. "Anatomie pathologique," 2: 52.

55. Ibid., p. 53.

56. Ibid., p. 51.

57. Rudolf Virchow, *Hundert Jahre allgemeiner Pathologie;* cf. L. J. Rather, *Disease, Life and Man*, p. 186. Virchow calls the doctrine of Laennec organicism, forgetting that by the term *organic* Laennec simply meant anatomic, i.e., for Laennec an organic lesion is an anatomical lesion involving an organ or a tissue.

58. Laennec, s.v. "Anatomie pathologique," 2: 51, 60.

59. Ibid., pp. 54-58.

60. Gaspard-Laurent Bayle and Jean-Bruno Cayol, *Dictionnaire,* s.v. "Cancer," "Cancer of the breast rarely attacks men; it is in women that it is most commonly observed, especially in those of forty to fifty-five years; it almost never begins before the twentieth year; it sometimes develops between twenty and thirty years, and often enough from thirty to forty; from the age of sixty years to the last stages of old age it becomes more and more uncommon. A woman, touching her breast, remarks there a small induration that is not normal but which causes her not the slightest discomfort; she is unable to say at precisely what period it began to be present; she is unaware of its cause or perhaps attributes it to a blow that she received in the past, to the pressure exerted by her corset, to milk that must have clotted in her breast while she was nursing one or another of her infants: for the rest she enjoys perfect health; it even seems to her that for some time now she has acquired more bloom and plumpness than she formerly possessed. But the induration of the breast increases by degrees: it had only the volume of a small hazel-nut when it first became apparent but already it appears equal to a duck's egg. In the beginning it was rounded, circumscribed, and rolled under the finger; now its surface is unequally bossed and the adjacent cellular tissue participates in the engorgement. The tumor has developed some attachments to the skin and perhaps also to the muscles. From time to time there occur painful twinges, sharp and transient, comparable to the prick of a needle; these twinges make themselves felt more particularly toward the evening or at night; otherwise it may be touched or even squeezed rather strongly without causing any pain. The lymph nodes of the axilla swell and are themselves not exempt from pain. As long as the breast tumor was indolent its progress was slow and almost insensible but since it became painful its growth has been more rapid: the twinges, from day to day more frequent and sharp, have reached the point of troubling and sometimes preventing sleep. After these latter symptoms we ought no longer designate the tumor a *scirrhus;* it is an *occult cancer,* such as is described by all authors. The patient (for we may henceforth call her by this name) begins to grow thin and lose her bloom; her complexion becomes a pale yellow; her appetite decreases; it is irregular and often very bizarre. The tumor, until recently only apparent to the touch, begins to protrude somewhat; the skin covering it, to which it is adherent, takes on a reddish, livid color; the superficial veins are more and more apparent; the nipple becomes obliterated little by little; soon it will no longer present as an eminence but as a more or less deep depression. A small fissure, from which a little serous fluid exudes, forms at the reddest place in the skin. From this time the disease acquires the name of *ulcerated cancer.* The margins of the fissure progressively separate, thicken, become everted, harden and take on from day to day a pallid color. The surface of the ulcer becomes covered with reddish vegetation that yields an ichorous or sanious pus, more or less abundant and often very fetid. The pain is at times lancinating, at other times it is a lively smarting, a sensation like that of a burn, a heavy pain, or an insupportable itching that nothing can assuage. While this hideous ulcer enlarges in all directions and irregularly eats away at all the surrounding parts, sparing neither arterial or venous vessels, it often gives rise to hemorrhage which is followed by a momentary diminution in suffering, but which does not fail to further weaken the patient. At the same time the general symptoms of cancerous cachexia continue to worsen; emaciation is extreme; the flesh is remarkably soft and in a state bordering on edema. The patient is often tormented by a sharp cough accompanied by burning heat behind the sternum; she is oppressed, she experiences invincible repugnance for food and obstinate constipation replaced from time to time by liquid diarrhea; at last she succumbs, exhausted by a hectic fever and by the most cruel torments. Such is the most usual course of cancer of the breast when no accident hinders or impedes it."

61. Laennec, s.v. "Anatomie pathologique," p. 59.

62. Laennec, s.v. "Encéphaloïdes," 12: 175.

63. Ibid., pp. 172-76.

64. Laennec, s.v. "Dégénération," 8: 201-208 and passim.

65. Laennec, s.v. "Anatomie pathologique," 2: 59.

66. Laennec, s.v. "Encéphaloïdes," 12: 174.

67. Laennec, s.v. "Dégénération," 8: 202-3.

68. Ibid., p. 205.

69. Ibid., p. 206. The terms *metaplasia* (*Metaplasie*) and *metamorphosis* (*Metamorphose*) were introduced as alternatives for *tissue-transformation* (*Gewebesumwandelung*) by Rudolf Virchow in *Die Cellularpathologie*, 4th ed., p. 70.

70. Laennec, s.v. "Cartilages accidentels," *Dictionnaire*, 4: 123.

71. William E. Horner, *Treatise on Pathology*, pp. xiii, 19.

72. August Chomel, *Élémens de pathologie générale*, p. 668.

73. In early-nineteenth-century France and Germany, as well as in England, the new humoralism was usually credited to Hunter and William Hewson. For a later assessment of Hunter's role see Virchow's Croonian Lecture of 1893, "The Place of Pathology among the Biological Sciences," in Rather, *Disease, Life and Man*, pp. 161-64.

74. Chomel, *Élémens*, p. 669.

75. Justus Liebig, *Thierchemie*. The English translation by William Gregory, *Animal Chemistry in its Application to Physiology and Pathology*, was published in New York in the same year.

76. Mueller, *Handbuch*. 1: 341-45. For the rival corpuscular theory see Rather, *Addison and the White Corpuscles*, ch. 2/1.

77. Liebig, *Animal Chemistry*, pp. 40-42.

78. Ibid., pp. 105, 106.

79. Franz J. Simon, *Animal Chemistry*, 1: 5. This is a translation by George E. Day of Simon's *Physiologische und pathologische Anthropochemie*. The term *protein* was suggested to Mulder by J. J. Berzelius, according to J. R. Partington, *A History of Chemistry*, 4: 319.

80. Johann F. Lobstein, *Traité d'anatomie pathologique*.

81. Ibid., 1: 360, 361.

82. Ibid., pp. 364, 365.

83. Ibid., pp. 365, 370, 471.

84. Ibid., pp. 393, 403.

85. Ibid., pp. 469, 470.

86. Robert Brown, "A Brief Account of Microscopical Observations," *Edinburgh New Phil. J.* 5 (1828): 358-71.

87. John Hughes Bennett, "Lectures on Molecular Physiology, Pathology and Therapeutics," *Lancet*, January-December 1863.

88. Lobstein, *Traité*, pp. 399, 403.

89. Ibid., pp. 401, 474-76.

90. Jean Cruveilhier, "Description anatomique de cancers de l'intestine grêle, de l'estomac, de la mammelle," *Bull. Soc. Anat. de Paris*, 2d ed. (1844), pp. 4-16.

91. Cruveilhier, "Essai sur l'anatomie pathologique en général."

92. Gabriel Andral, *Précis d'anatomie pathologique*. English translation by Richard Townsend and William West, *A Treatise on Pathological Anatomy*.

93. Andral, *Précis*, p. 501. Using the same phrases Andral also rejected both the concept and the term *inflammation:* "Created in the infancy of science, this quite metaphorical term ... *inflammation* has become an expression so vague, its interpretation so arbitrary, that it has lost all value; it is like a worn-out effaced coin which ought to be withdrawn from circulation" (ibid., p. 9). Andral's rejection of the concept of cancer can be read as the rejection of an abstract "malignancy" in favor of the particular events themselves, in all their variety. The same applies to his rejection of inflammation.

94. Ibid., pp. 166, 167. Some of the lesions would be classified by the modern histopathologist as reactive hyperplasias of connective tissue, others as true tumors. Elsewhere

Andral describes three forms of "accidental fibrous tissue," the cordlike, the membranous, and the tumorous (ibid., pp. 269-72).

95. Ibid., pp. 233, 234.

96. Ibid., pp. 167, 168.

97. The queries were first circulated in the form of a brochure and then reprinted in the *Edinburgh Med. Surg. J.* 2 (July, 1806): 382-89. The other queries are (1) What are the diagnostic signs of cancer? (3) Is cancer always an original and primary disease? (4) Are there any proofs of cancer being a hereditary disease? (5) Are there any proofs of cancer being a contagious disease? (6) Is there any well-marked relation between cancer and other diseases? If there be, what are those diseases to which it bears the nearest resemblance in its origin, progress, and termination? (7) May cancer be regarded at any period, or under any circumstances merely as a local disease? Or does the existence of cancer in one part afford a presumption that there is a tendency to a similar morbid alteration in other parts of the animal system? (8) Has climate or local situation any influence in rendering the human constitution more or less liable to cancer, under any form, or in any part? (9) Is there any particular temperament of body more liable to be affected with cancer than other? If there be, what is the nature of that temperament? (10) Are brute creatures subject to any disease resembling cancer in the human body? (11) Is there any period of life absolutely exempt from the attack of this disease? (12) Are the lymphatic glands ever affected primarily in this disease? (13) Is cancer, under any circumstances, susceptible of a natural cure? These queries may also be found in Philippe Pinel, *Nosographie philosophique,* 3: 351-52.

98. John Abernethy, "An Attempt to Form a Classification of Tumours According to Their Anatomical Structure," in *Surgical Observations.* On page 3 Abernethy mentions the questions posed by the society but does not give the entire list.

99. Ibid., p. 5.

100. Ibid., pp. 9-11.

101. Ibid., pp. 19, 20.

102. Ibid., pp. 12, 13.

103. Ibid., pp. 66-75. The remaining seven species are (1) "common vascular or organized sarcoma"; (2) "adipose sarcoma," an encapsulated subcutaneous fatty tumor concerning which Abernethy remarks that no other tumor can be "removed with so much celerity, with such apparent dexterity, or with such complete security against future consequences" (pp. 26-33); (3) "pancreatic sarcoma," so-called because of its resemblance in color, texture and lobulation to the pancreas—Abernethy's case appears to have been a fibro-adenomatous tumor of the breast in a young woman (pp. 33-42); (4) "cystic sarcoma," usually multicystic and most commonly met with in the ovary and testis (pp. 42-44); (5) "mastoid or mammary sarcoma"—one of Abernethy's instances was an unencapsulated, ultimately lethal, tumor of the thigh (pp. 44-47); (6) "tuberculated sarcoma," a tumor often involving the lymph nodes but thought not to be "scrofulous" by Abernethy (pp. 47-51); and (7) "medullary sarcoma," a tumor often found in the testis (pp. 51-66).

104. Ibid., pp. 98, 99.

105. John Burns, *Dissertations on Inflammation.*

106. William Hey, "Of the Fungus Haematodes," in *Practical Observations in Surgery,* pp. 153-83. In the text the tumor is sometimes called "fungous haematodes."

107. James Wardrop, *Observations on Fungus Haematodes or Soft Cancer.*

108. Ibid., pp. 191-95.

109. Ibid., pp. 187, 188.

110. Thomas Hodgkin, "On the Anatomical Character of Some Adventitious Structures," *Medico-Chirur. Trans.* 15/2 (1829): 265-338. (Hodgkin's paper on the morbid anatomy of the disease that bears his name appeared in 1832. It, too, contained no microscopic findings.)

111. Ibid., pp. 271, 293.

112. Ibid., pp. 266, 267. Andral, for example, calls trematodes, cestodes, and cystic entozoa

"organized morbid products endowed with individual life" (*Précis*, 1: 503).

113. Ibid., pp. 268-70.

114. Ibid., pp. 272-75.

115. Ibid., pp. 276-85. Hodgkin placed ovarian cysts containing "masses of hair and fat" in the category of nonproliferative foreign body cysts (ibid., pp. 268-70).

116. Ibid., pp. 294-308.

117. Ibid., p. 327.

118. Ibid., pp. 292, 293. In a later account of melanotic tumors Hodgkin credited Laennec with the first description of "melanosis" (*Lectures on the Morbid Anatomy of the Mucous and Serous Membranes* 1: 331-9). Merat's article on melanosis in 1819 mentions Dupuytren's claim to priority here (*Dictionnaire des sciences médicales*, s.v. "melanose," 32: 183-88).

119. Ibid., pp. 313-21.

120. Robert Carswell, *Pathological Anatomy*. Carswell was also the coauthor, with William Cullen, of "On Melanosis," a paper that appeared in *Trans. Medico-Chirur. Soc. of Edinburgh* 1 (1824): 264-84. The authors described cases of the disease in horses and human beings, calling it "invariably fatal" and distinguishing it from both cancer and fungus hematodes. Later Carswell wrote a review of the subject in Forbes, *Cyclopaedia of Practical Medicine*, 3: 284-303, where he distinguished true melanosis, i.e., melanoma, from other pigmented lesions of benign character. There he refers to an article by Laennec in the *Bulletins de l'École Méd. de Paris* of 1806 as the first account of true melanosis.

121. Carswell, *Pathological Anatomy*, see "Analogous Tissues" (unnumbered pages).

122. Ibid., Carswell discusses in this connection cysts of the subcutaneous tissue, ovarian cysts containing hair, urinary bladder cysts, etc.

123. Ibid., cf. "Heterologous Formations: Carcinoma." As we have seen Laennec did doubt that all tumors were "tissues."

124. Thomas Hodgkin, *Lectures*.

125. Ibid., p. 25.

126. Ibid., p. 180, 181.

127. Cf. Lecture 7, "On Parasitic Animals," in which cysticercus, echinococcus, and acephalocystis are discussed. The belief that cancers were true parasites rather than intrinsic lesions of structure was reviewed at length and defended in Richard Carmichael's *An Essay on the Effects of Carbonate and Other Preparations of Iron upon Cancer*.

128. Hodgkin, *Lectures*, pp. 344, 345. Broussais held that scirrhous and encephaloid tumors were not "new tissues" but "fluid animal matter fixed by some cause, and more or less altered, in delicate canals...and in areolae." He agreed with Andral that cancer was not a separate disease, but stated that Andral had borrowed this notion from his own school of "physiological medicine" (François Broussais, *Examen des doctrines médicales et des systemes de nosologie*, 4: 506, 507, 552, 553). Breschet held that cancer was always secondary to irritation or inflammation and represented the abnormal organization of exuded coagulable lymph (Gilbert Breschet and Guillaume Ferrus, *Dictionnaire de médecine*, 1822 ed., s.v. "cancer").

129. Samuel D. Gross, *Elements of Pathologic Anatomy*. Gross agreed that Hodgkin's theory held good in a limited number of instances (p. 181). He himself believed that cancers formed directly from exuded coagulable lymph, without going through a cystic stage.

130. Thomas Hodgkin and J. J. Lister, "Notice sur quelques observations microscopiques sur le sang et le tissu des animaux," *Ann. sci. nat.* 12 (1827): 53-68. Lister's name, except in one footnote, is spelt *Lyster* throughout.

131. Ibid., passim: "Muscle tissue is composed of bundles of fibers bound together by a cellular membrane...these fibers themselves consist of still smaller fibers...although there is no trace of globular structure to be found, innumerable very small but distinct and fine parallel striations or lines transversely marking these tiny fibers may be clearly perceived"; nerves "appear to be composed essentially of fibers"; arteries consist of "long, slender and very delicate fibers that do not at all display the transverse striations that we have considered the particular feature of muscle"; cellular membrane is "entirely composed of fibers."

Hodgkin says that he is "tormented by the idea that I would differ in opinion with my excellent and learned friend, Dr. Milne Edwards." The latter's *Mémoire sur la structure élémentaire des principaux tissus organiques des animaux* revived the globule theory.

132. Hodgkin, *Lectures,* p. 26. Hodgkin states that his "friend Joseph Lister, who has carried the powers of the microscope far beyond anything to which they had previously attained, has very minutely examined this" (the ultimate structure of membranes).

133. Oscar Hertwig (*Lehrbuch der Entwickelungsgeschichte,* ed ed., pp. 124, 125) and Rudolph Koelliker (*Entwickelungsgeschichte des Menschen und der hoeheren Thiere,* 2d ed., pp. 9, 10) give Wolff credit for discovering, as Koelliker puts it, "the entire newer doctrine of the formation of the body from several leaf-like primitive organs." Both also allow Wolff priority in respect to the claim that plant organs represent metamorphosed leaflike primordia.

134. In his essay "Zur Morphologie" Goethe cites Wolff's statement (in *De formatione intestinorum*) that "all parts of a plant, exclusive of the stem, can be referred back to the form of a leaf and are nothing but modifications of it" (*Gedenkausgabe,* ed. Ernst Beutlev 17: 96-100).

135. See E. S. Russell, *Form and Function,* for a history of early-nineteenth-century embryology, including translations from Karl Ernst von Baer's work; see also Jane Oppenheimer, *Essays in the History of Embryology and Biology.*

136. Christian Pander, *Beitraege zur Entwickelungsgeschichte des Huehnchens im Eye.*

137. Ibid., pp. 4, 5, 20. Table 10 contains a figure illustrative of the "globular layer of the germinal membrane at the highest magnification."

138. Ibid., pp. 5-12, passim.

139. Karl Ernst von Baer, *Uber Entwickelungsgeschichte der Thiere.*

140. Cf. the words of von Baer to this effect cited by Russell, *Form and Function,* p. 120.

141. Von Baer, *Entwickelungsgeschichte* 1: 153, 154.

142. Ibid., 2: 68 and note. Von Baer's *Fleischschicht* and *Gefaessschicht* correspond fairly closely, in origin and destination, to the mesodermal layer of later embryologists.

143. Ibid., 1: 155. The term *histology* was used, possibly for the first time, by A. J. F. K. Mayer in 1819 in his thesis "Ueber Histologie und eine neue Eintheilung der Gewebe des menschlichen Koerpers." The term *morphology* was used by Goethe (in his diaries) as early as 1796 but first appeared in print in 1800 (*Gedenkausgabe,* 17: 995). Goethe distinguished morphological from anatomical investigation—the former as holistic, the latter as analytic in approach. "We have already achieved," Goethe wrote, "an anatomical physiology through the precise study of structure...but...this manner of understanding and representing organic bodies does not satisfy all men, many of whom have a tendency to begin with the whole and to develop the parts from it." The chemist too, like the anatomist, approached the study of living matter through procedures "separative in character," according to Goethe (*Gedenkausgabe,* pp. 115-17).

144. Ibid., 1: 156.

145. Ibid., 78-92, passim.

146. Rudolf Virchow, "Cellular-Pathologie," *Arch. path. Anat. Phys. klin. Med.* 8 (1855): 7.

147. Von Baer, *Entwickelungsgeschichte,* 1st ed., p. 93.

148. Von Baer, "Die Metamorphose des Eies der Batrachier vor der Erscheinung des Embryo, und Folgerungen aus ihr fuer die Theorie der Erzeugung," *Arch. Anat. Phys. wiss. Med.* (1834), pp. 481-509.

3

1. One notable exception is furnished by the studies of English, Scotch, and German microscopists, at the turn of the nineteenth century, on the pathophysiology of inflammation. See L. J. Rather, "Virchow und die Entwicklung des Entzuendungsfrage im neunzehnten Jahrhundert," *Verh. 20 Int. Kongr. Gesch. Med.*

2. Saville Bradbury, *The Evolution of the Microscope.* See also David E. Wolfe, "Sydenham and Locke on the Limits of Anatomy," *Bull. Hist. Med.* 25/3 (1961): 193-220.

3. Marjorie H. Nicolson, *Science and Imagination,* esp. pp. 155-234.

4. Bruno Zanobio, "Micrographie illusoire et théories sur la structure de la matière vivante," *Clio Medica* 6 (1971): 25-40.

5. Cf. Ludwig Darmstaedter, *Handbuch zur Geschichte der Naturwissenschaften und der Technik,* 2d ed.; Charles Singer, *A History of Technology,* 4: 358, 359; and Bradbury, *Evolution.*

6. Joseph J. Lister, "On Some Properties in Achromatic Object Glasses Applicable to Improvement of the Microscope," *Phil. Trans. Roy. Soc.* 130 (1830): 187-200. Bradbury, *Evolution,* p. 190, quotes a remark by C. R. Goring in 1830 to the effect that the Amician reflecting microscope, corrected lenses, and the diamond lens had brought microscopy to the pinnacle of perfection. Goring himself contributed the diamond lens; see his paper "The Diamond Microscope," in the *Franklin Journal* 4 (1827): 208.

7. Gottlieb Gluge, "Recherches microscopiques sur le fluide contenu dans les cancers encéphaloïdes," *Compt. rend. Acad. Sci.* 4 (1837): 20, 21.

8. Everard Home, *A Short Tract on the Formation of Tumours.*

9. The first occasion was that of Mueller's address in celebration of the forty-second year of the foundation of the Friedrich Wilhelm Institut in Berlin, on August 2, 1836 (*Rede zur Feier des zwei und vierzigsten Stiftungstages des Koeniglichen medicinisch-chirurgischen Friedrich-Wilhelms-Instituts.*) Insofar as tumors were concerned, Mueller confined his attention here largely to enchondroma. He states, however, that the "finest elements" revealed by the compound microscope in all "funguses, from polyps and neuroma to medullary fungus...are fibers" (p. 27). The second occasion was that of his report "on the finer structure of morbid tumors" read before the general session of the Royal Prussian Academy of Sciences at Berlin on December 8, 1836 (*Bericht ueber die zur Bekanntmachung geeigneten Verhandlungen der Koeniglichen Preussischen Akademie der Wissenschaften zu Berlin,* pp. 107-113). This report was subsequently included *in toto* by Mueller in his review of advances in anatomy and physiology in 1835 [*sic*] ("Jahresbericht ueber die Fortschritte der anatomisch-physiologischen Wissenschaften im Jahre 1835"), published in the *Arch. Anat. Phys. wiss. Med.* (Berlin), 1836, see pp. ccxviii-xxiv.

10. Mueller also terms the fibrous tumor in question a *desmoid;* it is said to occur in the peritoneum, uterus, bones, brain, and dura mater.

11. Mueller, "Bericht ueber die zur Bekanntmachung geeigneten Verhandlungen," p. 107.

12. Ibid., p. 110.

13. In all likelihood these observations were made with the Schieck microscope described by Mueller in his monograph of 1838 on the fine structure of tumors.

14. Matthias Schleiden, "Beitraege zur Phytogenese," *Arch. Anat. Phys. wiss. Med.,* 1838, pp. 137-76.

15. Ibid., pp. 137, 138: "dieser eigenthuemliche kleine Organismus, die Zelle."

16. Robert Brown, "On the Organs and Mode of Fecundation in Orchids and Asclepiadae," *Trans. Linn. Soc.* 16 (1833): 685-738 (read on November 1st and 15th, 1831). Brown states that the "nucleus or areola" can be found in "some figures of epidermis in the recent works of Meyen and Purkinje, and in one case in Adolphe Brongniant's memoir on the structure of leaves...[but] so little importance seems to be attached to it, that the appearance is not always referred to in the figures in which it is represented." Aside from noting that certain pollens consist of cell nuclei, Brown assigned the nucleus no role in cell genesis.

17. For the story of this meeting see Robert Waterman's *Theodor Schwann, Leben und Werk,* pp. 98, 99.

18. Theodor Schwann, "Ueber die Analogie in der Structur und dem Wachstum der Thiere und Pflanzen," *Neue Notizen aus dem Gebiete der Natur und Heilkunde,* nr. 93 (January, 1838), cols. 33-37; "Fortsetzung der Untersuchung ueber die Uebereinstimmung in der

Structur der Thiere und Pflanzen," ibid., nr. 103 (February, 1838), cols. 225-29; "Nachtrag zu der Untersuchung ueber die Uebereinstimmung in der Structur der Thiere und Pflanzen," ibid., nr. 107 (April, 1838), cols. 21-23.

19. Schwann, "Ueber die Analogie," pp. 33, 34.

20. Ibid., pp. 35, 36.

21. Ibid., p. 35.

22. Schwann, "Fortsetzung der Untersuchung." The passage is worth quoting in full: "Cellular tissue [i.e., loose connective tissue] contains as its base a *gelatinous structureless mass which, however, steadily diminishes as a large number of peculiar corpuscles* [i.e., cells] *develop in it.* [emphasis added] In accordance with the level of their development they display very different appearances. They are at first round, opaque, granular cells with characteristic nuclei lying on the walls and containing one or two nucleoli. As they continue to develop they gradually assume cylindrical shape meanwhile retaining their nuclei. The ends of the small cylinders gradually lengthen and sharpen into numerous threads of some length that ultimately take on the appearance of cellular tissue [i.e., connective tissue] fibers."

23. Johannes Mueller, "Jahresbericht ueber die Fortschritte der anatomisch-physiologisch Wissenschaften im Jahre 1837," *Arch. Anat. Phys. wiss. Med.,* 1838, pp. xci-cxcviii; cf. pp. xciv-vi. In spite of the date given in the title, Mueller here reviewed several papers published in 1838.

24. Schwann, *Ueber die Analogie.*

25. Schwann, "Nachtrag zu der Untersuchung." Mueller's statement is as follows. "At all events, the pigment of melanosis is contained in distinct cells. Furthermore, cells with nuclei were seen in collonema. Cell nuclei were recognized on occasion in the cellular albuminous osteosarcoma. The albuminous cellular sarcoma, which is to be distinguished from the albuminous fibrous sarcoma, also belongs here. Its interior structure and chemical composition are analogous to that of the *decidua Hunteri,* which consists of large, plant-like cells provided with distinct nucleoli and large nuclei. Enchondroma has a similar structure but consists of cartilaginous matter. The tailed bodies (*geschwaenzten Koerper*) occasionally described in medullary fungus and in melanosis were found also in osteosarcoma and in a peculiar kind of benign sarcoma. They originate from nucleated cells."

26. Johannes Mueller, *Ueber den feinern Bau und die Formen der krankhaften Geschwuelste. In zwei Lieferungen. Erste Lieferung.* (The second fascicle never appeared.) The contents of Mueller's monograph are as follows: "General Remarks on the Finer Structure of Morbid Tumors," pp. 1-9; "Studies on the Finer Structure of Cancerous Tumors," pp. 10-30; "On the Development and Softening of Tumors," pp. 23, 24; "On Chemical Properties of Carcinomas," pp. 24, 25; "On the Nature of Cancer," pp. 25-30; "On Tumors that can be Confused with Cancer," pp. 31-60. Fifty-five figures are appended. Mueller's book is unique in representing a double advance: it is both the first full-scale application of the microscope to the study of tumors, and the first application of cell theory to oncology.

27. Ibid., pp. 5-8.

28. Ibid., pp. 3, 5, 6, 8, 14, 29, passim. Curiously enough, Mueller cites here in support of his claim that he had already become cognizant of the cellular structure of some tumors in 1836 the address that he had given on August 2, 1836 in Berlin, instead of the previously mentioned report to the Royal Prussian Academy of Sciences (see note 9). The address (*Rede zur Feier des zwei und vierzigsten Stiftungstages*) is even less calculated to support his claim. The only "cells" mentioned in it are, as before, tissue compartments visible to the naked eye, perhaps aided by a loupe. Microscopic corpuscles (*Koerperchen*) are mentioned only in passing. In general, Mueller seems doubtful of the value of the microscope alone in the study of tumors: "The compound microscope alone would certainly lead us here into error and one-sidedness, in the absence of parallel chemical studies. In all fungous growths (*Schwaemmen*) without exception it discloses fibers to us, and in a large number of benign and malignant fungous growths corpuscles as well; these, however, are extremely variable

in form and number in one and the same kind" (p. 23). In Table II, figures 3a and 3b, of the monograph the reader will find depictions of the tissue compartments or "cells" in alveolar carcinoma. Mueller's ambiguous use of the term *cell* did not escape notice at the time. Rudolph Virchow called attention to it in 1847 ("Zur Entwickelungsgeschichte des Krebses, nebst Bemerkungen ueber Fettbildung im thierischen Koerper und pathologischer Resorption," *Arch. path. Anat. Phys. klin. Med.* 1 [1847]: 97-204, see p. 117). See also ch. 3, notes 130, 131.

29. Mueller, *Ueber den feinern Bau*, p. 3. In support of his claim Mueller cites a footnote appended by him to a paper by Gluge in the *Arch. Anat. Phys. wiss. Med.*, 1837. But the footnote makes no mention of cells, Schwannian or otherwise.

30. Ibid., p. 3. How far many other microscopists of the time were from the view adopted by Schwann and Mueller may be judged from the list of microscopic components of normal tissue in Joseph Berres's *Anatomia microscopica corporis humani*. Using a Ploessl microscope equipped with achromatic-aplanatic lenses, Berres found normal tissues to consist of tiny spherules (*spherulae* or *Blaeschen*) and somewhat larger vesicles (*vesiculae*), all related in some not entirely clear fashion to a network of minute tubules and larger vessels.

31. Ibid., p. 7.

32. Ibid., p. 10.

33. Ibid., p. 23: "I am moreover far from believing that all cell globes of *carcinoma reticulare* and *simplex* arise in this fashion as germ cells within other cells and become free by rupture or dissolution of mother cells. The phenomenon is not common enough for this. The frequency with which one observes only several or more small corpuscles in the cell globes speaks rather clearly for the fact that new small cells arise just as easily, and perhaps more easily, outside of already present cell globes, as they develop from granules in the same way as they do within already present cells. These granules can be freed by the rupture or dissolution of a larger cell, but they can also arise independently of and outside of cells. For this is often the case in normal tissues. Epithelial cells, for example, certainly do not arise in other cells, although they must take their origin from a nucleus which remains present on their wall, since they correspond with other cells in this respect."

34. Mueller summed up his views on the nature of cancer under ten headings (ibid., pp. 25-30):

I. Carcinoma differs both in structure and inner nature from simple induration. II. Carcinoma also differs in nature from an ulceration of an indurated part. III. Carcinoma is not a heterologous tissue and the finest components of its tissue are not essentially different from the tissue components of benign tumors and primitive embryonic tissues. IV. Just as little does carcinoma contain (putrefaction aside) distinctive chemical components. V. Nevertheless, the peculiar kind of productive and destructive activity characteristic of carcinoma gives rise to general anatomical features that permit many, if not most, carcinomas to be recognized with the naked eye. VI. A general derangement of vegetative growth, or a local derangement of vegetative growth with a tendency to become generalized, is part of the development of cancer. VII. If there is indeed a general disposition to carcinoma present in most cases at the time they arise locally, it must nevertheless be admitted that carcinoma can also form from a local disposition, in consequence of which the general disposition then arises later, and that this local disposition can demonstrably be caused by certain influences. VIII. Certain tumors, which are in themselves completely non-cancerous, and which by nature remain completely localized, can, under certain circumstances, readily take on a local disposition to cancer. IX. On the other hand, many tumors different from cancer have no tendency, even after repeated mistreatment, toward a cancerous disposition, or, to speak more correctly, their tendency toward a cancerous disposition is at least no greater than that of other, healthy, tissues. X. Every form of cancer appears to occur in all age-groups and all organs, but some organs are more disposed toward cancer in certain age-groups.

35. Theodor Schwann, *Mikroskopische Untersuchungen ueber die Uebereinstimmung in der Struktur und dem Wachstum der Thiere und Pflanzen*, translated by Henry Smith as *Microscopical Researches into the Accordance in the Structure and Growth of Animals and Plants*. (One suspects that in substituting "Uebereinstimmung" for "Analogie" Schwann may have intended to distance himself from German romantic biology, where a rather free use of analogical reasoning was prevalent.)

36. Schwann, *Untersuchungen*, p. 196.

37. Ibid., p. 196.

38. Ibid., p. 197.

39. Ibid., p. 72.

40. Ibid., p. 74.

41. Ibid., p. 82. The term epithelium (*epi,* 'on,' *thēlē,* 'nipple') is said by Henry Alan Skinner to have been introduced around 1700 by Frederick Ruysch as a designation for the tissue layer covering the nipple and similar papillated areas (*The Origin of Medical Terms*). Arthur W. Ham, on the other hand, claims that it referred "not to the nipple of the breast but rather to the little papillae of connective tissue so frequently seen under epithelial membranes" (*Histology*, 3d ed., p. 192). Neither claim is documented. Bichat did not use the terms *epithelium* and *epithelial tissue*. His four covering tissue layers were designated epidermal, mucous, serous, and synovial.

42. Schwann, *Untersuchungen*, p. 85.

43. Ibid., p. 82.

44. Ibid., p. 83. Here Schwann states that not all epithelial cells are hexagonal plates; some are elongated strips, as Henle had observed in the case of the "epithelium of the vessels."

45. This is still true, in part, today. As Ham has correctly pointed out, tissues can be classified in accordance with three sometimes conflicting criteria: structural (including both the features of the individual cells and of their composite arrangement), functional, and embryological (the germ layer of origin of the tissue in question). In practice, a mixture of criteria is usually employed; hence the confusion that can arise. Using the morphological criterion alone, Ham classifies under the heading of epithelium all lining layers composed of flattened cells, including those of blood and lymph vessels, of synovial spaces, and of the pericardium, pleura, and peritoneum (*Histology*, pp. 190-92). The derivation of the proto-typical epithelial tissues from the ectodermal and endodermal germ layers seems, however, to have generated some reluctance on the part of histologists to apply the term epithelium to morphologically "epithelial" cells of mesodermal origin; hence the two overlapping terms *endothelium* and *mesothelium*—the first indicative of position, the second of origin (embryonic, mesodermal). These terms, too, are inconsistently applied in practice, e.g., the lining cells of the genito-urinary tract are largely of mesodermal origin but are customarily referred to as epithelial. Further, the cells of most exocrine and endocrine glands, regardless of their germ layer of origin or the fact that they are in no sense covering layers, are considered by modern histologists to be epithelial.

46. Schwann, *Untersuchungen*, p. 75. According to Schwann, Julius Vogel's studies of 1838 indicate that the lymph corpuscles are cells, although Vogel himself did not use the term.

47. Ibid., pp. 77-79. Schwann mentions Ludwig Gueterbock's discovery that the cell membranes of mucous corpuscles (*Schleimkoerperchen*) are dissolved by acetic acid and the nuclei break up into "two or three smaller corpuscles." Pus corpuscles behave similarly, and there is good reason to suppose, says Schwann, that pus and mucous corpuscles are closely related, if not identical, formations.

48. Ibid., pp. 85-87. Schwann states here that his idea of the cell differs from Henle's.

The latter had believed, prior to Schwann's affirmation of the identity of plant and animal cells, that epithelial cell growth was merely the result of an increase in volume, perhaps due to imbibition. But now, says Schwann, "we must ascribe a peculiar life (*eigenthuemliches Leben*) to animal cells as well as plant cells, and explain the expansion of animal cells as well as plant cells as growth by intussusception."

49. Ibid., p. 109. Schwann's earlier view of the matter appears on pp. 194-95, where he writes that the "pre-existence of the nucleus and the formation of a cell around it...[as well as] the formation of new cells within cells" are characteristic of the chorda dorsalis.

50. Ibid., pp. 112, 113.

51. Ibid., p. 134. In modern histological terminology *blastema* survives as a designation for an as yet undifferentiated mass of cells, while *cytoblastema* has dropped out of use. *Intercellular substance*, as now used, includes both fibrous and amorphous varieties and designates a cell product rather than a primary generative substance.

52. Ibid., p. 158.

53. Cf. L. J. Rather, "Some Relations between Eighteenth-Century Fiber Theory and Nineteenth-Century Cell Theory," *Clio Medica* 4 (1969): 191-202.

54. *Omnis cellula e cellula ejusdem naturae*, as Louis Bard was to say ("La spécificité cellulaire et l'histogénèse chez l'embryon," *Arch. physiol. norm. path.* 7/3 [1886]: 406-20).

55. Schwann, *Untersuchungen*, p. 108. No reason is given by Schwann for the assumption here that the "overall organismal plan," rather than some feature of the formative cytoblastema, determines the appropriate appearance of muscle and connective tissue cells.

56. L. J. Rather, *Addison and the White Corpuscles*, see "The Decline of the Blastema Theory," pp. 125-38, and "Subsequent Fate of the Blastema Theory in England, France, Germany and the U.S.S.R.," pp. 217-27.

57. Julius Vogel, "Gewebe (in pathologischer Hinsicht)," *Handwoerterbuch der Physiologie mit Ruecksicht auf physiologische Pathologie*, ed. Rudolf Wagner, 1: 789-859.

58. Ibid., pp. 810-13.

59. Ibid., p. 824. Vogel's point is not that the line of distinction is difficult to draw in practice (which it still is today), but that it does not exist.

60. Ibid., pp. 824, 830.

61. Ibid., pp. 824-29.

62. Julius Vogel, *The Pathological Anatomy of the Human Body*, trans. George E. Day (Philadelphia, 1847). All citations are from the American edition. Vogel's book also appeared in 1847 in French and Italian translations. With the overthrow of the blastema theory a few years later, the book became obsolete. (Rudolf Virchow's essay [1855] and book [1858] on cellular pathology, in which the blastema theory was discarded, will be discussed in Chapter 4.) Vogel's cell theory can justifiably be called Schwannian, although it should be noted that he disagreed with Schwann in a number of respects insofar as the precise manner of formation of cells from cytoblastemas was concerned. Further, he held that connective tissue fibrils took form directly from the blastema, without passing through the cell stage. "Schwann's theory requires considerable modifications before it can be applied to morbid tissues," writes Vogel, and even "all perfectly formed tissues do not originally possess a decided cellular formation." In the course of tissue development, cells may lose their "original cellular form," and this may occur as the result of cell fusion (as in the case of vessels, nerves, and muscle) or cell division (as in the case of cellular, i.e., connective tissue) (pp. 123-25). Cell division here means no more than the separation of cells into separate parts; it has nothing to do with cell multiplication, i.e., the production of new cells.

63. Ibid., pp. 189-91.

64. Ibid., p. 245.

65. Ibid., pp. 253-59, 379.

66. Ibid., pp. 266-78. The archetypal observational instance of the organization of a fluid "blastema" into a solid "tissue" was the clotting of drawn blood. This was also the basis of the

fiber theory of tissue structure and was in clear conflict with Schwann's account of the formation of fibers from cells. In 1842, for example, the well-known English microanatomist George Gulliver asked: "How is the origin of fibrils which I have depicted in so many varieties of fibrine to be reconciled with this [Schwann's] doctrine? And what is the proof that these fibrils may not be the primordial fibers of all animal textures?" ("On the Structure of Fibrinous Exudations or False Membranes," *London, Edinburgh, Dublin Phil. Mag. J. Sci.* 3d ser. 21 [October, 1842]: 241-46).

67. Vogel, *Pathological Anatomy*, pp. 112-14.

68. Karl von Rokitansky, *Handbuch der pathologischen Anatomie*, vol. 1, 1846; vol. 2, 1844; vol. 3, 1842. The four-volume English translation by William Edward Swaine, *A Manual of Pathological Anatomy*, was published in London, vol. 1, 1854; vol. 2, 1849; vol. 3, 1850; vol. 4, 1852.

69. Rokitansky, *A Manual of Pathological Anatomy*, 1: 88-93.

70. Ibid., pp. 81-82.

71. Ibid., pp. 170, 171.

72. Rudolf Virchow, "Rokitansky, *Handbuch der allgemeinen pathologischen Anatomie*," *Preuss. Med. Z.*, no. 49 (December, 1846), pp. 237, 238; no. 50 (December, 1846), pp. 243, 244. Cf. L. J. Rather, "Virchow's Review of Rokitansky's *Handbuch* in the *Preuss. Med. Z.* Dec. 1846," *Clio Medica* 4 (1969): 127-40, which contains a translation of Virchow's review. Some of Virchow's criticisms bear on Rokitansky's introduction (omitted in large part from Swaine's translation as being too speculative for English tastes) to the first volume of the *Handbuch*. Cf. L. J. Rather and Eva R. Rohl, "An English translation of the Hitherto Untranslated Part of Rokitansky's *Einleitung* to Volume I of the *Handbuch der allgemeinen Pathologie* (1846); With a Bibliography of Rokitansky's Published Works," *Clio Medica* 7 (1972): 215-28.

73. The real point at issue was a methodological one. Rokitansky's speculative procedure recalled the excesses of German romantic biology against which Virchow and others of his generation were reacting. Virchow's call for a stricter, "positivistic" procedure may be found in two of his early essays, "Standpoints in Scientific Medicine" (1847) and "Scientific Method and Therapeutic Standpoints" (1849) (see Rather, *Disease, Life, and Man*). In 1895, toward the end of his life, Virchow stated (somewhat misleadingly) that his attack on Rokitansky's system of general pathology had been necessary for the protection of medical science against a "false pathology of the humors," rather as if it had been an attack on humoral pathology in general (see "One Hundred Years of General Pathology," in *Disease, Life, and Man*).

74. In the new edition Rokitansky changed the title of the work from *Handbuch* to *Lehrbuch der pathologischen Anatomie*. The new edition was published in Vienna in 1855. In the same year Virchow's review of the revised version of volume 1 ("Die neue Auflage von Rokitansky's allgemeiner pathologischen Anatomie," *Wien. med. Woch.* no 26 [1855], pp. 4015; no. 27 [1855], pp. 417-21), appeared, together with his programmatic essay on cellular pathology ("Cellular-Pathologie," *Arch. path. Anat. Phys. klin. Med.* 8 [1855]: 1-38). For comments on Virchow's review of the new edition see Rather and Rohl, "An English Translation."

75. The essays "Zur Entwickelungsgeschichte des Krebses" [On the developmental history of cancer] and "Ueber die Reform der pathologischen und therapeutischen Anschauungen durch die mikroskopischen Untersuchungen" [On the reform of pathologic and therapeutic views by studies with the microscope], appeared in 1847 in the first volume (pp. 94-204 and 207-55, respectively) of the *Arch. path. Anat. Phys. klin. Med.* (Virchow's *Archiv*), founded and edited by Rudolf Virchow and Benno Reinhardt.

76. Virchow, "Ueber die Reform," pp. 207, 208. He states that at least part of the skepticism of practicing physicians was a consequence of the diagnostic errors committed by microscopic pathologists. Presumably the reference would be to tumor diagnosis. If so, there is historical irony here because Virchow himself, in 1888, contributed a misleading microscopic diagnosis in the case of the fatal ailment (which ultimately proved to be cancer of the larynx) of Kaiser

Friedrich III. See ch. 4, note 66.

77. Ibid., pp. 211-15.

78. Virchow, "Zur Entwickelungsgeschichte," pp. 110, 111. Since the walls of blood vessels were normally impermeable to solids, a blastema or "nutritive plasma" (*Ernaehrungsplasma*) was fluid at the time of its passage, according to Virchow, although subsequently it might coagulate.

79. Ibid., pp. 111-13. Jacob Henle had suggested in 1844 that a variant form of fibrin, one incapable of normal organization, was the "basis for the development of malignant tumors, tubercles and fungous growths" ("Bericht ueber die Arbeiten im Gebiet der rationellen Pathologie," *Z. rat. Med.* 2 [1844]: 265).

80. Virchow, "Zur Entwickelungsgeschichte," pp. 112-19. Virchow states that the "transformation of a fibrous clot into cancer, assumed by Hunter, Home and Abernethy, really seems to take place," but only insofar as *intravascular* fibrin coagula are concerned.

81. Virchow, "Ueber die Reform," p. 218.

82. Virchow, "Zur Entwickelungsgeschichte," p. 125.

83. Virchow, "Ueber die Reform," p. 218. Possibly Virchow did this because Schwann had begun by describing the intracellular formation of normal cells, à la Schleiden, and did not change his views (in print, at least) until after Mueller had claimed that tumor cells more often arose from an *extracellular* blastema.

84. Virchow, "Zur Entwickelungsgeschichte," p. 107. In stained smears of fluids containing cancer cells the occurrence of cells within cells is common enough to have some limited diagnostic value. The phenomenon has been labeled "cannibalism" (S. M. Farber et al., *Cytologic Diagnosis of Lung Cancer*, p. 40).

85. Ibid., p. 133.

86. In his Huxley Lecture of 1898, "Recent Progress in Medicine and Its Influence in Medicine and Surgery," Virchow stated that Schwann's cell theory of 1839 (in which cells were derived from an *extracellular* cytoblastema) amounted to a "resuscitation of the archaic doctrine of spontaneous generation" (see *Disease, Life, and Man*, p. 225). But the truth is that to Schwann (and to Virchow, at that time) it amounted to the formation of cells from a primary living substance, the cytoblastema. Not only was Schwann no believer in spontaneous generation, he had carried out experiments (almost as conclusive as those of Pasteur much later) designed to rule out that possibility. This he did before he developed the cell theory. Cf. Schwann's "Vorlaeufige Mitteilungen, betreffend Versuche ueber die Weingaehrung und Faeulnis," *Ann. Physik Chem.* 41 (1837): 184-94. See also ch. 4, note 1.

87. Virchow, "Ueber die Reform," p. 235.

88. Ibid., p. 236. Virchow states here that the end-result of the regenerative organization of a blastema, namely, an amount of tissue equivalent to that lost, can be regarded as a homologous scar (*homologe Narbe*). Heterologous development, as in the healing of an incised muscle, yields a "heterologous scar," composed of mere connective tissue.

89. Ibid. The only abnormal tissue named by Virchow capable of impressing its own character on a blastematous exudate is pus (considered here as a fluid tissue). But he could have said the same of any growing tumor, benign or malignant, since its growth was thought to depend on the appropriate organization of freshly supplied blastematous exudate.

90. Ibid., p. 238. This seems to be the force of Virchow's objection.

91. Robley Dunglison, *A Dictionary of Medical Science*, p. 590.

92. In one of the best-known essays included in the Hippocratic corpus, *On the Nature of the Human Being (Peri physios anthrōpou)*, *metastasis* is used in connection with the evacuation and shifting (*tēn kenōsin kai tēn metastasin*) of a superfluous or abnormal humor from one internal organ to another. Cf. *Hippocrates*, trans. W. H. S. Jones, 4: 12, 13. All but one of the seven references to metastasis in Littré occur in that essay. Cf. *Oeuvres complètes d'Hippocrate*, 10: 691. According to Galen (in his commentary on the Hippocratic aphorisms), diseases are

properly termed *metastasizing* whenever they move from one part of the body to another. Cf. Kuehn, *Claudii Galeni Opera Omnia*, 17/2: 790.

93. Mueller, *Ueber den feinern Bau*, p. 29.

94. Jacob Henle, "Von den Miasmen und Kontagien," in his *Pathologischen Untersuchungen*. Cf. George Rosen's translation "Jacob Henle: On Miasmata and Contagia," *Bull. Hist. Med.* 6 (1938): 907-83. In his introductory remarks Rosen claims that Henle's explanation of metastasis in neoplastic disease "shows clearly that Henle was already thinking along the lines of cellular pathology years before Virchow published his classic work." But Henle was an adherent of the blastema theory, and any "thinking along the lines" of cellular pathology that he might have engaged in (for which there is *no* convincing evidence) would have anticipated Vogel in 1845 rather than Virchow in 1858, for the distinguishing feature of Virchow's *Cellularpathologie* was its systematic rejection of the blastema theory in favor of the derivation of all cells from preexisting cells.

95. Cf. Rosen, "Jacob Henle," p. 951 for the reference to tubercle cells. Still more general is the basic thesis of Henle's essay, namely, that the seeds of disease are living organisms capable of reproducing themselves in the body of a host organism and of passing from one host to another directly (in contagious diseases) or indirectly (in miasmatic diseases). Tubercle cells and the cells of cancers, according to this line of thought, are semiindependent living organisms, derived from the host.

96. Ibid., p. 950. The resemblance is implied rather than directly stated.

97. Johannes Mueller, *On the Nature and Structural Characteristics of Cancer, and of Morbid Growths Which May Be Confounded With It*, trans. Charles West. The work was never, as far as I know, translated into French. It was given a detailed review by Louis Mandl in 1840 ("De la structure intime des tumeurs ou des productions pathologiques," *Arch. gén. méd.*, 3d ser., 8 [1840], 313-29), and Mandl's own studies of the histogenesis of tumors yielded results not essentially different from those of Mueller. Cf. Louis Mandl, *Anatomie microscopique*, vol. 2, *Histogénèse*, pp. 339-70.

98. Walter H. Walshe, *The Anatomy, Physiology, Pathology, and Treatment of Cancer*. Walshe's monograph was first published in W. B. Costello's *Cyclopaedia of Practical Surgery*, 1: 590-692.

99. Walshe, in *Cyclopaedia*, pp. 609, 610, 628.

100. Cf. Dunglison, *Dictionary*, p. 572.

101. In discussing the subject in his essay of 1840, Henle makes use of "a comparison pursued only in the interest of wit, rather than a genuine explanation," that of the so-called metaphorical thorn or *spina metaphorica* (as van Helmont termed it). For some comments on the history of this "thorn," from Galen's hypothetical *skolops* to the real thorn used by Metchnikov in his studies on inflammation in the larval starfish see L. J. Rather, *Addison and the White Corpuscles*, pp. 180, 181, 188, 189; see also Peter Niebyl, "The Helmontian Thorn," *Bull. Hist. Med.* 45 (1971): 570-95, for a full treatment of the topic. Henle needed it, he believed, to clarify the difference between his own understanding of the nature of "living contagions" and the belief, widespread among German physicians of the romantic period, that the concrete manifestations (i.e., the lesions) of disease were independent parasitic forms of life. The *cause* of the disease, not the *disease* itself, was transmitted by the disease-seed, said Henle, and he asks the reader to visualize a thorn embedded in the flesh of a finger. This thorn will give rise to inflammatory and suppurative disease, but it is neither the disease nor its product; it is the irritating *cause* of the disease. Suppose, then, that every least part of the thorn were capable of reproducing and multiplying, not only in the body of the patient immediately concerned but also in the bodies of other individuals. There the particles would multiply, meanwhile inciting the same disease, i.e., inflammation and suppuration: the disease will be the "same" because the inciting causal agent is the same. Generalizing on the basis of this traditional model, Henle proposed that the specificity of the known contagious and miasmatic diseases followed from the specificity of their—as yet

unknown—living causal agents. Henle then outlined the criteria (now called postulates and associated with the name of his most famous pupil, Robert Koch) for distinguishing between micro-organisms causative of disease and micro-organisms adventitiously present in diseased tissues. The only *spina manifesta* of this kind available to him at the time, as far as disease in human beings was concerned, was the itch-mite *Acarus scabiei* (although in animals he could point to the fungus, described by Agostino Bassi in 1837, responsible for muscardine in silkworms).

102. Bernard Langenbeck, "Ueber die Entstehung des Venekrebses, und die Moeglichkeit, Carcinoma vom Menschen auf Thiere zu uebertragen," *Jahrb. in-und auslaend. gesam. Med.* 25 (1840): 99-104. For a full translation of this paper see L. J. Rather, "Langenbeck on the Mechanism of Tumor Metastasis and the Transmission of Cancer from Man to Animal," *Clio Medica* 10 (1975): 213-25.

103. Langenbeck, "Entstehung des Venekrebses"; cf. Rather, "Langenbeck," p. 221.

104. Langenbeck, "Entstehung des Venekrebses," p. 103. In assessing the value of this evidence (of the rarity of primary lung cancer at the time) the reader should bear in mind that an enormous amount of gross pathological anatomical evidence bearing on cancer localization had been accumulated since the great days at the Charité in Paris (when Laennec could boast that "for twelve years...no death occurred without an autopsy"; cf. R. H. Laennec, *A Treatise on Diseases of the Chest,* facsimile of London edition of 1821, p. ix).

105. Ibid., p. 220.

106. Ibid., p. 223.

107. Julius Vogel pointed out in 1845 that Langenbeck had by no means proved the exclusive generation of secondary tumors from cells transmitted from primary tumors, commenting that this hypothesis had, however, become widely accepted. Vogel attempted to repeat Langenbeck's animal experiment, without success. See Vogel, *Pathological Anatomy,* pp. 283, 284. Rudolf Virchow, who might have been expected to welcome Langenbeck's claim in the light of his 1850s version of cellular pathology, was another notable skeptic. It is important to remember that Langenbeck did not claim that the transmission of cells was the *sole* mode of cancer metastasis.

108. The promised observations were, apparently, never published.

109. Langenbeck, "Entstehung des Venekrebses"; cf. Rather, "Langenbeck," pp. 218, 219. Injection experiments had long since familiarized pathologists with the existence of disrupted vessels in tumors. The notion that circulating objects became impacted in capillary vessels and gave rise to local disease had been current since the late seventeenth century. It was a crucial feature of Boerhaave's system of pathology.

110. Cf., for example, John Pearson, *Practical Observations on Cancerous Complaints,* who makes the following remark in regard to the question of whether cancer is a contagious disease: "A series of experiments might indeed speedily terminate our inquiries; but it may be presumed, that no man ever had, nor will have the unwarrantable temerity, to attempt the solution of this pathological doubt, by a method so repugnant to the laws of humanity." Pearson cites the words of Johannes Junker [Juncker] (1679-1759) to the effect that the contagious nature of cancer is suggested by many observations and that the contagion itself is a kind of ferment: "contagiosum esse cancrum, plures observationes persuadent; id quod potissimum a fermentescente ejus indole dependet, quam a seroso-lymphatica, et chyloso-salivali materia nanciscitur" (p. 23).

111. Langenbeck, "Entstehung des Venekrebses"; cf. Rather, "Langenbeck," p. 223.

112. Rather, "Langenbeck," p. 223. The tumor is referred to by Langenbeck as a *carcinoma medullare humeri.* Since no other information is given, it is impossible to guess what a modern pathologist might call it. In any case, it was not necessarily an osteogenic sarcoma. The disarticulation had been carried out two and a half hours prior to the injection.

113. Ibid., p. 224. Langenbeck refers his readers to some illustrations, but the article was published without them. Virchow stated in 1863 that he had examined Langenbeck's drawings

of the microscopic appearance of the pulmonary nodules, and found them, oddly enough, to suggest "spontaneous forms of cancer" in the dog rather than "human cancer elements" (Rudolf Virchow, *Die krankhaften Geschwuelste* [Berlin, 1863], 1: 87, 88). One might have expected mere infarcts or abscesses.

114. Ibid., 218, 222. Langenbeck writes:

"It is known that the development and growth of carcinomas, and probably that of all morbid formations maintaining a connection with the organism, depends on the simple growth of cells, and takes place in accordance with laws the same as those first pointed out by Schleiden in plants, by Schwann in normal animal tissues, and by Mueller in numerous morbid formations....An extraordinary correspondence between the development of plant and animal tissues has been demonstrated thereby. Yet the analogy gains still further support from my discovery of the fact that the germ-cells (*Keimzellen*) of a cancerous tumor...are able to develop independently into carcinomas in any part of the capillary vascular system, precisely as in the lower plants every cell separated from the plant can continue to grow independently." Langenbeck then compares cancer cells to fertilized egg cells: "Like the germ of the ovary, every single carcinoma cell must now appear as an organism endowed with life-force and developmental ability which, even though robbed of all organic connection with its primal native soil, can nevertheless continue to develop independently as long as it finds itself in the neighborhood of and under the influence of living organic tissue—however, a cancer cell differs essentially from a cell of the ovary in that it requires no more than contact with and the enlivening effect of living organic substance, whereas the constrained life-force of the latter can come into living effectivity only under the influence of a specified external stimulus, the male generative substance" (p. 41).

115. Cf. ch. 3, note 7. Later, however, Gluge did come to regard these bodies, or ones like them, as cancer cells. In his *Pathologische Histologie* (Jena, 1850), translated by Joseph Leidy as *Atlas of Pathological Histology* (Philadelphia, 1853), Gluge states that the "characteristic cancer cells...average about the .02 mil. in diameter, and possess finely granular contents, with a round or oval nucleolated nucleus as large as or larger than a pus-corpuscle. Sometimes cancer cells are double the ordinary size, or more, and not unfrequently contain several nuclei, or even other cells, constituting parent or endogenous cells" (p. 70).

116. Cf. ch. 3, note 9, and text.

117. For Mueller this did not mean that cancers were not microscopically distinguishable from benign tumors and normal tissues. Hence Walshe was making a mere verbal point in stating, three years later, that although the microscopical *elements* of cancers were not heterologous, Mueller's claim that *cancers* were not heterologous formations did not follow, since the heterology of cancer was constituted by the "mode of combination and arrangement of the ultimate physical elements of the diseased growth" (Treatment of Cancer, p. 62).

118. Cf. Mueller, *Ueber den feinern Bau*, p. 7, where Mueller states that tailed corpuscles are "not formations peculiar to medullary carcinoma...very often they are not present, and, on the other hand, they occur just as often in non-cancerous tumors." Yet a few years later we find Karl Friedrich Hecker, in a report on the microscopic features of a malignant tumor of the nasal mucosa, stating that the "tailed corpuscles described by J. Mueller as characteristic of medullary carcinoma could not be found" ("Bericht ueber die Ereignisse in der chirurgisch-opthalmologischen Klinik zu Freiburg," *Arch. phys. Heilkunde* 3 [1844]: 261). Writing in 1847, Virchow noted a "widespread misunderstanding" of the significance of Mueller's tailed corpuscles ("Zur Entwickelungsgeschichte," p. 98). Another instance of this misunderstanding (not mentioned by Virchow) may be found in a case report by James Simpson in 1841. With reference to a tumor of the uterine cervix in which cells with large nuclei and multiple nucleoli were found, Simpson adds that there were "none of the caudate

or spindle-shaped bodies described by Mueller as often existing in morbid encephaloid structures" ("Case of Amputation of the Womb Followed by Pregnancy; with Remarks on the Pathology and Radical Treatment of the Cauliflower Excrescence from the Os Uteri," *Edinburgh Med. Surg. J.* 55 [1841]: 104-12).

119. Adolph Hannover, "Bericht ueber die Leistungen in der skandinavischen Literatur im Gebiete der Anatomie und Physiologie in den Jahren 1841-43," *Arch. Anat. Phys. wiss. Med.,* 1844, pp. 18, 19. Hannover refers here to his paper (in Danish) of 1843. It is worth noting that Walshe's monograph (*Treatment of Cancer*) includes some good drawings of large cells with double nuclei and prominent nucleoli found in cancers.

120. Philipp F. H. Klencke, *Untersuchungen und Erfahrungen im Gebiete der Anatomie, Pathologie, Mikrologie und wissenschaftlichen Medicin.* Vol. 1, *Der Nervus Sympathikus in seiner morphologischen und physiologischen Bedeutung.* Vol. 2, *Mikroskopisch-pathologische Beobachtungen ueber die Natur des Contagion* (Leipzig, 1843).

121. Ibid., 2: 121-23. Vogel (Pathological Anatomy, p. 282) was not averse to Klencke's views on cancer cells, but he pointed out some of the difficulties involved in the conception of cancer as a contagious disease. In our own day immunopathologists have found that in a large number of diseases, possibly including cancer, cells that are foreign, or "not-self," arise and are subsequently dealt with by the organism in somewhat the same manner as are invading bacterial organisms.

122. Hermann Lebert, *Physiologie pathologique,* 2: 254-60. In the *Atlas* of twenty-two plates supplementing his *Traité d'anatomie pathologique* (pp. 5-16) is an account of Lebert's procedure for the anatomical investigation of excised tumors. After a careful gross dissection of the tumor (perhaps aided by a loupe) microscopic observations were made on fresh, unstained, hand-cut sections and on fluid expressed by pressure or scraped off the surface, placed between glass slides and cover slips. Dilute acetic acid helped to emphasize nuclear detail, and tincture of iodine was used to stain the cells. Preliminary treatment with hydrochloric acid permitted bony tissues to be examined in the same manner. Lebert recommended the Oberhaueser microscope, equipped with Hachet objectives, and an ocular micrometer calibrated in units of 1/1000 mm. He mentions the successful employment by Donné of the daguerrotype, but preferred freehand drawings made with a *chambre claire,* or "camera lucida."

123. Lebert believed that cancer cells were continually being generated from a cancer blastema at the tumor site. The mature cells eventually broke down into a granular mass. Although the cancer blastema was capable of generating normal stromal connective tissue, it was possible, he said, that the stroma might arise from the "simple hypertrophy of connective tissue" (*tissu cellulaire*) in the organ involved (p. 260).

124. Vogel, *Pathological Anatomy,* pp. 267-69. Among the cells occasionally present in malignant lesions were some with thick, doubly-contoured walls. Vogel's description of the gross lesion in this case, together with the drawing given of these cells, suggests a fungal disease.

125. Charles Sédillot, *Recherches sur le cancer,* reprinted in Sédillot, *Contributions à la chirurgie,* 1: 448-617. Commenting on the use of the microscope, Sédillot states that "we ought not delay in imitating them [the Germans] and in demanding from the microscope the last resources of its power in the diagnosis of cancer" (p. 455).

126. In his *Recherches,* Sédillot attributes all microscopic observations to Émile Kuess. The first account of the use of Kuess's punch biopsy instrument appeared in 1847 in the *Gaz. méd. de Strasbourg* (not available to me). This article was then reported in *L'Union médicale,* April 1, 1847, p. 158, and in the *Month. J. Med. Sci.* 7 (1847): 853. (In both reports Kuess's name is incorrectly given as Kuen.) The instrument appears to have been used on three occasions, with complete success.

127. Heinrich Meckel's *Habilitationsschrift* (Halle, 1845), "De pseudoplasmatibus in genere et de carcinomate in specie," appeared in the *Amtlicher Bericht ueber die 24sten Versammlung*

Deutscher Naturforscher und Aerzte im September 1846, pp. 162-63. Meckel's description of cancer cells is not particularly precise, but it is notable for introducing an adjective that has since remained in use: cancer cells, he writes, are at times "drawn out into the most manifold and bizarre (*bizarrsten*) extensions."

128. Virchow, "Zur Entwickelunggeschichte," p. 108. On this same page, interestingly enough (in view of his later attempt to derive epithelial cancer cells from the reservoir of undifferentiated connective tissue cells), Virchow notes the frequent resemblance of cancer cells to epidermal cells and to epithelial cells in general.

129. Virchow seems to have regarded the large, atypical cells found in cancers as functionally specific elements, even though not always identifiable as such on the basis of purely anatomical criteria. He assigned all other cellular elements of tumors, together with connective tissue fibers and small blood vessels, to the tumor stroma (*Krebsgeruest*). He discounted the alternative view that they were residua of invaded normal tissues, although he admitted that such residua might be detected during the "crude" stage of cancer, i.e., before the cancer blastema had undergone full organization (pp. 96, 97, 133, 134). The views of other histopathologists on the stroma are worth recalling here: Lebert had suggested that the supporting connective tissue framework of a tumor might, in some instances at least, be a product of local connective tissue hypertrophy (see note 123); Sédillot found this supposition unnecessary and claimed to have seen cancer cells undergoing transformation into ordinary fibers, indistinguishable from those normally present (*Recherches,* p. 525); and Heinrich Meckel ("De pseudoplasmatibus," pp. 162, 163), divided all cancers into two components, the *Krebssaft* or cancer-juice, composed of specific cancer cells, and the stroma, composed of normal connective tissues. All these views, it should be observed, relate back to the distinction drawn by Greek anatomists between the *strōma* — literally, the strewn bed or framework — of an organ and its parenchyma, or essential, fluid or semifluid constituent.

130. In 1836, at the commencement of his interest in the fine structure of tumors, Mueller expressed his doubt as to the value of the microscope in the absence of parallel chemical studies (cf. note 28). In his monograph of 1838 he states that "it is thus easy to see that the applied diagnosis of tumors cannot rest on the use of such subtle aids. . . . Microscopical and chemical analysis ought therefore never become the means of medical diagnosis; to desire this or suppose it likely would be laughable" (p. 2).

131. Carl Bruch, *Die Diagnose der boesartigen Geschwuelste,* pp. xiii, xiv, 277, 278, 318, 330, 340. Bruch cites numerous articles on the microscopic structure of tumors written in the mid-1840s — a few adversely critical of Mueller's work, but most representing attempts to apply it in surgical practice. He notes (p. 223) that Mueller's concept of the cell is ill-defined (*unbestimmt*) and includes vesicles of noncellular (in the new, strict sense) character. Bruch admits that he has never seen a cancer blastema but presumes that its existence is transitory (p. 225). He believes that nuclei can exist as such; hence, the cell is not, as Schwann supposes, the common basis of all tissues but is, rather, a secondary formation (p. 289). And he agrees with Henle that most fibers form directly from a blastema rather than by the metamorphosis of cells, as described by Schwann (p. 296).

132. John Hughes Bennett, *On Cancerous and Cancroid Growths.* Bennett's description of his procedure in the examination of surgically removed tumors is given here in full:

> The following is the method which, for some years, I have employed in the examination of morbid growths, and which I recommend to the young pathologist. The specimen should always be recent; the addition of alcohol causing coagulation of the albuminous compounds, and altering the form of the corpuscular elements. In the first place the external physical characters of the growth should be accurately examined, and as much learned of the history of the case as is possible. A section should then be made, and the appearance of the cut surfaces carefully examined. These should be squeezed, to see if they yield any fluid; if not, the surface should be

gently scraped. A drop of fluid or pulpy substance so obtained, should now be placed between glasses, and examined with an achromatic microscope under a power of 250 linear diameters. After the appearances of the more fluid parts have been observed, water should first be added, then acetic acid, and the effect of each re-agent studied. Water generally causes the cell formations to enlarge by endosmosis, and enables the manipulator to separate coherent masses, and examine each corpuscle, perfectly isolated. It is only in this way that the numerous molecules and granules floating in the blastema can be separated from those within the cell, which now may be seen revolving in the fluid with its contents. Acetic acid has the remarkable property of dissolving and rendering very transparent many of the albuminous compounds. The walls of most recent cell formations are, in this way, rendered transparent, or caused to disappear; and the nucleus, which was formerly obscure, is rendered clear and well defined. The action of acetic acid on cell structures is of the utmost importance in a diagnostic point of view, and the having omitted to describe its effects has vitiated the account of many otherwise good observations. I would recommend the young pathologist to repeat these demonstrations several times before terminating this part of the inquiry, and further to study the effects of ether and of liquor potassae, diluted with an equal part of water. In every case, whenever the cut surface of the tumour presents differences in structure, colour, or consistence, the same manipulations and observations must be repeated on the fluid or pulpy substance from each altered portion. Having now examined the fluid parts of the growth, the solid parts must be investigated. For this purpose a thin slice should be removed, placed between glasses, and inspected under the microscope, and in like manner successively treated with water and acetic acid. A thin slice may be obtained with a sharp knife, or a pair of curved scissors; but by far the best means is the double-bladed knife of Valentin. This instrument, indeed, may be considered almost indispensable to the histologist, especially where large sections are required, and where it is of importance not to derange the relation of the elementary structures to each other. A transparent section thus obtained, enables the observer to see the fibrous stroma of the growth, the arrangement of the ultimate filaments, the relation to those of the cells, granules, molecules, or mineral particles, he has previously examined; the arrangement of the blood vessels, etc., etc. Several sections should always be made, and attentively inspected from various parts of the tumours; of course, taking care to include in these every variety of appearance and structure it may present. The observation is now complete. To keep a record of it, however, it is necessary that a note be immediately taken of the appearances observed, with and without re-agents, and that the different structures be accurately drawn. This requires some little skill in drawing, and especially in copying from the field of the microscope. I cannot, however, too strongly recommend the early and constant practice of drawing what is seen not only because mere words often utterly fail in giving a correct idea of the object described, but because such practice necessitates a much more careful examination of the object itself (ibid., pp. 1-2).

133. Cf. Ibid. pp. vii, viii; also pp. 221-2, where he writes: "The only physical proof we can arrive at of the existence of cancer, is by means of the microscope; not that this instrument is in itself capable, even in the most expert hands, of doing any thing, but, conjoined with a knowledge of the symptoms, progress of the case, form and appearance of the morbid growth, it offers us an additional and most valuable means of prosecuting our inquiries. It is from a union of all of these circumstances, combined with a minute examination of the growth, under such magnifying powers as will clearly display its cells and other primary elements, that we ought to found a diagnosis, and not from one or the other separately." Bennett, like almost all oncologists, disagreed with Mueller's estimate of the value of the

microscope in the practical diagnosis of tumors. According to Bennett, Mueller had given two quite opposing estimates of the value of the microscope in the study of tumors. Bennett overlooks, however, the fact that Mueller's opposite estimates concerned the research value and the practical value, respectively, of the instrument (see notes 28, 130).

134. Cf. Bruch's remarks two years earlier. Bennett states (*On Cancerous and Cancroid Growths*, p. 162) that "it is not by analysing large masses of morbid structure, including as they do, granules, cells, filaments and salts, mingled together, that any light will be thrown on the chemistry of cancer; but rather by first separating, with the aid of the microscope, the minute structural elements entering into the composition of the growth, and then endeavouring, by chemical manipulations under the same instrument, to ascertain the exact nature of each."

135. Ibid., p. 145. How Bennett reached the conclusion that Mueller and Virchow considered normal and cancerous tissues indistinguishable under the microscope remains unexplained. The view that normal and cancerous tissues were microscopically indistinguishable was, however, unequivocally upheld by Thomas Watson, the third edition of whose book, *Lectures on the Principles and Practice of Physic*, Bennett cites to this effect. Oddly enough, Dr. Francis Condie, the annotator of the second edition of Watson's book (Philadelphia, 1845), had already pointed out (p. 139) that Watson's view of the matter was incorrect — in the light of Mueller's findings.

136. Bennett, *On Cancerous and Cancroid Growths*, pp. 145-49.

137. Bernard Peyrilhe, *A Dissertation on Cancerous Diseases*, pp. 92-102.

138. Jean-Louis Alibert, *Clinique de l'Hôpital Saint-Louis, ou traité complet de maladies de la peau*, pp. 197-99. "Chimney-sweepers' cancer," referred to on page 199, is apparently equivalent to "soot-wart." Hence the lesion is a *carcine* rather than a true cancer. Pott, on the other hand, described it as a cancer, capable of spreading to the regional lymph nodes and interior abdomen (*The Chirurgical Works of Percival Pott, F.R.S.: A New Edition*, 3 vols. (London, 1779), s.v. "Cancer Scroti," 3: 225-29).

139. John Hunter had supposed that certain tumors arose in and from the skin (see ch. 1, n. 123 and text).

140. Alexander Ecker, "Ueber den Bau der unter dem Namen 'Lippenkrebs' zusammengefassten Geschwuelsten der Lippe," *Arch. phys. Heilkunde* 3 (1844): 380-84.

141. Ibid. The reference is to table 24 of Julius Vogel's *Icones histologiae pathologicae.*

142. Georges-François Mayor, "Examen microscopique de deux tumeurs cutanées," *Bull. soc. anat. Paris* 19 (1844): 218-25.

143. Émile Kuess, in Sédillot, *Recherches*, pp. 485, 486.

144. Mayor, *Sur les tumeurs épidermiques et sur leurs relations avec l'affection cancéreuse.*

145. Lebert used the term *cancroid* in his *Physiologie pathologique*. The term itself was credited to Jean-Louis Alibert by Hannover, who rejected it in favor of *epithelioma* (Adolph Hannover, *Das Epithelioma*, see pp. 6, 7). In Alibert's treatise on skin diseases (cf. note 138) only the term *carcine* is used in this connection.

146. Bennett, *On Cancerous and Cancroid Growths*, pp. 190-92, 216. For Bennett, *cancroid* seems to be equivalent to *homologous tumor* in the terminology of his time, and to *benign tumor* in current terms. He states, however, that certain kinds of cancroids sometimes undergo cancerous transformation.

147. Ibid., pp. 148, 149.

148. Ibid., pp. 147, 148. Kuess's description of the "multiplications des cellules par division" in cancers is rather vague; at first he had taken the fragmentation of cells visible in squeeze-preparations of cancer fragments to be the result of trauma (in Sédillot, *Recherches* p. 505). In his opinion cancer cells could arise either from a blastema or within preexisting cancer cells (p. 524).

149. Rudolf Virchow, *Die medicinische Reform*, no. 51 (June 22, 1849), pp. 271, 272. Virchow's remarks appear in the minutes (May 14) of the Society for Scientific Medicine. On

this occasion he distinguished the alveolar structure of cancer from that of cancroid: cancer alveoli had their own walls, composed of connective tissue, whereas cancroids "consisted entirely of cells," i.e., they had no walls of their own.

150. Rudolf Virchow, "Ueber Kankroide und Papillargeschwuelste," *Verh. phys. med. Gesell. in Wuerzburg* 1 (1850): 106-11.

151. Ibid., p. 108. Virchow gave credit to Frerichs for having first described cancroid alveoli in 1849, in a cancroid of the lip. Frerichs, however, believed that the epithelial cells were of dual origin, arising in part from the overlying epidermis and in part from the underlying connective tissue (Friedrich Theodor Frerichs, "Ueber die destruirenden Epithelialgeschwuelste," *Jenaische Ann. Phys. Med.*, 1849, p. 9).

152. It is of course possible that the tumor described by Virchow as a tibial cancroid was in fact a metastatic deposit from an undetected primary cancer located elsewhere; given Virchow's familiarity with metastasis, and the peculiarly characteristic location of the lesion in question, this seems unlikely.

153. Hermann Lebert, *Traité pratique des maladies cancéreuses.*

154. Ibid., p. 596.

155. Ibid., pp. 101, 611, 615-21.

156. Ibid., pp. 598, 599, 603.

157. Adolph Hannover, *Das Epithelioma.*

158. Ibid., pp. 3, 4, 7, 26.

159. Ibid., pp. 12, 24, 33-37.

160. Ibid., p. 51.

161. Ibid., p. 21.

4

1. Before developing the cell theory, Schwann had carried out a series of carefully designed experiments that spoke as conclusively against spontaneous generation as did the later and now far better known experiments of Louis Pasteur. Cf. Marcel Florkin, "Le journal des expériences de Théodore Schwann sur la génération spontanée, la fermentation alcoolique et la putréfaction," *Bull. Acad. Roy. Méd. Belgique* 17 (1952): 164-67; Theodor Schwann, "Vorlaeufige Mittheilung, betreffend Versuche ueber die Weingaehrung und Faeulnis," *Ann. Physik Chem.* 11 (1837): 184-94. In the same way that the free formation of cells made it impossible in principle to trace the cells of a mature organism back to the primal cell of that organism, spontaneous generation made it impossible in principle to trace the evolutionary development of present-day organisms to their primitive precursors in the remote past. Addressing this topic in 1898, Rudolf Virchow remarked that Schwann had in effect revived the "archaic doctrine of spontaneous generation...at a time when Darwin was already at work proving that new species arose by the modification of preexisting forms." Schwann's acceptance of the free formation of cells had implied that "every form of organic tissue or organism, every formation of new cells, must be separated from the preceding by a definite gap (*hiatus*), and that each new-formation must be considered a discontinuous vital process" (from Virchow's Huxley Lecture of 1898, "Recent Progress in Science and Its Influence on Medicine and Surgery," in Rather, *Disease, Life and Man*).

2. Karl von Baer, "Die Metamorphose," *Arch. Anat. Phys. Med.*, 1834, pp. 481-509.

3. Theodor Schwann, *Untersuchungen*, pp. 61, 62.

4. Cf. Jacob Henle, "Theodor Schwann. Nachruf," *Arch. mikr. Anat.* 21 (1882): i-xlix. Henle comments (p. xxi) that in the 1830s the "dogma of the development of the firm (*das Festen*) from the fluid (*dem Fluessigen*) had struck root too deeply in animal physiology for doubt of the free formation of cells to find a place." He notes also that Schwann, in his

comments on cleavage in the egg, had come close to the solution of the problem of cytogenesis.

5. Karl B. Reichert, "Bericht ueber die Fortschritte," *Arch. Anat. Phys. wiss. Med.,* 1841, pp. clxii-xxvii. The opening sentences of Reichert's review of recent progress in microscopic anatomy show how Schwann's histogenetic thesis was received by some of his colleagues:

> Well-known investigators have published findings which limit or modify the principle of cell formation as the developmental principle common to the most varied elementary parts of plant and animal organisms. Indeed, some have gone so far that this principle—which Oken, Mayer and, in particular, Raspail and Dutrochet expressed as an idea, in the absence of full awareness of its forms, which other observers, without having been permeated by the genial idea, knew, if only in part, in its forms, and which was, finally, achieved in both form and idea by Schwann and Schleiden in so masterful a fashion—that this principle, I say, has been brought into question as a whole; they have sought to explain it in terms of physical processes, or to eliminate it and to replace it with elements, such as the cell nucleus and intercellular substance, previously held to be inessential in the formation of tissues.

6. Ibid., pp. clxvi, clxvii.

7. Rudolf Koelliker, *Entwickelungsgeschichte der Cephalopoden.*

8. Cf. Rather, *Addison and the White Corpuscles,* pp. 135, 136.

9. Reichert, "Bericht ueber die Fortschritte," *Arch. Anat. Phys. wiss. Med.,* 1854, pp. 1-80.

10. For example, T. H. Huxley's statement, in 1853, that "vital phenomena are not necessarily preceded by organization" ("The Cell Theory," *British and Foreign Med. Chir. Rev.* 12 [1853]: 221-43) echoed John Hunter's claim of seventy years earlier that "life" was prior to "organization" (cf. ch. 1, n. 119 and accompanying text). For the later history of the blastema theory, see Rather, *Addison and the White Corpuscles,* Appendix C, pp. 217-27.

11. Remak's collected papers (1851-55) on embryology were published in Berlin in 1855 under the title *Untersuchungen ueber die Entwickelung der Wirbelthiere.* This work presents cellular embryology for the first time from the standpoint that all cells arise from other cells; it bears the same relationship to previous works on the subject that Virchow's cellular pathology was to bear toward the earlier cellular pathology of Julius Vogel.

12. Robert Remak, "Ueber extracellulare Entstehung thierischer Zellen," *Arch. Anat. Phys. wiss. Med.,* 1852, pp. 47-57.

13. Ibid., p. 57.

14. Robert Remak, "Ein Beitrag zur Entwickelungsgeschichte der krebshaften Geschwuelste," *Deutsche Klinik,* 1854, pp. 170-74. Langenbeck is mentioned in this paper as Remak's chief source of supply of tumor material.

15. Ibid., p. 172.

16. Reichert, "Bericht ueber die Fortschritte," *Arch. Anat. Phys. wiss. Med.,* 1854, pp. 1-80. Like Remak, he equated "free formation" with "spontaneous generation" (ibid., p. 3).

17. Henle, in 1882, attributed the premature close of Schwann's brilliant period of scientific productivity to a language difficulty; after leaving Berlin in 1839 to fill the chair in anatomy at Louvain, Schwann chose to write only in French, a language he had not yet mastered. Cf. "Theodor Schwann. Nachruf," p. xliii. Although Schwann taught at Louvain and, subsequently, at Liège until 1878, his work on the isolation of pepsin, the experimental disproof of spontaneous generation, and the cell theory fell between 1836 and 1839, when he was associated with Johannes Mueller.

18. Rudolf Virchow, *Handbuch der speciellen Pathologie und Therapie,* vol. 1. For Addison's rejection of the blastema theory, see Rather, *Addison and the White Corpuscles,* esp. pp. 125, 151, 200, 201.

19. Virchow, *Handbuch,* 1: 329, 330, 335.

20. Virchow reported to the Wuerzburg Physical-Medical Society in 1850 that "tubercle arises. . .from a *metamorphosis of organized elements* and in no way from an exudate" (*Verh. physik. med. Gesell. in Wuerzburg,* 1 [1850]: 83-87). His statement is somewhat misleading, for he still believed that the organized elements, in the main connective tissue cells, themselves arose from an exudate.

21. Compare Henle's claim that the evidence on the basis of which Schwann's belief in the free formation of cells was overthrown was faulty and insufficient ("Theodor Schwann. Nachruf," pp. xxxvii, xxxviii).

22. Rudolf Virchow, "Cellular-Pathologie," *Arch. path. Anat. Phys. klin. Med.* 8 (1855): 1-39. Virchow's words are: "Ich formulire die Lehre von der pathologischen Generation, von der Neoplasie im Sinne der Cellular-pathologie einfach: *Omnis cellula a cellula.*" For a translation of the essay see Rather, *Disease, Life, and Man,* pp. 71-101.

23. The controversy over these issues involved an ideological moment, apparent in Virchow's statement that *"generatio aequivoca,* particularly when it is conceived of as self-arousal, is downright heresy or devil's work, and when we, of all people, defend not only the inheritance of generations on the whole but the legitimate succession of cell forms as well this is truly trustworthy testimony" ("Cellular-Pathologie," p. 23). The point is that Virchow and his fellow believers in the "mechanistic interpretation of life" (the title of an essay by Virchow, published in 1858) would have been happier with the view that they found themselves forced to reject. In the later controversy between Félix Pouchet and Louis Pasteur before the French Academy on the topic of spontaneous generation, Pasteur, as a faithful son of the Catholic Church, found himself on the right side. Pouchet, too, was supported by those who regarded spontaneous generation as "indispensable for a natural-scientific explanation of the origin of life" (Erik Nordenskiöld, *The History of Biology,* p. 434).

24. Virchow, *Cellular-Pathologie,* pp. 16, 38. Virchow's cellular pathology, like Bichat's tissue pathology, does not fall entirely under the heading of pathological anatomy. Histo-chemistry was an integral part of Bichat's doctrine. So too the chemistry of the cell for Virchow, who stated in 1855 that the functional capacity of cells depended on their "molecular composition," on "physical and chemical alterations of their content." The subsequently one-sided development of cellular pathology was a consequence of the technical imbalance in favor of anatomical over chemical procedures, characteristic of the late nineteenth century and persisting well into the twentieth. Cf. L. J. Rather, "Rudolf Virchow's View on Pathology, Pathological Anatomy, and Cellular Pathology," *A.M.A. Arch. Path.* 82 (1966): 197-204.

25. August Foerster, *Handbuch der pathologischen Anatomie,* vol. 1, *Allgemeine pathologischen Anatomie.*

26. Ibid., p. 78. Foerster quotes here the following postulates, which he attributes to Virchow: "All pathological formations are either degenerations, transformations or repetitions of typical physiological structures"; and *"omnis cellula a cellula."* A bibliographical reference to the essay itself is lacking.

27. Ibid., pp. 77-78.

28. Ibid., p. 77.

29. Ibid., p. 85.

30. Ibid., pp. 84-85.

31. Ibid., p. 85.

32. Ibid., pp. 174-78.

33. Ibid., pp. 180-181.

34. Ibid., p. 207.

35. Ibid., p. 208. On p. 216 Foerster clarifies the matter by stating that the combination of papillary tumor with carcinoma can come about in a twofold manner: firstly, "when a carcinoma develops from a primary, simple or destructive papillary tumor, secondly when a

simple carcinoma acquires a villous or papillary character due to the papillary outgrowth of its stromal meshwork."

36. Ibid., p. 173.

37. Ibid., p. 229.

38. This distinction between "undifferentiated" and "dedifferentiated" cells is implied but not stated by Foerster.

39. A sarcoma, according to Foerster, is a tumor "predominantly made up of embryonal connective tissue elements, here growing as such in an unrestrained [*schrankenlos*] manner, without development into mature connective tissue." On the one hand, sarcomas are related to tumors composed of mature connective tissue elements; on the other, they are closely related to carcinomas, not only because of their like manner of "unrestrained nuclear and cell formation" but also because of their tendency to recur after superficial removal and to disseminate themselves throughout the body (*Handbuch*, p. 219).

40. Cf. ch. 3, n. 149-61 and corresponding text.

41. Rudolf Virchow, "Ueber Perlgeschwuelste (Cholesteatoma Joh. Mueller's)," *Arch. path. Anat. Phys. klin. Med.*, 8 (1855): 371-415.

42. Ibid., p. 414.

43. Ibid., p. 415.

44. Rudolf Virchow, *Die Cellularpathologie in ihrer Begruendung auf physiologische und pathologische Gewebelehre*, 1st ed. p. 355. Emphasis added. A facsimile version of this work was published in 1966 by Georg Olms, Hildesheim. The passage, in slightly different form, will be found on p. 441 of the Dover facsimile of the English translation (first published in 1863) of the second edition, *Cellular Pathology As Based upon Physiological and Pathological Histology*.

45. Cf. ch. 2, notes 30-41 and text.

46. Virchow, *Die Cellularpathologie*, pp. 37-41; *Cellular Pathology*, pp. 69-73. This account is of course no more than Virchow's summation of a long and complicated series of studies and controversies. The investigators had at their disposal neither aniline dyes nor modern microtomes (neither of which was introduced until several decades later). Much of the work was carried out on fresh, relatively unstained tissues. Cf. Rather, *Addison and the White Corpuscles*, Appendix B., pp. 211-16.

47. Virchow, *Die Cellularpathologie*, pp. 25, 26; *Cellular Pathology*, pp. 55, 56.

48. Virchow, *Die Cellularpathologie*, pp. 30, 31; *Cellular Pathology*, pp. 60, 61.

49. Virchow, *Die Cellularpathologie*, pp. 35, 36, 354, 355; *Cellular Pathology*, pp. 66, 67, 440, 441.

50. Remak, *Untersuchungen*, pp. 60, 78, 102, 103.

51. Virchow, *Die Cellularpathologie*, pp. 427-30; *Cellular Pathology*, pp. 527-30.

52. See ch. 3 for Langenbeck's work.

53. Cf. ch. 3, note 113.

54. Robley Dunglison, *Dictionary*, p. 992. The notion of an infectious "ferment" was an inheritance from the iatrochemists; it is most clearly stated in the seventeenth century by Thomas Willis. Cf. L. J. Rather, "Pathology at Mid-Century: A Reassessment of Thomas Willis and Thomas Sydenham," in ed. A. G. Debus, *Medicine in Seventeenth Century England*, pp. 71-112.

55. Virchow, *Die Cellularpathologie*, p. 196; *Cellular Pathology*, pp. 253, 254. Virchow points out here that the lungs are less commonly involved than the liver after the development of a primary breast cancer, contrary to what would be expected if the transfer followed the laws of embolism. On pp. 407 and 408 (*Cellular Pathology*, p. 505) he repeats these comments, adding however that he must "still admit that spread via the vessels possibly depends on a dispersion of cells from the tumors themselves." On p. 168 (*Cellular Pathology*, p. 221) he remarks that when the axillary glands become involved subsequent to cancer of the breast

we must suppose that they have taken up a poisonous substance (*giftigen Stoffes*) from the tumor and that, as in the analogous case of syphilis, after for a time protecting the remainder of the body, the axillary glands then serve as a secondary source for the further spread of that substance.

56. Virchow's collected papers on thrombosis and embolism are conveniently available in his *Gesammelte Abhandlungen zur wissenschaftlichen Medicin* (Frankfurt, 1856; 2d ed., Berlin, 1862). Laennec, Cruveilhier, and Rokitansky, among others, had shown that pulmonary infarcts were frequently associated with blockage of the corresponding arterial branch. At the autopsy table and by means of experiments on animals, Virchow clearly demonstrated that pulmonary arterial blockage in such instances most often resulted from the lodgement of thrombus material thrown off (*emballōn*) from a thrombosed peripheral vein. See Rudolf Beneke, in Ludwig Krehl and Felix Marchand's *Handbuch der allgemeinen Pathologie*, vol. 2, pt. 2, for a historical review of early work on thrombosis and embolism.

57. Virchow, *Die Cellularpathologie*, p. 400; *Cellular Pathology*, pp. 495, 496.

58. Virchow, *Die Cellularpathologie*, pp. 418-24; *Cellular Pathology*, pp. 517-24.

59. Virchow, *Die Cellularpathologie*, pp. 357-59; *Cellular Pathology*, pp. 443-45. Virchow gave Robert Breuer credit for first describing cell division, citing the latter's inaugural dissertation, "Meletemata circa evolutionem ac formas cicatricum" in which the author's serial microscopic studies on the healing of wounds in a variety of tissues were described. According to Breuer, a cytoblastema was present only during the first two or three days; it disappeared after having given rise to cells with distinctly visible nuclei of various shapes. From the third to the fifteenth day the endogenous formation of new nuclei and of new cells was evident, the nuclei first dividing into two or more parts and the cells then breaking up into corresponding parts (*inter tertium ad quindecimum usque diem . . . in cellula primaria nova nuclei formatio cernebatur, nuclei bipartitione aut divisione multiplici cellulas ipsas in partes convenientes dissolvebant*). According to Breuer, once the primary cells have formed from the cytoblastema, new cells are thereafter formed only by nuclear (and cell) division, more rarely by nuclear "disjunction" (*Primis cellulis formatis nova ipsarum formatio nunquam cytoblastemate primario fit. Generatio verum endogena fit divisione aut rarius sejunctione nucleorum*). (The difference between *divisione* and *sejunctione* is not made clear.) Nuclei, described as either opaque or transparent or divided in the middle (*nucleum aut opacum, aut transparentem, aut in centro divisum*), are said to be surrounded by delicate cell envelopes (*involucra*), which break up and disappear when acetic acid is added (*Fines horum globulorum, quamquam tenuissimi, valde distincti sunt, involucrum acido acetico instillatio inflatum, rumpitur et disparet*). Breuer says these cells resemble those described by Gluge as *globuli producti inflammatorii* or *Entzuendungsproduktkugeln*. Undoubtedly many of the cells seen by Breuer were polymorphonuclear leucocytes, and some of them may have been regarded by him as nuclei undergoing division.

60. Virchow, *Die Cellularpathologie*, pp. 410, 411; *Cellular Pathology*, pp. 507, 508.

61. Virchow, *Die Cellularpathologie*, p. 361; *Cellular Pathology*, p. 447.

62. Virchow, *Die Cellularpathologie*, pp. 54-56; *Cellular Pathology*, pp. 88-91.

63. Virchow, *Die Cellularpathologie*, pp. 57-60, 361; *Cellular Pathology*, pp. 92-96, 447. In this connection Virchow notes that histological substitution (*histologische Substitution*) is a phenomenon of common occurrence in the animal kingdom, e.g., one animal has smooth muscle where another has striped; the human sclera consists of connective tissue, that of fish, of cartilage, and so on. "Histological substitution" also occurs under physiological or pathological circumstances in one and the same animal: cylindrical epithelium or ciliated epithelium may be replaced by squamous epithelium, soft epithelium by epidermis (as in the case of vaginal prolapse). Physiological substitution, says Virchow, involves tissues of the same kind (homologous tissues), whereas under pathological circumstances a heterologous tissue may be substituted (*Die Cellularpathologie*, pp. 63, 64; *Cellular Pathology*, pp. 99, 100).

Virchow, we see, is still seeking his term *metaplasia,* as well as emphasizing the plasticity of tissues.

64. Virchow, *Die Cellularpathologie,* pp. 428, 429; *Cellular Pathology,* p. 529.

65. Virchow, *Die Cellularpathologie,* pp. 417, 418; *Cellular Pathology,* pp. 514, 515.

66. Cf. ch. 3, n. 76. Virchow's paper on hyperplastic, nonmalignant epithelial laryngeal growths, designated by him "pachydermia" ("Ueber Pachydermia laryngis," *Berlin. klin. Woch.,* August 8, 1887, pp. 585-89), was occasioned by his involvement in the fatal illness of Friedrich III. Early in 1887 the then Crown Prince first showed signs of the laryngeal lesion that was to bring about his death in 1888. After unsuccessful treatment with a galvano-cautery the German surgeons in charge, Ernst von Bergmann and Karl Gerhardt, concluded in May, 1887, on clinical grounds, that the lesion was probably an epithelioma of malignant nature and advised partial laryngectomy. The Crown Prince being reluctant, advice was sought from the English laryngologist Morell Mackenzie, who asked that a biopsy specimen of the lesion be submitted to microscopic analysis. After examining three successively removed bits of tissue, Virchow found no evidence of cancer and concluded that the lesion was an instance of pachydermia. The operation was therefore not performed. Friedrich III died in June, 1888, by which time the evidence of cancer was unmistakable. Cf. Arend Buchholtz, *Ernst von Bergmann,* 3d ed., pp. 460-504, s.v. "Die Krankheit Kaiser Friedrichs," wherein the terms *Epitheliom* and *Pachydermie* [*sic*] may be found.

67. Rudolf Virchow, *Die krankhaften Geschwuelste.* Only the first twenty-five of the promised thirty lectures appeared in print.

68. Virchow, *Die krankhaften Geschwuelste,* 1: 3. "Wollte man auch Jemand auf das Blut pressen, das er sagen sollte, was Geschwuelste eigentlich seien, so glaube ich nicht, dass man irgend einen lebenden Mensch finden wuerde, der in der Lage waere, dies sagen zu koennen."

69. Ibid., 1: 3, 4. Virchow's account of the historical development of medical thought in respect of the nature of tumors (in the narrower sense) and inflammatory masses is as follows. The older physicians included both under the heading "inflammatory tumors" (*entzuendlichen Geschwuelste*). Because some of these tumors were benign in their clinical behavior, and other malignant, the older physicians spoke of *inflammatio maligna* and *inflammatio benigna.* Two ways of classifying tumors became evident, one "anatomical" and the other "physiological," depending on whether priority was accorded to anatomical structure or to clinical behavior. For practical purposes physicians preferred the latter; they wished also to known the tendency (*Neigung*) of a given tumor, discovered in its early stages, to behave in a benign or malignant manner. This information, insofar as it was available, was at first obtainable only by correlating tumor behavior with tumor structure. Later, attempts were made to distinguish benign from malignant tumors by chemical means; attempts doomed to failure, according to Virchow, because the difference between them was quantitative rather than qualitative (ibid., pp. 5-7).

A great step forward was made toward the end of the eighteenth century, when it was discovered that certain tumors contained tissues, or combinations of tissues, resembling those normally present in the body. John Abernethy, whose *Surgical Observations* was published in German translation (Halle, 1809) by J. F. Meckel, called attention to "pancreaslike" and "breastlike" sarcomas (*pancreasartigen . . . brustdruesenartigen Sarkom*). Bichat's doctrine of tissues then had its effect. Dupuytren (*Bull. Ecole Méd. de Paris* 2 [1805]: 15-17) divided tumors into two groups, those that more or less resemble normal tissues and those that deviate from them. The latter came to be regarded by some workers as parasitic or *sui generis* formations, an idea that, says Virchow, recalls William Harvey's statement in his *De generatione animalium* that cancers, sarcomas, melicerides, and other such tumors are nourished and grow by their own vegetative power, as they weaken and waste away the genuine parts. Since the behavior of parasitic worms in the body of a human host, especially in their cystic stage of development, was not understood, it was possible for John Adams, among others, to espouse the parasitic theory of tumors until well into the nineteenth century. Most investigators, however, preferred to follow Lobstein's development of Hunter and Hewson's notion of the plastic lymph into the idea that homeoplastic tumors arose from "euplastic," and heteroplastic (mostly malignant tumors) from "kakoplastic" lymph. Not until the school of Doellinger began its work in the field of embryology and Schwann and Mueller, using the microscope, identified the ultimate units of both tumors and normal tissues as cells did the possibility of classifying tumors on an anatomical-genetic basis (*anatomisch-genetischen Grundlagen*), i.e., histogenetically, become feasible (ibid., pp. 14-20). Some still entertained the hope that chemists would turn up a specifically cancerous substance in malignant tumors or that microscopists would be able to identify a specifically cancerous, sarcomatous or tuberculous cell. Such investigations should be pursued, but it was unlikely that absolute distinctions would be forthcoming (ibid., pp. 24-26).

Virchow believed that his own "anatomical-genetic" solution to the problem of tumor histogenesis had brought medical thought back in a circle, or rather a spiral, to the notion of the fundamental identity of inflammatory and neoplastic tumors. The difference between the old idea and the new is that all tumors were then thought to result from the mere transfer of humoral substances from one part of the body to another; now they are to be understood as developmental cellular processes. Every tumor is constantly in a state of change (*in jedem Augenblick etwas Werdendes ist*) and has its characteristic life history (*Lebensgeschichte*) or developmental history (*Entwickelungsgeschichte*). Failure to grasp this point leads, says Virchow, to errors in tumor classification, successive stages in the life history of one and the same tumor being mistaken for different tumors (ibid., pp. 73, 74).

70. Ibid., 1: 49. Although Virchow pointed out (pp. 6, 7) that a classification of tumors into malignant and benign was as unscientific as would be a classification of plants into poisonous and edible, he recognized that both procedures were useful in practice.

71. Ibid., 1: 50-52.

72. Ibid., 1: 54-56.

73. Remember that only a small minority of pathologists at this time identified "pus" cells with blood leucocytes. The notion of cells wandering about the body had unfavorable connections with the *cellules vagabondes* and the "intercalatory" theory of tissue nutrition, espoused and subsequently discarded by René Dutrochet and later revived by William Addison. Cf. Rather, *Addison and the White Corpuscles*, pp. 8, 59-68, 155-66.

74. Rudolf Virchow, "Opinion sur la valeur du microscope," *Gaz. hebdomadaire méd. chirur.*, pp. 124-26. The letter is dated February 7, 1855.

75. Eugène Michel, "Du microscope, de ses applications à l'anatomie pathologique, au diagnostic et au traitement des maladies," *Mém. Acad. Roy. de Méd.* (Paris) 21 (1857): 241-442.

76. Ibid., pp. 248, 249, 330, 331.

77. Carl Thiersch, *Der Epithelkrebs, namentlich der Haut* (Leipzig, 1865). Thiersch reported some preliminary findings at the thirty-sixth Congress of German scientists and physicians at Speyer on September 17, 1861. The report, as printed, is brief and inconclusive.

78. Ibid., pp. 90-98.

79. Ibid., pp. 58-60.

80. Ibid., p. 61.

81. Ibid., pp. 41, 66, 67. Thiersch cites Virchow's paper of 1850 (ch. 3, n. 150) and refers to a "primary epithelial cancer of the mandible" reported by Carl Otto Weber (*Chirurgische Erfahrungen und Untersuchungen*, p. 343).

82. Thiersch, *Epithelkrebs*, pp. 42, 43; 66, 67.

83. Ibid., pp. 42, 43. The reference is to Sir James Paget's *Lectures on Surgical Pathology*, 2: 447, 448. According to Paget, there was "no appearance of cancer, or wart of any kind, on the scrotum or penis," yet "abundant epithelial cancer cells" were found in grumous matter expressed from the diseased inguinal nodes.

84. Thiersch, *Epithelkrebs*, p. 43. Thiersch thought it likely that the cancerous degeneration (*Entartung*) of dermoid cysts was responsible for the tumors described by Langenbeck.

85. Ibid., pp. 45-58. Thiersch did not hold that the "transplantation hypothesis" was applicable to all forms of cancer. In the case of melanotic cancer of the skin (*melanotischer Krebs*), his microscopic findings led him to believe that the starting point of secondary deposits was to be sought in "a disturbance of chemical conversion, whereby the parenchymal fluid of the papillae first receives a coloration, to which the histogenetic proliferation succeeds as a secondary process" (ibid., p. 77).

86. Ibid., pp. 78, 79. A history of the role of ideology in nineteenth-century biology remains to be written. See n. 206.

87. Wilhelm His, "Beobachtungen ueber den Bau des Saeugethier-Eierstockes," *Arch. mikr. Anat.* 1 (1865): 151-202.

88. Ibid., pp. 160-63.

89. Theodor Billroth, *Die allgemeine chirurgische Pathologie und Therapie in 50 Vorlesungen.* Lectures 46-50 are devoted to neoplastic diseases (*Geschwulstkrankheiten*). On pp. 579, 580 Billroth states that cells can arise only from preexistent cells, and that of all cells in the body the connective tissue cells are most disposed toward division. Hence, they are the original source of tumors and new-formations of all kinds, e.g., inflammatory new-formations. Sarcomatous diseases (*Sarkomkrankheiten*) differ from carcinomatous diseases (*Carcinomkrankheiten*) in that they run a less rapid course and seldom involve the neighboring lymph nodes (p. 586). Billroth prefers the term *epithelial carcinoma* (*Epithelialcarcinom*) to *cancroid*, since the lesions in question arise "in consequence of the clusterlike proliferation of connective tissue cells, just as do other cancers"; the pseudoacinous, glandlike formations present in certain epithelial cancers do not arise, as he had once believed, from the epithelium of sweat glands, sebaceous glands, or the rete Malpighii (pp. 670, 677). It would be difficult otherwise to explain their presence in primary epithelial carcinoma of the tibia (one instance of which Billroth had seen) and other sites remote from normal glandular epithelium (pp. 675, 677). Billroth's views on the subject of cancroid are very close to those of Virchow, except that he considers epithelial pearls (*globules épidermiques, Epidermiskugeln*) to be formations "quite peculiar to epithelial carcinoma" (p. 677), whereas Virchow described them in benign growths. Billroth's belief in the influence of mental or emotional disturbances on the course of cancerous diseases is worth noting (p. 683).

90. Billroth, "Kritische und erlaeuternde Bemerkungen zu dem Werke von Professor C. Thiersch in Erlangen," *Arch. klin. Chirur.* 7 (1866): 848-59.

91. Ibid., p. 850-51.

92. Billroth, *Die allgemeine chirurgische Pathologie*, p. 656.

93. Billroth, "Kritische und erlaeuternde Bemerkungen," p. 855.

94. Ibid., pp. 852-53.

95. Friedrich von Recklinghausen, "Ueber Eiter- und Bindegewebeskoerperchen," *Arch. path. Anat. Phys. klin. Med.* 28 (1863): 157-97.

96. Cf. Wilhelm Preyer, "Ueber amoeboide Blutkoerperchen," *Arch. path. Anat. Phys. klin. Med.* 30 (1864): 417-44, for a contemporary review of studies by Ernst Haeckel, Max Schultze, Virchow, von Recklinghausen, and others on the movements of ameboid cells, including the engulfing of particulate matter.

97. Von Recklinghausen, "Bindegewebeskoerperchen," p. 187.

98. Julius Cohnheim, "Ueber Entzuendung und Eiterung," *Arch. path. Anat. Phys. klin. Med.* 40 (1867): 1-79.

99. Julius Cohnheim, *Neue Untersuchungen ueber die Entzuendung* (Berlin, 1873).

100. Cf. Rather, *Addison and the White Corpuscles*, Appendix C pp. 217-27. In *Leçons sur les humeurs normales et morbides du corps de l'homme* (Paris, 1874), Robin accepted Cohnheim's view of inflammation, with the reservation that in nonvascular tissues white cells arose from a blastema (pp. 378-83).

101. Charles Robin, "Mémoire sur les divers modes de la naissance de la substance organisée en général," *J. anat. phys.*, 1864, pp. 152-83; ibid., 1865, pp. 113-52.

102. André-Victor Cornil, "Mémoire sur les tumeurs épithéliales du col de l'utérus," *J. anat. phys.*, 1864, pp. 472-507. The citations are from p. 496.

103. Ibid., 1865, pp. 266-76, 476-96. Thiersch is referred to on p. 491.

104. Louis Řanvier and André-Victor Cornil, "Contributions à l'étude de développement histologique des tumeurs épithéliales," *J. anat. phys.*, 1866, pp. 271-86. The authors refer to the cases of supposedly primary cancroid of bone described by Rudolf Virchow ("Ueber Kankroide") and by Carl Otto Weber (in his *Chirurgische Erfahrungen und Untersuchungen*, p. 343) and state that their case falls into a different category, since it was associated with an osteomyelitic sinus.

105. The terms *ectoderm, endoderm*, and *mesoderm* were in use in this sense by 1875. Cf. Jane Oppenheimer, "The Non-Specificity of the Germ-Layers," *Quart. Rev. Biol.* 15 (1940): 1-27.

106. Wilhelm His, *Die Haeute und Hoehlen des Koerpers.* The passage reads as follows: "The layer of cells covering serous and vascular spaces is usually designated *epithelium.* The same term is applied to the inner surfaces of articular membranes and the reverse side of the horny skin. But all cell layers facing the interior spaces of the middle germ layer have among themselves so much in common, and, from the time of their first appearance, differ so strikingly from layers of cells arising from the two peripheral germ layers that we would do well, in the interest of physiological understanding, to distinguish them by means of a special term, whether we contrast them as *false [unaechte] epithelia* with the *true*, or call them *endothelia*, in order to express their relationship to the inner surfaces of the body with this term" (pp. 17, 18). Later, the term *mesothelium* replaced *endothelium*, except in the case of blood and lymph vessels. Commenting on these two terms in 1899, Felix Marchand observed that the etymological meaning had been almost wholly lost, insofar as Frederik Ruysch's use of *thêlê* (nipple or papilla) was concerned ("Ueber die Beziehungen der pathologischen Anatomie zur Entwickelungsgeschichte, besonders der Keimblattlehre," *Verh. deutsch. path. Gesell.*, 1899, pp. 38-107). Cf. ch. 3, note 41, on the term *epithelium.*

107. Thiersch, *Epithelialkrebs*, p. ii.

108. Oskar Wyss, "Die heterologen (boesartigen) Neubildungen der Vorsteherdruese," *Arch. path. Anat. Phys. klin. Med.* 35 (1866): 378-412.

109. Bernard Naunyn, "Ueber die Entwicklung der Leberkrebse," *Arch. Anat. Phys. wiss. Med.*, 1866, pp. 717-33.

110. Ibid.

111. Carl Otto Weber, "Ueber die Entwickelung des Epithelkrebses in inneren Organen, nebst Bemerkungen ueber die Structur der Leber und Lunge," *Arch. path. Anat. Phys. klin. Med.* 29 (1864): 163-89.

112. Ibid. Weber refers here to the *growth*, not the *accumulation*, of transported pus corpuscles.

113. Edwin Klebs, "Bemerkungen ueber Larynx-Geschwuelste," *Arch. path. Anat. Phys. klin. Med.* 38 (1867): 202-20, cf. p. 213.

114. Ibid., p. 214.

115. Ibid., p. 217.

116. Ibid., pp. 216, 217.

117. Ibid., pp. 213, 216, 217.

118. Theodor Langhans, "Ueber Krebs und Cancroid der Lunge, nebst einem Anhang ueber Corpora amylacea in der Lunge," *Arch. path. Anat. Phys. klin. Med.* 38 (1867): 497-543.

119. Ibid., pp. 550, 551. Langhans states here that only *one* (table 6, fig. 5) illustration in Thiersch's book carries conviction.

120. Ibid., p. 535.

121. Ibid., p. 511.

122. Ibid., pp. 527, 534, 535.

123. Ludwig Buhl, "Wahre recidivirendes Myom (Rhabdomyom Zenker's)," *Z. Biol.* 1 (1865): 263-72.

124. Ibid., pp. 270, 271. Buhl refers to p. 74 of Friedrich Zenker's *Ueber die Veraenderungen der willkuerlichen Muskeln im Typhus.*

125. Ibid., p. 263. Buhl refers to August Weismann's paper "Ueber das Wachsen der quergestreiften Muskeln nach Beobachtungen am Frosch." *Z. rationelle Med.* vol. 3, ser. 9 (1861): 263-84. For Weismann's theory see August Weismann, *Das Keimplasma: Eine Theorie der Vererbung,* esp. pp. 76, 77.

126. Carl Otto Weber, "Ueber die Betheiligung der Muskelkoerperchen und der quergestreiften Muskeln an den Neubildungen nebst Bemerkungen ueber die Lehre von der Specificitaet der Gewebselements," *Arch. path. Anat. Phys. klin. Med.* 39 (1867): 254-69, esp. pp. 267, 268. See also Weber, s.v. "Ueber die Neubildung quergestreiften Muskelfasern, insbesondere die regenerative Neubildung derselben nach Verletzungen," ibid., pp. 216-53, esp. pp. 221, 222.

127. Wilhelm Waldeyer, "Die Entwickelung der Carcinome," *Arch. path. Anat. Phys. klin. Med.* 41 (1867): 470-523.

128. Ibid., p. 470.

129. Ibid., pp. 471-76.

130. Ibid., p. 484.

131. Ibid., pp. 470-84, 510-16. On p. 489 Waldeyer credits Cornil with having described the *begleitende* proliferation of small cells as an "essential attribute of malignant epithelial tumors." The modern histopathologist would be inclined to identify these small cells as lymphocytes, possibly reactive, the more so in view of Waldeyer's statement (p. 501) that in skin cancer the *einleitende* form is very frequently absent, whereas the *begleitende* form is always present as a small-cell accumulation bordering the margins of the cancer.

132. Ibid., pp. 485-87, 496.

133. Ibid., pp. 505-9.

134. Ibid., p. 514.

135. Ibid., pp. 503, 504, 516-18.

136. Ibid., pp. 483, 500, 512.

137. Ibid., pp. 502-5.

138. Differential staining (*Farbenanalyse*) with aniline dyes was introduced by Paul Ehrlich in 1877 and employed by him in the study of white cells in blood smears. See Rather, *Addison and the White Corpuscles,* pp. 211-16. Goldmann, in 1892, applied Ehrlich's procedures (for the first time, he says) in pathological histology. (E. E. Goldmann, "Beitrag zu der Lehre von dem 'malignen Lymphom,'" *Centrb. allg. path. Anat.* 3 [1892]: 665-90).

139. At the first session of the *Deutsche Gesellschaft fuer Pathologie,* in 1898, Virchow warned his colleagues that pathology was being developed in a one-sided, morphological direction. To look at a glass slide and say "endocarditis" was, he commented, like looking at a burnt-out match and saying "fire." At the twenty-fifth session, in 1930, Robert Roessle repeated Virchow's warning and commented that it had been of no avail: pathology was still developing one-sidedly along the line of least resistance. Cf. L. J. Rather, "Rudolf Virchow's Views on Pathology, Pathological Anatomy, and Cellular Pathology," *Arch. Path.* 82 (1966): 197-204.

140. See Norman F. Moon, "Adamantinoma of the Appendicular Skeleton. A Statistical Review of Reported Cases and Inclusion of Ten New Cases," *Clin. Orth.* 43 (1965): 189-213. Moon assembled ninety-one cases from the world literature since 1900.

141. Wilhelm Waldeyer, "Die Entwickelung der Carcinome," *Arch. path. Anat. Phys. klin. Med.* 55 (1872): 67-159. This is the second and concluding half of Waldeyer's essay on the

histogenesis of carcinoma. Cf. pp. 140-42; 148, 149.

142. Richard Volkmann, "Die Krankheiten der Bewegungsorgane," in *Handbuch der allgemeinen und speciellen Chirurgie,* ed. Franz von Pitha and Theodor Billroth (Stuttgart, 1865-1882), vol. 2, bk. 2/1. Cf. pp. 467, 468.

143. In 1859 Robin called attention to a peculiar fibrous tumor arising from the tooth follicle and marked by the presence of "star-shaped fibroplastic bodies furnished with two to five pale prolongations on the periphery of the nucleus, as in the dental pulp and the enamel organ of the fetus" (Charles Robin, "Sur une variété particulière de tumeur fibreuse provenant du follicule dentaire," *Bull. acad. méd.* 24 [1858-59]: 1205-11). In 1862 he again discussed this tumor, "formed at the expense of the tissue of the dental bulb," and commented on the presence of "corps fibro-plastiques étoilés. . .comme dans la pulpe dentaire et l'organe de l'émail chez le foitus" (Robin, "Mémoire sur une espèce de tumeur formée aux dépens du tissue des bulbes dentaires," *Compt. rend. soc. biol.* vol. 4, ser. 3 (1862): 199-221. (The reader will by now be familiar with the meaning of Robin's phrase "at the expense of," i.e., the tumor cells are *not* thought to be derived directly from those of a tooth germ but by way of an intermediary blastema.

The histogenesis of dental tumors was treated in great detail by Malassez in 1885; he, too, called attention to and beautifully illustrated cells of a "forme étoilée ou adamantine" in certain of these tumors (Louis-Charles Malassez, "Sur le rôle des débris épithéliaux paradentaires," *Arch. Phys.* 5 [1885]: 309-40; ibid. 6 [1885]: 379-449). In 1887 Albarran reported an "adamantine epithelioma" involving the maxillary sinus; he derived it from paradental epithelial debris. The following comment by Albarran is of interest: "We shall not pause at the hypothesis that epithelium forms at the expense of connective tissue, for even if certain epithelial elements perhaps have a mesodermal origin, we cannot admit that epithelium so clearly of ectodermal nature, and of a differentiation so clearly marked as adamantine epithelium, can originate all of a piece in the midst of connective tissue" (L. Albarran, "Épithélioma adamantin du sinus maxillaire," *Compt. Rend. Soc. Biol.* vol. 4, ser. 8 (1887): 618-21; Épithélioma adamantin du maxillaire supérieure," ibid. 4 [1887]: 667-71). The phrase "at the expense of" here probably no longer implies an intermediary blastema; we see also that the mesodermal origin of true epithelium is now admitted as a possibility.

For additional older literature on the subject of dental adamantinomas and related tumors see Oskar Roemer, "Die Pathologie der Zaehne," in *Handbuch der speziellen pathologischen Anatomie und Histologie,* ed. Friedrich Henke and Otto Lubarsch (Berlin, 1928), vol. 4, bk. 2, pp. 489-92.

144. Otto Hildebrand, "Ueber das tubulaere Angiosarkom oder Endotheliom des Knochens," *Deutsche Z. Chirur.* 31 (1900-1901): 263-81. Hildebrand spells the name *Sudhof.* See note 146 for Carola Maier's comment on Sudhoff's case. See also Léon Thévenot, "Des endothéliomes des os," *Rev. Chirur.* 21 (1900): 756-79, and William T. Howard, Jr., and George W. Crile, "A Contribution to the Knowledge of Endothelioma and Perithelioma of Bone," *Ann. Surg.* 42 (1905): 358-93.

145. Carola Maier, "Ein primaeres Plattenepithelcarcinom der Ulna," *Beitr. z. klin. Chirur.* 26 (1900): 513-36.

146. Ibid. As *possible* instances she mentions: (1) Karl Sudhoff ("Ueber das primaere multiple Carcinom des Knochensystems," *Inaug. Diss.,* Erlangen, 1875) describes a thirty-two-year-old man with multiple carcinomas of the skeleton, no primary tumor found at autopsy. (2) Otto Lubarsch (*Ergeb. allg. Path. Anat.* [1895], vol. 2, bk. 2, p. 443) cites a tumor of the sacrum resembling under the microscope a carcinoma cylindroepitheliale adenomatosum of the gut, explained by Lubarsch as a tumor arising from "epithelial germs" displaced from the primitive gut to the medullary cavity during embryonic development. (3) Kumar ("Zur Pathologie des Schultergelenks," *Wien. med. Blaett.,* no. 41) described a case of medullary cancer of the head of the humerus with metastases in the lung. Maier, however, commented

that a "primary carcinoma of the lung could well have been present, although such a tumor is unusual." (4) *Virchow-Hirsch Jahresbericht* (1879, 1: 270) gives an account of two cases reported by W. J. Walsham in *St. Barth. Hosp. Rep.* 15 (1879): 111-18. Walsham's paper, entitled "On the Osseous Tumours of Bone Formerly Called Osteoid Cancers," is an account of two specimens from the museum at St. Bartholomew's: (1) a thirty-two-year-old man with "osteoid cancer" of the lower end of the femur and a "hard cancer impregnated with earthy salts" in the pleura; (2) a twenty-four-year-old man with "osteoid cancer" of the lower end of the humerus and tumor deposits in the right lung, liver, and kidneys. Walsham thought that both were instances of primary carcinoma of bone. He states that those who hold with Thiersch and Waldeyer that carcinoma is essentially an epithelial growth "deny that primary carcinoma does or ever can occur in bone" and affirm that in all cases so reported the real primary has been overlooked.

147. Ibid. Maier refers to Cohnheim as the proponent of the "embryonal germ" displacement theory and to Hugo Ribbert as the proponent of the rival or supplementary theory she herself prefers in this instance.

148. Bernhard Fischer (Fischer-Wasels), "Ueber ein primaeres Adamantinom der Tibia," *Frankfurt. Z. Path.* 12 (1913): 422-41.

149. Ibid. p. 437. Fischer's complete statement of his theoretical position, based on the latest developments in experimental embryology, is as follows:

The nature of embryonal development is such that progressive cell division goes hand in hand with progressive differentiation of cells, i.e., the potencies of individual cells for tissue formation become ever more restricted throughout the course of embryonal development. Specifically, experimental investigations (Thomas Morgan, Hans Driesch) on sea-urchin eggs have shown that at the moment when ectoderm and endoderm have been formed—at the gastrula stage, that is—the potency of cells of these two germ layers is at once restricted, in such a way that from then on they are capable of forming elements and derivatives of their own germ layer only, whereas in the blastula stage all cells of the germ are still capable of forming both ectoderm and endoderm. Despite this restriction in the gastrula stage, all components of the endoderm are still capable of forming all tissues in general arising from endoderm, and the same is of course true for the outer germ layer. Thus, the primary rudiment of the gut can form rudiments of pancreas not only where the pancreas arises, but anywhere along the entire course of the intestinal canal as well. But once the pancreas is fully formed, the prospective potency of the remaining endodermal cells of the intestinal canal for forming pancreas is lost.

Mutatis mutandis, the same would apply to epidermal cells: once the tooth-germ or dental rudiment had been formed, the remaining epidermal cells would lose the "potency" for forming dental tissue.

150. C. S. Richter, "Ein Fall von adamantinomartiger Geschwulst des Schienbeins," *Z. Krebsforsch.* 32 (1930): 272-79.

151. Arnold Lauche, "Zur Kenntnis von Pathologie u. Klinik der Geschwuelste mit synovialmembranartigem Bau (Synovialome oder synovial Endothelio-Fibrome und Sarkome)," *Frankfurt. Z. Path.* 59 (1947): 2-29. Lauche cited Brunner's medical dissertation (Zurich, 1936), stating that the work had been directed by E. Uehlinger.

152. J. Douglas Hicks, "Synovial Sarcoma of the Tibia," *J. Path. Bact.* 67 (1954): 151-61. The new case was that of a tibial tumor, diagnosed by X-ray as a "bone cyst," in a seventy-year-old woman; under the microscope the tumor proved to be a "well-differentiated fibrosarcoma with synovial and squamous development." The other case was that of a tibial tumor in a twenty-one-year-old woman. The tumor had recurred several times. Finally, the patient was treated by "excision of the lower two-thirds of the tibia, boiling it and replacing

it." After five years there had been no recurrence of tumor. See note 144 for literature on endothelioma of bone.

153. H. Lederer and A. J. Sinclair, "Malignant Synovioma Simulating 'Adamantinoma of the Tibia,'" *J. Path. Bact.* 67 (1954): 163-68.

154. G. W. Changus, J. S. Speed, and Fred Stewart, "Malignant Angioblastoma of Bone: A Reappraisal of Adamantinoma of Long Bone," *Cancer* 10 (1957): 540-49.

155. F. Gloor, "Das sogenannte Adamantinom der langen Rohrenknochen," *Arch. path. Anat. Phys. klin. Med.* 336 (1963): 489-502.

156. J. Albores Saavedra, D. Díaz Gutiérrez, and M. Altamirano Dimas, "Adamantinoma de la tibia. Observaciones ultraestructurales," *Rev. Méd. Hosp. Gen. México* 31 (1968): 241-52. Tonofibrils and desmosomes are shown in their electron micrographs.

157. Juan Rosai, "Adamantinoma of the Tibia. Electron Microscopic Evidence of its Epithelial Origin," *Am. J. Clin. Path.* 51 (1969): 786-92. Note the implied inference from cell type to cell of origin, made on the assumption *omnis cellula a cellula ejusdem naturae.*

158. Ibid., p. 791.

159. Harlan J. Spjut, et al., *Tumors of Bone and Cartilage,* AFIP Atlas of Tumor Pathology, 2d ser. (Bethesda: 1971) fasc. 5, pp. 315-23. Spjut reviewed Rosai's light microscope sections and electron micrographs.

160. W. G. MacCallum, *A Textbook of Pathology,* 6th ed., p. 1025. The statement occurs in all editions, from the first (1916) through the seventh (1940).

161. Leslie Foulds, *Neoplastic Development,* 1: 139. "The undertones of retrospection inherent in histogenetic classifications of tumours," writes Foulds, "are distasteful to myself; if strictly applied the classification can be misleading or worse. . . when used moderately, as by [Rupert] Willis for example, they are less objectionable although, in my view, not particularly helpful" (1: 95).

162. A. von Albertini, *Histologische Geschwulstdiagnostik.* The concept of histogenesis has a threefold character, according to von Albertini: (1) the tissue of origin of a given tumor; (2) the tissue *Anlagen,* or pathological rests, from which certain tumors are thought to take origin; and (3) the lineage (*Herkunft*) of the tumor cells. The first of these three refers to "histogenesis in the narrower sense"; the notion that tumor tissue arises *de novo* or is derived from an undifferentiated mesenchymal stem cell being inacceptable, we must consider, as a working hypothesis (*Arbeitshypothese*), that a given tumor arises from tissue resembling it at the site where the tumor first makes its appearance in the body. The second of the three is, according to von Albertini, largely a theoretical problem, the supporting data being meager. The third, on the other hand, presents us with an actual problem, that of the cytogenesis of the tumor cells. And, says von Albertini, hematology has taught us how cautious we must be in drawing conclusions in regard to cell lineages. Hematology, moreover, "has the great advantage over the study of tumors in that the cell types in question are more or less constant and standardized. And yet it seems impossible for the various investigators to reach agreement regarding cell lineages; not even for the array of granulocytes has this been achieved, let alone for the rarer cell forms, such as plasma cells, monocytes, and so on. If this is not possible even in the case of so-called normal cells, how should it be possible in the first instance with respect to inconstant tumor cells and their countless variants! The cause of this difficulty, in the final analysis, is that it is in general not possible to set forth the precise lineage of a tumor cell" (pp. 4, 5). Returning to the subject in 1956, von Albertini again emphasized the frequently overlooked distinction between an objective histological description and the subjective interpretation, the "histogenetic hypothesis," drawn from the data (von Albertini, "Allgemeine Systematik der Geschwuelste," in vol. 6/3 of *Handbuch der allgemeinen Pathologie,* ed. F. Buechner, E. Letterer, and F. Roulet, cf. pp. 4, 5).

Rupert Willis, whom von Albertini (*Handbuch,* 6: 5) calls "a rather unreserved defender of histogenetic classification," stated in the first edition (1948) of his book on tumors that

MacCallum's criticism of the histogenetic basis of tumor classification was "groundless." Citing it in part, he comments: "Such a statement from an experienced pathologist is incomprehensible." On the contrary, "the evidence for the origin of tumours from their specific normal counterparts is, for most classes of neoplasms, precise and conclusive; 'good guesses' are unnecessary" (Rupert Willis, *Pathology of Tumours,* 1st ed., p. 12). Although this passage does not appear in the fourth (1967) and last edition of the book, Willis remained convinced of the validity of his position. The way in which he states it, however, shows a certain lack of comprehension of the issues raised by MacCallum and von Albertini and, later, by Foulds. "Unquestionably," Willis wrote in 1967, "the fundamental basis of scientific classification is histogenetic, *that is according to the tissues from which tumours arise and of which they consist"* [emphasis added]. He went on to say that a tumor should be named and classified according to the nature of the tissue from which it is derived, at the same time expressing his agreement with F. B. Mallory, citing the latter's statement that "tumors are classified like normal tissues on a histologic basis. . . . The type of cell is the one important element in every tumor. From it the tumor should be named." Willis recognized that "by metaplasia a tumour may come to consist, partly or wholly, of tissue or tissues unlike its tissue of origin." He believes, nevertheless, that uncertainty regarding the tissue of origin "now obtains with only a few kinds of tumours." On the other hand, Willis rejects attempts to classify tumors on what he calls an "embryological basis." To try to do so lays a "wholly unwarrantable emphasis on the germ-layer derivation of the tissues from which tumours arise. . . . *Indeed the germ-layers, the status of which has of recent years greatly declined even for the embryologist, are devoid of significance for the pathologist."* He quotes with approval James Ewing's assertion that oncology is not a department of embryology, but a separate chapter in the biology of the cell *(Pathology of Tumours,* 4th ed., pp. 9-14).

Willis's views on adamantinoma of the tibia may be of interest to the reader. He rejects the view that the tumors are in fact synoviomas or angiosarcomas; while noncommittal with respect to the various hypotheses for their epithelial derivation, he states that the eight examples he examined were, like many of the reported instances, "plainly epithelial" (ibid., pp. 288, 289).

163. Wilhelm Waldeyer, "Die Entwickelung der Carcinome," *Arch. path. Anat. Phys. klin. Med.* 55 (1872): 67-159. See p. 141.

164. Ibid., pp. 70-73. Writing in 1870, Classen had argued that the small round cells found adjacent to growing carcinomas (Waldeyer's *begleitende Bindegewebswucherung*) were on their way to becoming epithelial cancer cells. Their source was the lymph stream. He (and others, including Klebs) had observed transitions from simple lymphoid cells to epithelial cancer cells. The development of a primary epithelial carcinoma probably took place as follows, according to Classen: "In a hyperemic zone—usually one that has been hyperemic for years—covered by a layer of epithelium or epidermis, arise masses of small round cells which in all likelihood have moved out of the vessels, and, in any case, primarily follow the course of blood vessels, until they begin to loosen up the meshes of the connective tissue stroma, as they grow into epithelial forms." Of the Waldeyer-Thiersch epithelial theory, Classen acutely remarked: "The theory is not drawn from experience; on the contrary, experience has had to bring itself in line with the theory of specific cell descent." And with respect to Waldeyer's rejoinder to Weber's call for a reagent to distinguish true epithelial cells from connective tissue cells—namely, that keratinization of epithelial cells amounted to such a reagent—Classen noted that keratinization served only to distinguish the *later* developmental stages of the cells in question ("Ueber ein Cancroid der Cornea und Sclera, ein Beitrag zur Entwickelungsgeschichte der Carcinome," *Arch. path. Anat. Phys. klin. Med.* 50 [1870]: 56-79).

165. Ibid., pp. 73-76. Although Waldeyer agreed in principle with Virchow's postulate that all cells were derived from preexistent cells he was not convinced that complete cells,

i.e., single, nucleated cells, alone had this capability: "Nevertheless, as far as we know at present, new tissue always presupposes a similarly constituted germinal tissue (*Keimgewebe*), the "germinal matter" or "bioplasm" of L. Beale, whether this be in the form of complete, separate cells or as formless, diffuse protoplasm with nuclei scattered throughout" (cf. n., p. 73).

166. Ibid., pp. 74-77. Waldeyer's book on the embryology of the ovary, *Eierstock und Ei*, is mentioned here. His's revision of Remakian germ-layer doctrine first appeared in his *Untersuchungen ueber die erste Anlage des Wirbelthierleibes*. Sixteen years later His gave an account—"Die Lehre vom Bindesubstanzkeim (Parablast). Rueckblick nebst kritischer Besprechung einiger neuerer entwickelungsgeschichtlicher Arbeiten," *Arch. Anat. Entwickelungsgeschichte*, 1882, pp. 62-108—of the course of his thought since his first attempt, in 1865, to correlate histology and embryology (*Die Haeute und Hoehlen des Koerpers*). In 1865 he had derived connective tissue in all its forms, blood, and smooth and striated muscle from the middle germ layer, and coined the term *endothelium* to distinguish the epitheliallike cells of the vascular system and serous cavities from the true epithelium stemming from the outer and inner germ layers. Shortly afterward he abandoned this view of things for his doctrine of the archiblast and parablast. He now held that true epithelium, glands (not including the so-called lymph glands), muscle, and nerves were derivatives of the archiblast, while all other cells and tissues, including of course endothelium, were of parablastic, that is, extraembryonal, origin. From the beginning he had been convinced that epithelial cells could not be derived from connective tissue cells ("Die Lehre," pp. 61-67, 107).

A full account of developments in embryology during the second half of the nineteenth century is beyond the scope of the present book. In 1885 Waldeyer brought the subject up to date in his relatively brief but clear and complete review, "Die neúreren Forschungen im Gebiete der Keimblattlehre," *Deutsche med. Woch.* 85 (1885): 305-16. As he had done in 1872, Waldeyer again rejected His's claim that the so-called parablastic tissues were *not* derived from the cleavage cells of the egg by way of the three recognized germ layers. Waldeyer's explanation of His's findings in that review is as follows: In meroblastic eggs, as he, E. Ray Lankester, and others have observed, particles of the mass of cells formed by cleavage of the original egg cell extend from the periphery of the developing germ into the white yolk, or *Nahrungsdotter*, as germ-processes (*Keimfortsaetzen*). It was from these extensions of the germinal mass (His's archiblast) into the white yolk, rather than from the white yolk itself, that blood and connective tissues developed.

167. Waldeyer, "Die Entwickelung der Carcinome," pp. 78, 85, 151, 152.

168. Ibid., pp. 79, 83. Von Recklinghausen ("Ueber Eiter- und Bindegewebskoerperchen") devised a moist chamber attached to the microscope objective above and the glass slide below for his studies on "wandering" cells. Max Schultze, in 1865, added to this a microscope stage heated by an alcohol flame ("Ein heizbarer Objekttisch und seine Verwendung bei Untersuchungen des Blutes," *Arch. mikr. Anat.* 1 [1865]: 1-42). Presumably Waldeyer used something of the sort in his own studies. Despite Waldeyer's lack of success, the technique was perfectly adequate (given the right observational material) for the purpose. In the latter half of the 1870s Walther Flemming used it to describe in detail the sequences of mitotic division in living, unstained dermal epithelial cells of the larval salamander. See Rather, *Addison and the White Corpuscles*, for reproductions of the original illustrations from papers by Recklinghausen, Schultze, and Flemming.

169. Ibid., p. 79. At a hint from Virchow, Cohnheim, in 1867, credited (incorrectly) William Addison with the first description, in 1849, of white cell emigration ("Ueber Entzuendung," pp. 57, 58). The passage of white cells through intact vascular walls had, however, been fairly accurately described and depicted by Augustus Waller in 1846. Waller's work was recalled, in connection with that of Cohnheim, by English and Austrian investigators in 1868. See Rather, *Addison and the White Corpuscles*, for details.

170. Ibid., pp. 79, 80. The already considerable literature on the subject of the supposed metamorphoses of emigrated white cells was reviewed in 1869 by Arnold Heller in his dissertation, "Untersuchungen ueber die feineren Vorgaenge bei der Entzuendung" (Erlangen, 1869). For comments on Heller's dissertation, see Rather, "Virchow und die Entwicklung," pp. 170, 171; and Rather, *Addison and the White Corpuscles,* pp. 167-69. These claims amounted to a revival of the idea, championed by William Addison in the 1840s, that tissue growth, maintenance, and repair were mediated by colorless, "embryonal" blood cells, which passed from the blood into the tissues as needed and underwent appropriate transformations.

171. Ibid., pp. 141-45.

172. Ibid., pp. 145, 146.

173. Ibid., p. 144. Waldeyer refers here to a *Handbuch der pathologischen Anatomie* (p. 104), presumably by Maier. The reference may be to Maier's *Lehrbuch der allgemeinen pathologischen Anatomie.*

174. Waldeyer, pp. 142, 143. The citation is credited to Rudolf Maier's "Zwei Faelle von Cylinder-Epitheliom, etc.," *Jenaische Z. Med. Naturw.* 6/3: 456ff.

175. Waldeyer, pp. 146-48.

176. Cf. ch. 4, n. 164.

177. Waldeyer, "Die Entwickelung der Carcinome," pp. 152-55.

178. Ibid., pp. 131-33, 136, 151.

179. Julius Cohnheim, *Neue Untersuchungen ueber die Entzuendung,* p. 84. The reference is to Klebs's *Beitraege zur pathologischen Anatomie der Schusswunden.*

180. Julius Cohnheim, *Vorlesungen ueber allgemeine Pathologie,* 1: 247.

181. For these and other developments in bacteriology at the time see William Bulloch, *The History of Bacteriology.*

182. Cf. Max Neuburger, *Die Lehre von der Heilkraft der Natur im Wandel der Zeiten;* also Rather, *Addison and the White Corpuscles,* pp. 179-93, and "Some Aspects of the Theory and Therapy of Inflammation: From William Harvey to Clemens von Pirquet," *Proceedings of the 22d International Congress of the History of Medicine,* 1: 8-12.

183. Rudolf Virchow, *Handbuch der speciellen Pathologie und Therapie* (Berlin, 1854), 1: 46-94. Cf. L. J. Rather, "Virchow und die Entwicklung," pp. 165, 166.

184. Cohnheim, *Vorlesungen* (Berlin, 1877), 1: 191-306.

185. Cohnheim, *Vorlesungen,* 2d ed. (Berlin, 1882), 1: 232-367. See also *Addison and the White Corpuscles,* pp. 172-78.

186. For the literature and further comment on this subject see Rather, *Addison and the White Corpuscles,* pp. 179-93.

187. In Cohnheim's *Vorlesungen* (1877), 1: 685, the following statement is made: "If now, in conclusion, we want to set forth the significance of tumors for the organism, you will recall that I have specially emphasized the fact that *they are eo ipso incapable of any work, any function.* A tumor, consequently, can never be of use to its bearer, and so much the more can it be of harm."

188. Julius Cohnheim, "Congenitales, quergestreiftes Muskelsarcom der Nieren," *Arch. path. Anat. Phys. klin. Med.* 65 (1875): 64-69.

189. Cohnheim, *Vorlesungen* (1877), 1: 622-28. Cohnheim's words here are of interest. For coverage of the retention tumors he refers his readers to Virchow's "great work" on tumors. He then adds: "But if we separate these from the true tumors, there remain only those that have been regarded, since ancient times, as the genuine [*eigentlichen*] pseudoplasms, neoplasms, or growths [*Pseudo- oder Neoplasmen oder Gewaechse*]. We have, however, on grounds that I have developed for you in detail...decided to withdraw separately still another highly important group of new formations, namely, the infectious tumors, from the other growths, and thus once again considerably to narrow the field." In a narrower sense, the term *infectious tumors* applied especially to syphilis, tuberculosis, leprosy, glanders, and "lupus."

Cohnheim believed that the histogenesis of the infectious tumors was bound up with the inflammatory process. He stated, however, that the source of the cells of these tumors was not yet clear; the "emigration hypothesis" did not necessarily account for them all, and it remained an open question "whether the infectious tumors are more closely related to the infectious inflammations or to the infectious hypertrophies, or whether an as yet still unknown intermediary position between the two must be reserved for them, in accordance with their nature" (pp. 618, 619).

190. Ibid., pp. 633-35. Cohnheim makes reference here neither to his own explanation of the presence of striated muscle fibers nor to Remak's derivation of tibial cancroid from an embryonal *Abschnuerung* of epidermis, but to Georg Albert Luecke's account of the histogenesis of dermoid (*Dermoide*) tumors of the subcutaneous tissues, orbit, mouth region, testes, and ovaries. Luecke had postulated the occurrence, during embryonic life, of outer germ-layer inclusions in certain of these tissues, which later became the starting point for the dermoids; he himself was simply broadening the scope of Luecke's hypothesis to cover *all* tumors. Luecke's hypothesis, which appeared in his essay "Die Lehre von den Geschwuelsten in anatomischer und klinischer Beziehung," in von Pitha and Billroth's *Handbuch der allgemeinen und speciellen Chirurgie*, vol. 2/1, was, like that of Remak before him, an explanation of the structure rather than the growth of a certain kind of tumor, i.e., it was a morphological rather than an etiological hypothesis. Luecke's remarks on dermoids of the genital organs are revealing: "Since the investigations of His have shown that testes and ovaries belong to the outer germ layer, the occurrence there of dermoids is no longer surprising; the genesis of teeth can also be explained at need. Yet it must freely be admitted here that at the moment we are in no position to understand the complex relations that must enter in so as to include these dermoids of the testes and ovaries. We might perhaps say that in the complicated path the organs named take in their development, still other germs than those of epithelium are included and participate in the well-known migration" (p. 127).

191. Cohnheim, *Vorlesungen* (1887), 1: 635-54. Here Cohnheim adduces several additional arguments of the same character in favor of his hypothesis. It explains the slight atypia of *all* tumor tissues (since the embryonal rudiments grow in the absence of the usual embryonal controls), and the frequency of occurrence of tumors at body orifices where tissues of different germ layer origin meet (since the chances for *Abschnuerungen* are thereby increased), etc.

192. Ibid., p. 637.

193. Friedrich Wilhelm Zahn, "Sur le sort des tissus implantés dans l'organisme," Congrès internationale des sciences médicales, Geneva, September 9-15, 1877, *Compt. rend. mém.* (1878), pp. 658-64.

194. Ibid. Which tumors, Zahn did not say. The relevance of his experiments to Virchow's doctrine of tumor genesis was, presumably, that the undifferentiated cells of the connective tissue from which Virchow derived tumors were "embryonal" in character.

195. Julius Cohnheim and Hermann Maas, "Zur Theorie der Geschwulstmetastasen," *Arch. path. Anat. Phys. klin. Med.* 70 (1877): 161-71. If the tissue implants could grow within the pulmonary blood vessels, the authors saw no problem posed by further growth following breakdown of the vessel walls. They found that the bits of tissue became vascularized, grew briefly and produced bone, but were quickly resorbed. Their conclusion was that displaced cells became subject to an inherent destructive capability (*Zerstoerungsfaehigkeit*) of the organism, which, however, differed in intensity in different organs and tissues. In this way they attempted to explain the vagaries of cancer metastasis and the fact that, in their opinion, all attempts to transplant cancers into healthy animals by injection had "so far been, without exception, unsuccessful."

It is worth noting that Zahn mistakenly believed that Virchow had confirmed Langenbeck's claim to have transferred a human tumor to a dog by injection. Zahn writes ("Sur le sort des tissus") that "les recherches macroscopiques et microscopiques, faites par Langenbeck lui-même, controlées plus tard par Virchow, confirmèrent indubitablement la nature carci-nomateuse de ces nodules." Langenbeck believed, however, that the transplanted tumor cells had proliferated; Virchow, at best, that the injected material had incited a spontaneous cancer in the animal. Cf. ch. 3, note 113.

196. G. Leopold, "Experimentelle Untersuchungen ueber die Aetiologie der Ge-schwuelste," *Arch. path. Anat. Phys. klin. Med.* 85 (1881): 283-324. Cohnheim, who had come to Leipzig in 1878 as professor of pathological anatomy, gave Leopold the cue for these experiments (p. 323).

197. Ibid., pp. 288-90. Leopold gives no details concerning the antiseptic precautions; he notes merely that it is "of course understood that all experiments were carried out with the most careful possible antiseptic precautions" (p. 289). Only two rabbits died, one from peritonitis, the other from panophthalmitis. Joseph Lister—son of Joseph Jackson Lister, who had helped develop achromatic microscope objectives and had worked with Thomas Hodgkin on the fine structure of tissues (see ch. 2, n. 130, 131, and text)—published his papers on the antiseptic principle in surgery in 1867; his procedures were used during the Franco-Prussian War.

198. Ibid., pp. 310, 311.

199. Julius Cohnheim, *Vorlesungen* (1882), 1: 737-58.

200. Leopold dealt with this problem along suggestively Thierschian lines. He writes ("Experimentelle Untersuchungen," p. 320): "This being so, then the only questions that arise are why the embryonal germs can remain latent so long and how they are suddenly stimulated to enormous growth. I suppose that the latency depends on an undisturbed equilibrium, which reigns for a time between the tissues of the embryonal germ and the neighboring tissues, and that when this is disturbed, whether due to decreased resistance on the part of the neighboring tissues or to especially strong stimulation and greatly increased blood flow to the embryonal germs in consequence of trauma or inflammation, every barrier to the great proliferative character of its cells is overthrown."

201. The phrase "aberrant germs" (*verirrte Keime*), as used in the nineteenth century, referred to displaced, persisting embryonal cells of all kinds, serving as potential sources for tumors, tumorlike malformations, and ectopic tissues generally; for the later meaning of the phrase, see note 215.

202. Rudolf Virchow, *Die Cellularpathologie*, 4th ed. (Berlin, 1871), pp. 570, 571.

203. Ibid., p. 70. Strictly speaking, *metaplasia* refers to *tissue* rather than *cell* transforma-tion.

204. Rudolf Virchow, "Krankheitswesen und Krankheitsursachen," *Arch. path. Anat. Phys. klin. Med.* 79 (1880): 185-228. Cf. pp. 193-95.

205. Ibid., pp. 191, 192. Franz Boll, author of *Das Prinzip des Wachstums: Eine anatomische Untersuchung*, the work to which Virchow refers, was professor of comparative anatomy and physiology at Bonn. Carl Hasse's brief monograph, *Die Beziehungen der Morphologie zur Heilkunde*, argues (on an entirely a priori basis) that "every pathological new-formation must, accordingly, like every normal new-formation, proceed from formative embryonal constituents, and will only arise where a preceding increase over the normal measure of the embryonal formative material of the tissue elements has at some time taken place, whether in consequence of inheritance, whether in consequence of the effect of altered external influences (alterations in the intake of nutritive substances in the broadest sense of the term—stimuli, trauma, infection), concerning which experiment must be decisive. This increase, this state of excess...has the result that, while the surrounding region passes through the normal course of formation of the tissue, a part remains at starting point and, beginning its independent life in opposition to the surrounding region as a foreign formation, presents itself as the germ of a tumor, as Cohnheim rightly calls it" (pp. 12, 13).

206. Virchow, "Krankheitswesen und Krankheitsursachen," pp. 189, 190. The first part of Virchow's essay had appeared earlier in the year ("Krankheitswesen und Krankheitsursachen," *Arch. path. Anat. Phys. klin. Med.* 79 [1880]: 1-19). The occasion was the publication of Edwin Klebs's *Ueber Cellularpathologie und Infektionskrankheiten*, in which the bacteriologically oriented Klebs had declared cellular pathology an insufficient foundation for general pathology. Virchow, in reply, attempted to explain the difference between etiology and pathogenesis. Further, he discusses the several variants of the germ theory of disease then current, mentioning Hans Buchner's *Die Naegeli'sche Theorie der Infectionskrankheiten in ihren Beziehungen zur medicinischen Erfahrung*, Lionel Beale's *Disease Germs*, John Drysdale's *The Germ Theories of Infectious Diseases*, and even Francesco Redi's *De animis vivis quae in corporibus animalium vivorum reperiuntur observationes*. Although Virchow prefers Klebs's "Pilztheorie" to the others, e.g., Beale's theory of bioplasms, he believes all go beyond the evidence and fail to recognize the important distinction between *Krankheitsursachen* and *Krankheitswesen*. Zahn's work on tissue transplantation is mentioned, Virchow noting that he himself had tried, without success, to implant a human tumor (a choroid melanoma) in the conjunctiva of a rabbit. The ideological background of Virchow's thought becomes evident at one point: transplantation experiments have shown clearly that cells are capable of independent life outside of their original milieu; this proves, says Virchow, that the alliance of cells in the organism is not unitarian or totalitarian (*einheitlicher*) but social or confederate (*gesellschaftlicher, genossenschaftlicher, socialer*) in character. He reminds his readers that in 1852 he had stated that "every cell is, as such, a closed unity, which has taken into itself the basis and principle of its life, bearing within itself the laws of its existence, and which has a definite degree of autonomy in respect to the rest of the world" (pp. 185, 186).

207. Rudolf Virchow, "Ueber Metaplasie," *Arch. path. Anat. Phys. klin. Med.* 97 (1884): 410-30. The paper was read at the International Medical Congress in Copenhagen.

208. Ibid., pp. 415, 416, 428-30. Virchow comments disparagingly here on those who have assigned *absolute metaplasia* to emigrated white cells.

209. This dispute was closely allied to an older one, that between preformationists and epigeneticists in the field of embryology. Hence the opposed positions were by no means occupied on the one side exclusively by pathologists, and on the other by embryologists. In 1899, for example, pathologists who made dogmatic use of germ-layer theory were dealt with rather severely by an embryologist and warned that the theory had little or no application to the study of tumors (Hermann Klaatsch, "Ueber den jetzigen Stand der Keimblattfrage, mit Ruecksicht auf die Pathologie," *Muench. med. Woch.* 46/1 [1899]: 169-72). A little later, a pathologist defended the opposing point of view, in despite of Klaatsch (Felix Marchand, "Ueber die Beziehungen der pathologischen Anatomie zur Entwickelungsgeschichte, besonders der Keimblattlehre," *Verh. deutsch. path. Gesell.*, 1899, pp. 38-107).

In an address to pathologists in 1901, C. S. Minot, an embryologist, held that embryology was "the basis on which pathological science must be erected." Each germ layer, said Minot, produced its own group of tissues and no other. "Apparent exceptions," such as the stratified, cornified epithelium of endodermal origin lining the oesophagus, and the stratified, cornified epithelium of ectodermal origin constituting the epidermis, presented us "with only a resemblance," i.e., they differed in origin and, therefore, in nature. Minot regarded it as "more than probable that all pathological tissues are as strictly governed by the law of the specific value of germ layers as are the normal tissues" (Charles Sedgwick Minot, "The Embryological Basis of Pathology, *Science* 13 [1901]: 481-98).

In 1918 G. W. Nicholson described sebaceous glands in a lesion of the cervix as products of the mesodermal layer (rather than as products of a displaced ectodermal "germ"), concluding with these words: "Should the case help to upset our ideas of the limitation, and indeed of the specificity of the germinal layers, so be it. Even were all zoologists satisfied with these laws, which is not the case, morbid anatomists not infrequently come across appearances which justify the suspicion that such laws are but man-made after all" ("Sebaceous glands in the cervix uteri," *J. Path. Bact.* 43 [1918]: 252-54).

In 1940 Jane Oppenheimer, an embryologist and historian of biology, remarking that it was of interest to trace historically "the dogged attempt of the human mind to cling to a fixed idea," gave an account of germ-layer doctrine in all its aspects, from Christian Pander to the latest work by experimental embryologists. She concluded with the statement that "the doctrine of the absolute specificity of the germ-layers...must be abandoned" ("The Non-specificity of the Germ-layers," *Quart. Rev. Biol.* 15/1 [1940]: 1-27). In 1947 an embryologist, Gavin Rylands De Beer, again called for "abandonment of the germ-layer theory in its classical form," adding that pathology would benefit thereby ("The differentiation of neural crest cells into visceral cartilages and odontoblasts in *Amblyostoma,* and a re-examination of the germ-layer theory," *Proc. Roy. Soc. (B)* 134 [1947]: 377-98). Two years later it was rejected by a pathologist, E. S. J. King ("Squamous epithelium in bursae: the import of the non-specificity of the germ-layers," *Austral. New Zeal. J. Surg.* 19/2 [1949]: 208-20).

Meanwhile, the germ-layer doctrine continued to occupy its place in introductory textbooks of embryology and to be tacitly accepted by pathologists, at times even by those who professed to be sceptical of it. As late as 1969, Foulds, in a discussion of so-called myothelial proliferation in the human breast, notes that the "proposition that cells of epithelial origin can produce connective tissues is uncongenial to those pathologists who hold to a rigid interpretation of 'the specificity of the germ layers' long after embryologists have abandoned it" (Foulds, *Neoplastic Development,* 1: 144).

210. Louis Bard, "Anatomie pathologique générale des tumeurs, leur nature et leur classification physiologique," *Arch. phys. norm. path.* 5 (1885): 247-65. A tumor, Bard states, is a new-formation or neoplasm, but not all new-formations are tumors (i.e., "true" tumors): "The progress of general pathology allows us, first of all, to separate from them all inflammatory processes, whatever their origin and external form. Syphilitic gummata and tuberculous nodules, no more than the processes of encystment of trichina or echinococcus, ought no longer be described under the heading of tumor. Nor, moreover, do we accept cysts formed by dilatation or retention of secretory products among the number of tumors" (p. 248).

211. Ibid., pp. 249, 250, 252-55, 257. Bard later abandoned the notion that tumors of mixed cellular composition arise from a *bouquet cellulaire.* He proposed instead that they arise from single cells, his *cellules nodales,* which have been segregated somewhere along the course of embryonic development before they give rise to their diverse progeny. Persisting in the adult organisms, these cells would, if they underwent neoplastic development, be capable of yielding descendants of different species. At the same time Bard rejected Cohnheim's attempt to trace *all* tumors back to embryonic cell rests, since, according to his own way of thinking, embryonic cells must inevitably yield tumors of mixed cellular composition ("Des tumeurs a tissus multiples," *Lyon Méd.* 58 [1888]: 5-15).

212. Louis Bard, "La spécificité cellulaire et l'histogénèse chez l'embryon," *Arch. phys. norm. path.* 7 (1886): 406-20. Bard's revised version is sometimes cited as *omnis cellula e cellula ejusdem generis.* (See Rather, *Addison and the White Corpuscles,* for Virchow's use of *a* and *e* in his aphorism.) Bard notes here that the few who still hold with Robin that cells are secondary formations in blastemas also take no proper account of cell and tissue specificity.

213. Walther Flemming, "Beitraege zur Kenntnis der Zelle und ihrer Lebenser-scheinungen," *Arch. mikr. Anat.* 16 (1879): 302-436. Flemming used aniline dyes in his studies, but in addition he described all phases of mitotic division in living unstained cells. See Rather, *Addison and the White Corpuscles,* fig. 6, for a reproduction of an illustration from the above article by Flemming.

214. Bard, "La spécificité," pp. 410-13.

215. Moritz Nussbaum, "Zur Differenzierung des Geschlechts im Tierreich," *Arch. mikr.*

Anat. 18 (1880): 1-121. Waldeyer rejected His's derivation of the genito-urinary apparatus from the ectoderm in 1870. According to Waldeyer, the germinal epithelium (*Keimepithel*) originated *in situ* from mesodermal elements (*Eierstock und Ei*, pp. 113, 114). In 1900 J. Beard described the migration of germ-cells from an extraembryonal site of origin (in the skate, *Raja batis*) to the rudimentary gonads. He generalized his findings to include all vertebrates and then attempted to account for extragonadal dermoid cysts and teratomas (which were "embryomas" to him) in human beings as the products of "vagrant or lost primary germ cells." These, he said, were the real representatives of the "hypothetical 'verirrte Keime' of the pathologists" ("The Morphological Continuity of the Germ Cells in *Raja batis,*" *Anat. Anzeig.* 18 [1900]: 465-85). Commenting on the widespread popularity enjoyed by Beard's notion, Emil Witschi stated in 1948 that, as far as human embryos were concerned, no convincing or even suggestive evidence in its favor was actually available ("Migration of the Germ Cells of Human Embryos from the Yolk Sac to the Primitive Gonadal Folds," *Contr. Embryol. Carnegie Inst.* 32 [1948]: 67-80). Again, in 1954, A. Duncan Chiquoine maintained that there were "no observations to support such a widespread distribution of lost germ cells" ("The Identification, Origin, and Migration of the Primordial Germ Cells in the Mouse Embryo," *Anat. Rec.* 118 [1954]: 135-45).

In 1960, however, Beatrice Mintz stated that in mice and chicks "substantial numbers" of primordial germ cells do become lost while migrating from the yolk sac to the germinal ridges. One such cell (identified by special stain) in the brain wall of a 22-somite chick embryo is illustrated in her paper "Formation and Early Development of Germ Cells." Mintz's findings have been cited by Simson et al. in support of the germ cell origin of suprasellar germinomas (L. Simson, I. Lampe and M. R. Abell, "Suprasellar Germinomas," *Cancer* 22 [1968]: 533-44).

216. Cf. ch. 4, note 125 and text. Weismann began to publish on this subject in the early 1880s, but he did not fully elaborate his theory of determinants until some years later.

217. Rudolph Koelliker, "Das Karyoplasma und die Vererbung, eine Kritik der Weismann'schen Theorie von der Kontinuitaet des Keimplasma," *Z. wiss. Zool.* 44 (1886): 228-38. Koelliker refers here specifically to Weismann's *Ueber die Vererbung, Die Kontinuitaet des Keimplasmas als Grundlage einer Theorie der Vererbung,* and *Die Bedeutung der sexuellen Fortpflanzung fuer die Selektionstheorie.*

218. Carl Wilhelm Naegeli, *Mechanisch-physiologische Theorie der Abstammungslehre.*

219. Ibid., pp. 25, 26, 65. Wilhelm Waldeyer subsequently termed the threadlike bodies *chromosomes* ("Ueber Karyokinese und ihre Beziehung zu den Befruchtungsvorgaengen," *Arch. mikr. Anat.* 32 [1888]: 1-22). For more on early molecular biology see L. J. Rather, "Alchemistry, the Kabbala, the Analogy of the 'Creative Word,' and the Origins of Molecular Biology." Cited in ch. 1, n. 86.

220. Rudolph Koelliker, "Die Bedeutung der Zellkerne fuer die Vorgaenge der Vererbung," *Z. wiss. Zool.* 42 (1885): 9-46. Some of the arguments used against Weismann by Koelliker in the following year ("Das Karyoplasma und die Vererbung") recall those on which Johannes Mueller based his much earlier claim that the somatic cells of mature organisms possessed "the power to form the whole," but that this power underwent suppression (*Hemmung*) in the course of embryonic development. *Cf.* Mueller's *Handbuch der Physiologie des Menschen,* 2: 614-17.

BIBLIOGRAPHY

BOOKS AND ARTICLES CITED

Abernethy, John. *Surgical Observations*. London, 1804.

Addison, Joseph. *Works*. 6 vols. London, 1882. "Meditations on Animal Life," in vol. 4.

Aguirre, Emiliano. "Paleopathología y medicina prehistórica." In *Historia Universal de la Medicina*, vol. 1, pp. 7-31. Edited by Pedro Laín-Entralgo. 7 vols. Barcelona: Salvat Editores, 1972-75.

Albarran, L. "Épithélioma adamantin du sinus maxillaire." *Compt. rend. Soc. Biol.* 4 (1887): 618-21.

_____. "Épithélioma adamantin du maxillaire supérieure." *Compt. rend. Soc. Biol.* 4 (1887): 667-71.

Alberti, Michael. *Introductio in medicinam universam*. Halle, 1718-21.

Albertini, A. von. *Histologische Geschwuelstdiagnostik*. Stuttgart: Thieme, 1955.

_____. "Allgemeine Systematik der Geschwuelste." In *Handbuch der allgemeinen Pathologie*. Edited by R. Buechner, E. Letterer, and F. Roulet. 11 vols. Berlin: Springer, 1956. Vol. 6, pt. 3, pp. 1-17.

Albores-Saavedra, J.; Díaz-Gutiérrez. D.; and Altamirando-Dimas, M. "Adamantinoma de la tibia: Observaciones ultraestructurales." *Rev. Méd. Hosp. Gen. México* 31 (1968): 241-52.

Alibert, Jean-Louis. *Clinique de l'Hôpital Saint-Louis, ou traité complet des maladies de la peau*. Paris, 1833.

Andral, Gabriel. *Précis d'anatomie pathologique*. 3 vols. Paris, 1829.

_____. *A Treatise on Pathological Anatomy*. Translated by Richard Townsend and William West. 2 vols. Dublin, 1829-31.

Aristotle. *De partibus animalium*. Translated by William Ogle. London, 1912.

_____. *Historia animalium*. Translated by D'Arcy Wentworth Thompson. London, 1910.

_____. *Parts of Animals*. Translated by A. L. Peck. London: Heinemann, 1937.

_____. *Problemata*. Translated by E. S. Forster. London: Oxford University Press, 1927.

Aselli, Gasparo. *De lactibus, sive lacteis venis, quarto vasorum necessariorum genere, novo invento, dissertatio*. Milan, 1627.

Astruc, Jean. *Tractatus de tumoribus et ulceribus ex Gallico sermone versus*. Venice, 1766.

_____. *Traité des tumeurs et des ulcères*. 2 vols. Paris, 1759.

Baer, Karl Ernst von. *Ueber Entwickelungsgeschichte der Thiere: Beobachtungen und Reflexionen*. 2 vols. Koenigsberg, 1824, 1837.

_____. "Die Metamorphose des Eies der Batrachier vor der Erscheinung des Embryo, und Folgerungen aus ihr fuer die Theorie der Erzeugung." *Arch. Anat. Phys. wiss. Med.* (1834), pp. 481-509.

Baillie, Matthew. *The Morbid Anatomy of Some of the Most Important Parts of the Body.* 2d ed. London, 1797.

Bard, Louis. "Anatomie pathologique générale des tumeurs, leur nature, et leur classification physiologique." *Arch. phys. norm. pathol.* 5 (1885): 247-65.

_____. "Des tumeurs à tissues multiples." *Lyon Méd.* 58 (1888): 5-15.

_____. "La specificité cellulaire et l'histogenèse chez l'embryon." *Arch. phys. norm. pathol.* 7 (1886): 406-20.

Bayle, Gaspard-Laurent, and Cayol, Jean-Baptiste. S.v. "Cancer," in *Dictionnaire de sciences médicales,* 1813 ed.

Beale, Lionel. *Disease Germs.* London, 1870.

Beard, J. "The Morphological Continuity of the Germ Cells in Raja batis." *Anat. Anzeiger* 18 (1900): 465-85.

Beneke, Rudolph. "Die Embolie." In *Handbuch der allgemeinen Pathologie.* Edited by Ludwig Krehl and Felix Marchand. 5 vols. Leipzig, 1908-24. Vol. 2, bk. 2, pp. 300-371.

_____. "Die Thrombose." In *Handbuch der allgemeinen Pathologie.* Edited by Ludwig Krehl and Felix Marchand. 5 vols. Leipzig, 1908-24. Vol. 2, bk. 2, pp. 130-299.

Bennett, John Hughes. "Lectures on Molecular Physiology, Pathology, and Therapeutics." *Lancet,* January-December, 1863.

_____. *On Cancerous and Cancroid Growths.* Edinburgh, 1849.

Berres, Joseph. *Anatomia microscopica corporis humani.* Vienna, 1837.

Bichat, François-Xavier. *Anatomie générale, appliquée à la physiologie et la médicine.* 4 vols. Paris, 1801.

_____. *Anatomie pathologique. Dernier cours de Xavier Bichat, d'après un manuscrit autographe de P. A. Béclard.* Paris, 1826.

_____. *General Anatomy Applied to Physiology and Medicine.* Translated by George Hayward from the French edition of 1801. Boston, 1822.

_____. *Traité des membranes, nouvelle édition, augmentée d'une notice historique sur la vie et les ouvrages de l'auteur, par M. Husson.* Paris, 1802.

_____. *Treatise of the Membranes.* Translated by J. G. Coffin from the French edition of 1802. Boston, 1813.

Billroth, Theodor. *Die allgemeine chirurgische Pathologie und Therapie in 50 Vorlesungen.* Berlin, 1863.

_____. "Kritische und erlaeuternde Bemerkungen zu dem Werke von Professor C. Thiersch in Erlangen." *Arch. klin. Chirur.* 7 (1866): 848-59.

Biographisches Lexikon der hervorragenden Aerzte aller Zeiten und Voelker. 3d. ed. 6 vols. Berlin, Munich: Urban and Schwarzenberg, 1962.

Boerhaave, Hermann. *Opera omnia.* Venice, 1747.

Bordeu, Théophile. *Recherches sur le tissu muqueux.* Paris, 1790.

Bradbury, Saville. *The Evolution of the Microscope.* London: Edward Arnold, 1967.

Breschet, Gilbert, and Ferrus, Guillaume-Marie-André. S.v. "Cancer," in *Dictionnaire de médecine,* 1822 ed.

Breuer, Robert. "Meletemata circa evolutionem ac formas cicatricum." Bratislava, November 24, 1843.

Broussais, François. *Examen des doctrines médicales et des systèmes de nosologie.* 3d ed. Paris, 1834.

Brown, Robert. "A Brief Account of Microscopical Observations Made in the Months of June, July and August, 1827, on the Particles Contained in the Pollen of Plants; and on the General Existence of Active Molecules in Organic and Inorganic Bodies." *Edinburgh New Phil. J.* 5 (1828): 358-71.

_____. "On the Organs and Mode of Fecundation in Orchids and Asclepiadae." *Trans. Linn. Soc.* (London) 16 (1833): 685-738.

Bruch, Carl. *Die Diagnose der boesartigen Geschwuelste.* Mainz, 1847.

Buchholtz, Arend. *Ernst von Bergmann.* 3d ed. Leipzig, 1913.

Buchner, Hans. *Die Naegeli'sche Theorie der Infectionskrankheiten in ihren Beziehungen zur medicinischen Erfahrung.* Leipzig, 1877.

Buhl, Ludwig. "Wahre, recidivirendes Myom (Rhabdomyom Zenker's)." *Z. Biol.* 1 (1865): 263-72.

Bulloch, William. *The History of Bacteriology.* London: Oxford University Press, 1938.

Burns, John. *Dissertations on Inflammation.* Edinburgh, 1800.

Burton, Robert. *The Anatomy of Melancholy.* 16th ed. London: B. Blake, 1836.

Caelius Aurelianus. *On Acute Diseases and Chronic Diseases.* Edited and translated by I. E. Drabkin. Chicago: University of Chicago Press, 1950.

Carmichael, R. C. *An Essay on the Effects of Carbonate and Other Preparations of Iron upon Cancer.* 2d ed. Dublin, 1809.

Carswell, Robert. *Pathological Anatomy: Illustrations of the Elementary Forms of Diseases.* London, 1833-38.

Carswell, Robert, and Cullen, William. "On Melanosis." *Trans. Medico-Chirur. Soc. of Edinburgh* 1 (1824): 264-84.

Castelli, Bartolomeo. *Lexicon medicum Graeco-Latinum.* Geneva, 1746.

Celsus. *De medicina.* Translated by W. G. Spencer. 3 vols. London: Loeb Classical Library, 1933.

Changus, G. W.; Speed, J. S.; and Stewart, F. "Malignant Angioblastoma of Bone: A Reappraisal of Adamantinoma of Long Bone." *Cancer* 10 (1957): 540-49.

Chiquoine, A. Duncan. "The Identification, Origin, and Migration of the Primordial Germ Cells in the Mouse Embryo." *Anat. Rec.* 118 (1954): 135-45.

Chomel, August. *Élémens de pathologie générale.* 3d ed. Paris, 1841.

Choulant, L. *Bibliotheca medico-historica.* Leipzig, 1842.

Classen, A. "Ueber ein Cancroid der Cornea und Sclera, ein Beitrag zur Entwickelungsgeschichte der Carcinome." *Arch. path. Anat. Phys. klin. Med.* 50 (1870): 56-79.

Cohnheim, Julius. "Congenitales, quergestreiftes Muskelsarcom der Nieren." *Arch. path. Anat. Phys. klin. Med.* 65 (1875): 64-69.

_____. *Neue Untersuchungen ueber die Entzuendung.* Berlin, 1873.

_____. *Pathologie.* 2 vols. Berlin, 1877-80; 2d ed. 2 vols., Berlin, 1882.

_____. "Ueber Entzuendung und Eiterung." *Arch. path. Anat. Phys. klin. Med.* 40 (1867): 1-79.

_____. *Vorlesungen ueber allgemeine Pathologie.* 2 vols. Berlin, 1877-80; 2d ed. 2 vols. Berlin, 1882.

Cohnheim, Julius, and Maas, Hermann. "Zur Theorie der Geschwulstmetastasen."

Arch. path. Anat. Phys. klin. Med. 70 (1877): 161-71.

Cooper, Astley. *Principles and Practice of Surgery.* 3 vols. London, 1836.

Cornil, André-Victor. "Mémoire sur les tumeurs épithéliales du col de l'uterus." *J. anat. phys.* 1864, pp. 472-507, 627-59.

————. "Mémoire sur les tumeurs épithéliales du col de l'uterus," *J. anat. phys.,* 1865, pp. 266-76, 476-96.

Costello, W. B. *Cyclopaedia of Practical Surgery.* 4 vols. London, 1841.

Cruveilhier, Jean. "Description anatomique de cancers de l'intestine grêle, de l'estomac, de la mammelle. Quel est l'élément que est le plus spécialement le siège de la dégénération cancéreuse?" *Bull. Soc. Anat. de Paris,* 2nd ed. Paris, 1844. pp. 4-16.

————. *Essai sur l'anatomie pathologique en général.* Paris, 1816.

Curtis, John G. *Harvey's Views on the Use of the Circulation of the Blood.* New York, 1915.

Dalton, John C. *Doctrines of the Circulation.* Philadelphia, 1884.

Daremberg, Charles. *Oeuvres anatomiques, physiologiques, et médicales de Galien.* 2 vols. Paris, 1854.

Darmstaedter, Ludwig. *Handbuch zur Geschichte der Naturwissenschaften und der Technik.* 2d ed. Berlin, 1908.

De Beer, G. R. "The differentiation of neural crest cells into visceral cartilages and odontoblasts in *Amblystoma,* and a re-examination of germ-layer theory." *Proc. Roy. Soc. of London,* ser. B, 134 (1947): 377-98.

Dictionnaire de médecine. 21 vols. Paris, 1821-28.

Dictionnaire des sciences médicales. 60 vols. Paris, 1812-22.

Dictionnaire historique de la médicine ancienne et moderne. 4 vols. Paris, 1828-39.

Drysdale, John. *The Germ Theories of Infectious Diseases.* London, 1878.

Dunglison, Robley. *A Dictionary of Medical Science.* 3d ed. Philadelphia, 1842.

Dupuytren, G. *Bull. École Méd. de Paris* no. 2 (1805), pp. 13-24.

Eble, Burkard. *Versuch einer pragmatischen Geschichte der Anatomie und Physiologie, 1800-1825.* Vienna, 1836.

Ecker, Alexander. "Ueber den Bau der unter dem Name 'Lippenkrebs' zusammengefassten Geschwuelsten der Lippe." *Archiv f. physiol. Heilkunde* 3 (1844): 380-84.

Edwards, Milne. *Mémoire sur la structure élémentaire des principaux tissus organiques des animaux.* Thesis, University of Paris, 1823.

Engelmann, W. *Bibliotheca medico-chirurgica et anatomico-physiologica.* Leipzig, 1848.

Ersch, J. S. *Literatur der Medizin.* Leipzig, 1822.

Falloppio, Gabriele. *Opera omnia.* 2 vols. Frankfurt, 1600.

Farber, Seymour; Rosenthal, Milton; Alston, Edwin F.; Benioff, Mortimer A.; McGrath, Allen K., Jr. *Cytologic Diagnosis of Lung Cancer.* Springfield: Charles C Thomas, 1950.

Fernel, Jean. *Universa medicina.* 6th ed. Frankfurt, 1607.

Ferrario, E. V.; Poynter, F. N. C.; and Franklin, K. J. "William Harvey's Debate with Caspar Hofmann on the Circulation of the Blood." *J. Hist. Med. Allied Sci.* 7 (1960): 7-21.

Fischer, Bernhard. "Ueber ein primaeres Adamantinom der Tibia." *Frankfurt. Z. Path.* 12 (1913): 422-41.

Fleming, Donald. "Galen on the Motions of the Blood in the Heart and Lungs." *Isis* 46 (1955): 14-21.

Flemming, Walther. "Beitraege zur Kenntnis der Zelle und ihrer Lebenserscheinungen." *Arch. mikr. Anat.* 16 (1879): 302-436.

Florkin, Marcel. "Le journal des expériences de Théodore Schwann sur la génération spontanée, le fermentation alcoolique, et la putréfaction." *Bull. Acad. Roy. Méd. de Belgique* 17 (1952): 164-67.

Foerster, August. *Handbuch der pathologischen Anatomie.* vol. 1. *Allgemeine pathologischen Anatomie.* 2 vols. Leipzig, 1855.

Forbes, J. F., ed. *Cyclopaedia of Practical Medicine.* 4 vols. Philadelphia, 1859.

Foster, Sir Michael. *Lectures on the History of Physiology during the Sixteenth, Seventeenth, and Eighteenth Centuries.* Cambridge, 1901.

Foulds, Leslie. *Neoplastic Development.* 2 vols. London and New York: Academic Press, 1969-75.

Frerichs, Friedrich Theodor. "Ueber die destruirenden Epithelialgeschwuelste." *Jenaische Ann. Phys. Med.* 1 (1849): 3-15.

Fuchs, Leonhard. *Institutiones medicinae.* Basel, 1594.

Galen. *Galen on the Natural Faculties.* Translated by A. J. Brock. London: Heinemann, 1952.

————. *Opera omnia.* Edited by C. G. Kuehn. 20 vols. in 22. Leipzig, 1821-33.

————. *Ueber die krankhaften Geschwuelste.* Translated by Paul Richter. Leipzig, 1913.

Garrison, F. H. *An Introduction to the History of Medicine.* 4th ed. Philadelphia: W. B. Saunders, 1929.

Garrison, F. H. and Morton, L. T. *Medical Bibliography.* 2d ed. New York: Argosy Book Stores, 1954.

Gaub, Jerome. *Anfangsgruende der medicinischen Krankheitslehre.* Linz, 1785.

————. *Institutiones pathologiae medicinalis.* 2d ed. Leiden, 1775.

Gendron, Claude-Deshaies. *Recherches sur la nature et la guérison des cancers.* Paris, 1700.

Gloor, F. "Das sogenannte Adamantinom der langen Rohrenknochen." *Arch. path. Anat. Phys. klin. Med.* 336 (1963): 489-502.

Gluge, Gottlob. *Pathologische Histologie.* Jena, 1850. Translated by Joseph Leidy as *Pathological Histology.* Philadelphia, 1853.

————. "Recherches microscopiques sur le fluide contenu dans les cancers encéphaloïdes." *Compt. rend. Acad. Sci.* 4 (January-June, 1837): 20, 21.

————. "Ueber Crystallformen in gesunden und kranken Fluessigkeiten, mit dem Mikroskope beobachtet." *Arch. Anat. Phys. wiss. Med.,* 1837, pp. 463-67.

Goethe, J. W. *Zur Morphologie.* 1817. Reprinted in *Gedenkausgabe.* Edited by Ernst Beutlev. Zurich: Artemis Verlag, 1952.

Goldman, E. E. "Beitrag zu der Lehre von dem 'malignen Lymphom.'" *Centrb. allg. path. Anat.* 3 (1892): 665-90.

Goring, C. R. "The Diamond Microscope." *Franklin Journal* 4 (1827): 208.

Grew, Nehemiah. *The Anatomy of Plants.* First published in 1671. Introduction by

Conway Zirkle. New York: Johnson Reprint Co., 1965.

Gross, Samuel D. *Elements of Pathologic Anatomy.* 2 vols. Boston, 1839.

Gulliver, George. "On the Structure of Fibrinous Exudations or False Membranes." *London, Edinburgh, Dublin Phil. Mag. J. Sci.,* 3d ser. 21 (1842): 241-46.

Haller, Albrecht von. *Bibliotheca anatomica.* 2 vols. Zurich, 1774; reprint ed., Hildesheim: Georg Olms, 1969.

_____. *First Lines of Physiology.* Edinburgh, 1786.

_____. *Primae lineae physiologiae.* Edinburgh, 1767.

Ham, Arthur W. *Histology.* 3d ed. Philadelphia: Lippincott, 1957.

Handbuch der allgemeinen Pathologie. Edited by Ludwig Krehl and Felix Marchand. 5 vols. Leipzig, 1908-1924.

Handbuch der allgemeinen und speciellen Chirurgie. Edited by Franciscus J. Pitha and Theodor Billroth. 4 vols. in 13. Stuttgart and Erlangen, 1865-82.

Handbuch der speciellen pathologischen Anatomie und Histologie. Edited by Friedrich Henke and Otto Lubarsch. 13 vols. Berlin. 1928.

Hannover, Adolph. "Bericht ueber die Leistungen in der skandinavischen Literatur im Gebiete der Anatomie und Physiologie in den Jahren 1841-43." *Arch. Anat. Phys. wiss. Med.,* 1844, pp. 1-49.

_____. *Das Epithelioma, eine eigenthuemliche Geschwulst, die man im allgemeinen bisher als Krebs angesehen hat.* Leipzig, 1852.

Harvey, William. *The Works of William Harvey.* Translated by Robert Willis. London 1847; reprint ed., New York and London: Johnson Reprint, 1965.

_____. *Opera omnia.* London, 1776.

Hasse, Carl. *Die Beziehungen der Morphologie zur Heilkunde.* Leipzig, 1879.

Hecker, Karl Friedrich. "Bericht ueber die Ereignisse in der chirurgisch-ophthalmologischen Klinik zu Freiburg." *Arch. phys. Heilkunde* 3 (1844): 241-77.

Heller, Arnold. *Untersuchungen ueber die feineren Vorgaenge bei der Entzuendung.* Berlin, 1873.

Henle, Jacob. "Bericht ueber die Arbeiten im Gebiete der rationellen Pathologie." *Z. rat. Med.* 2 (1844): 1-411.

_____. "Theodor Schwann: Nachruf." *Arch. mikr. Anat.* 21 (1882): i-xlix.

_____. "Von den Miasmen und Kontagien." In *Pathologischen Untersuchungen.* Berlin, 1840.

Herodotus. *With an English Translation by A. D. Godley.* London: Heinemann, 1921.

Hertwig, Oscar. *Lehrbuch der Entwickelungsgeschichte.* 3d. ed. Jena, 1890.

Hey, William. *Practical Observations in Surgery.* Philadelphia, 1805.

Hicks, J. Douglas. "Synovial Sarcoma of the Tibia." *J. Path. Bact.* 67 (1954): 151-61.

Hildebrand, Otto. "Ueber das tubulaere Angiosarkom oder Endotheliom des Knochens." *Deutsche Z. Chirur.* 31 (1900): 263-81.

Hippocrates. Translated by W. H. S. Jones. 4 vols. London: Heinemann, 1953-57.

_____. *Oeuvres complètes d'Hippocrate.* Translated by E. Littré. 10 vols. Paris, 1839-61.

His, Wilhelm. "Beobachtungen ueber den Bau des Saeugethier-Eierstockes." *Arch. mikr. Anat.* 1 (1865): 151-202.

_____. *Die Haeute und Hoehlen des Koerpers.* Basel, 1865.

_____. "Die Lehre vom Bindesubstanzkeim (Parablast). Rueckblick nebst kritischer Besprechung einiger neuerer entwickelungsgeschichtlicher Arbeiten." *Arch. Anat. Entwickelungsgeschichte,* 1882, pp. 62-108.

―――. "Ueber die Entdeckung des Lymphsystems." *Z. Anat. Entwickelungsgeschichte* 1 (1876): 129-43.

―――. *Untersuchungen ueber die erste Anlage des Wirbelthierleibes.* Leipzig, 1868.

Hodgkin, Thomas. *Lectures on the Morbid Anatomy of the Mucous and Serous Membranes.* 2 vols. London, 1836.

―――. "On the Anatomical Character of Some Adventitious Structures." *Medico-Chirur. Trans.* 15 (1829): 265-338.

Hodgkin, Thomas, and Lister, J. J. "Notice sur quelques observations microscopiques sur le sang et le tissu des animaux." *Ann. sci. nat.* 12 (1827): 53-68.

Hoffmann, Friedrich. *Fundamenta medicinae.* Halle and Magdeburg, 1703.

Home, Everard. *A Short Tract on the Formation of Tumours, and the Peculiarities That Are Met With in the Structure of Those That Become Cancerous.* London, 1830.

Hooke, Robert. *Micrographia.* London, 1665.

Horner, William E. *Treatise on Pathology.* Philadelphia, 1829.

Horst, Gregor. *Gregorii Horstii, senioris...operum medicorum...cura Gregorii Horstii junioris.* 3 vols. Gouda, 1661.

Howard, William T., and Crile, George W. "A Contribution to the Knowledge of Endothelioma and Perithelioma of Bone." *Ann. Surg.* 42 (1905): 358-93.

Hunter, John. *The Works of John Hunter, F.R.S.* Edited by J. F. Palmer. 4 vols. London, 1835-37.

―――. *A Treatise on the Blood, Inflammation, and Gun-Shot Wounds.* London, 1794.

Huxley, T. H. "The Cell Theory." *British and Foreign Medico-Chirur. Rev.* 12 (1853): 221-43.

Jevon, F. R. "Harvey's Quantitative Method." *Bull. Hist. Med.* 36 (1962): 462-70.

Keele, Kenneth D. *William Harvey.* London: Nelson, 1965.

King, E. S. J. "Squamous epithelium in bursae: the import of the non-specificity of the germ-layers." *Australian and New Zealand J. Surg.* 19 (1949): 208-20.

Klaatsch, Hermann. "Ueber den jetzigen Stand der Keimblattfrage, mit Ruecksicht auf die Pathologie." *Muench. med. Woch.* 46 (1899): 169-72.

Klebs, Edwin. *Beitraege zur pathologischen Anatomie der Schusswunden.* Leipzig, 1872.

―――. "Bemerkungen ueber Larynx-Geschwuelste." *Arch. path. Anat. Phys. klin. Med.* 38 (1867): 202-20.

―――. *Ueber Cellularpathologie und Infektionskrankheiten.* Prague, 1878.

Klencke, Philipp F. H. *Untersuchungen und Erfahrungen im Gebiete der Anatomie, Pathologie, Mikrologie und wissenschaftlichen Medizin. Erster Band. 1. Der Nervus Sympathikus in seiner morphologischen und physiologischen Bedeutung. 2. Mikroskopisch-pathologische Beobachtungen ueber die Natur des Contagion.* Leipzig, 1843.

Klibansky, Raymond; Panofsky, Erwin; and Saxl, Fritz. *Saturn and Melancholy.* New York: Basic Books, 1964.

Koelliker, Rudolf. "Das Karyoplasma und die Vererbung: eine Kritik der Weismann'schen Theorie von der Kontinuitaet des Keimplasma." *Zeitschr. wiss.*

Zool. 44 (1886): 228-38.

————. "Die Bedeutung der Zellkerne fuer die Vorgaenge der Vererbung." *Zeitschr. wiss. Zool.* 42 (1885): 9-46.

————. *Entwickelungsgeschichte der Cephalopoden.* Zurich, 1844.

————. *Entwickelungsgeschichte des Menschen und der hoeheren Thiere.* 2d ed. Leipzig, 1879.

Laennec, René H. *A Treatise on Diseases of the Chest.* London 1821; facsimile reprint ed., New York: Hafner, 1962.

————. S.v. "Anatomie pathologique," in *Dictionnaire des sciences médicales,* 1812 ed.

————. S.v. "Cartilages accidentels," in *Dictionnaire des sciences médicales,* 1812 ed.

————. S.v. "Dégénération," in *Dictionnaire des sciences médicales,* 1814 ed.

————. S.v. "Encéphaloïdes," in *Dictionnaire des sciences médicales,* 1815 ed.

Laín-Entralgo, Pedro, ed., *Historia universal des la medicina.* 7 vols. Barcelona: Salvat Editores, 1972-75.

Lamarck, J. B. *Histoire naturelle des animaux sans vertèbres.* 2d ed. Paris, 1835.

Langenbeck, Bernard. "Ueber die Entstehung des Venenkrebses und die Moeglichkeit, Carcinoma vom Menschen auf Thiere zu uebertragen." *Jahrb. in- und auslaend. gesam. Med.* 25 (1840): 99-104.

Langhans, Theodor. "Ueber Krebs und Cancroid der Lunge, nebst einem Anhang ueber Corpora amylacea in der Lunge." *Arch. path. Anat. Phys. klin. Med.* 38 (1867): 497-543.

Lauche, Arnold. "Zur Kenntnis von Pathologie u. Klinik der Geschwuelste mit synovialmembranartigem Bau (Synovialome oder synovial Endothelio- Fibrome und -Sarkome)." *Frankfurt. Z. Path.* 59 (1947): 2-29.

Laughlin, William. "Acquisition of Anatomical Knowledge by Ancient Man." In *Social Life of Early Man,* edited by Sherwood L. Washburn. Viking Fund Publications in Anthropology, no. 31. New York: Viking Fund, 1961.

Lebert, Hermann. *Physiologie pathologique.* 2 vols. Paris, 1845.

————. *Traité d'anatomie pathologique.* 2 vols. and atlas. Paris, 1857-61.

————. *Traité pratique des maladies cancéreuses et des affections curables confondues avec le cancer.* Paris, 1851.

Lederer, H., and Sinclair, A. J. "Malignant Synovioma Simulating 'Adamantinoma' of the Tibia." *J. Path. Bact.* 67 (1954): 163-68.

Le Dran, François. "Mémoire avec un précis de plusieurs observations sur le cancer." *Mém. Acad. Roy. Chirur.* (Paris) 7 (1757): 224-310.

Lemnius, Levinus. *The Touchstone of the Complexions . . . Containing most easy rules and ready tokens, whereby everyone may perfectly try and thoroughly know as well the exact state, habit, disposition and constitution of his body outwardly as also the inclinations, affections, emotions and desires of his mind inwardly: First written in Latin by Levine Lemnie, and now Englished by Thomas Newton.* London, 1581.

Leopold, G. "Experimentelle Untersuchungen ueber die Aetiologie der Geschwuelste," *Arch. path. Anat. Phys. klin. Med.* 85 (1881): 283-324.

Liebig, Justus. *Animal Chemistry in Its Application to Physiology and Pathology.* Translated by William Gregory. New York, 1842.

_____. *Thierchemie, oder die organische Chemie in ihrer Anwendung auf Physiologie und Pathologie*. Braunschweig, 1842.

Lister, Joseph J. "On some properties in achromatic object glasses applicable to improvement of the microscope." *Phil. Trans. Roy. Soc.* 130 (1830): 187-200.

Littré, Émile. *Oeuvres complètes d'Hippocrate traduction nouvelle avec le texte grec en regard*. 10 vols. Paris, 1839.

Lobstein, Johann F. *Traité d'anatomie pathologique*. Paris, 1829.

Luecke, Georg Albert. "Die Lehre von der Geschwuelsten in anatomischer und klinischer Beziehung." In *Handbuch der allgemeinen und speciellen Chirurgie*, vol. 2, bk. 1. Edited by Franciscus J. Pitha and Theodor Billroth. 4 vols. in 13. Stuttgart and Erlangen, 1869.

Macartney, James. *A Treatise of Inflammation*. London, 1838.

MacCallum, W. G. *A Textbook of Pathology*. 6th ed. Philadelphia, 1936.

Maier, Carola. "Ein primaeres myelogenes Plattenepithelcarcinom der Ulna." *Beitr. z. klin. Chirur.* 26 (1900): 513-66.

Maier, Rudolf. *Lehrbuch der allgemeinen pathologischen Anatomie*. Leipzig, 1871.

Majno, Guido. *The Healing Hand*. Cambridge, Mass.: Harvard University Press, 1975.

Malassez, Louis-Charles. "Sur le rôle des débris épithéliaux paradentaires." *Arch. Phys.* 5 (1885): 309-40; 6 (1885): 379-449.

Malpighi, Marcello. *Opera omnia*. Leyden, 1687.

Mandl, Louis. *Anatomie microscopique. Vol. 2: Histogénèse*. Paris, 1848-57.

_____. "De la structure intime des tumeurs ou des productions pathologiques." *Arch. gén. méd.* ser. 3, 8 (1840): 312-29.

Marchand, Felix. "Ueber die Beziehungen der pathologischen Anatomie zur Entwickelungsgeschichte, besonders der Keimblattlehre." *Verh. deutsch. path. Gesell.*, 1899, pp. 38-107.

Mayer, A. F. J. K. *Ueber Histologie und eine neue Eintheilung der Gewebe des menschlichen Koerpers*. Thesis, University of Bonn, 1819.

Mayor, Georges-François. "Examen microscopique de deux tumeurs cutanée," *Bull. soc. anat. de Paris* 19 (1844): 218-55.

_____. *Sur les tumeurs épidermiques et sur leurs relations avec l'affection cancéreuse*. Paris, 1846.

Meckel, Heinrich. "De pseudoplasmatibus in genere et de carcinomate in specie." In *Amtlicher Bericht ueber die 24sten Versammlung Deutscher Naturforscher und Aerzte im September 1846*, pp. 162-63. Kiel, 1847.

Merat de Vaumartoise, François. S.v. "Mélanose," in *Dictionnaire des sciences médicales*, 1819 ed.

Michel, Eugène. "Du microscope, de ses applications à l'anatomie pathologique, au diagnostic et au traitement des maladies." *Mém. de l'Acad. Royale de Médecine* (Paris) 21 (1857): 241-442.

Minot, Charles Sedgwick. "The Embryological Basis of Pathology." *Science* 13 (1901): 481-98.

Mintz, Beatrice. "Formation and Early Development of Germ Cells." In *Symposium on the Germ Cells and Earliest Stages of Development*, pp. 1-24. Edited by Silvio Ranzi. Fondazioni A. Baselli. Milan: Instituto Lombardo, 1961.

Montfalcon, Jean-Baptiste. S.v. "Tissu," in *Dictionnaire des sciences médicales*, 1821 ed.

Moodie, Roy L. *Paleopathology: An Introduction to the Study of Ancient Evidence of Disease.* Urbana, Ill.: University of Illinois Press, 1923.

Moon, Norman F. "Adamantinoma of the Appendicular Skeleton: A Statistical Review of Reported Cases and Inclusion of Ten New Cases." *Clin. Orth.* 43 (1961): 189-213.

Mueller, Johannes. *Handbuch der Physiologie des Menschens.* 2 vols. Koblenz, 1833-40.

————. "Jahresbericht ueber die Fortschritte der anatomisch-physiologischen Wissenschaften im Jahre 1835." *Arch. Anat. Phys. wiss. Med.,* 1836, pp. ccxviii-xxiv.

————. "Jahresbericht ueber die Fortschritte der anatomisch-physiologischen Wissenschaften im Jahre 1837." *Arch. Anat. Phys. wiss. Med.,* 1838, pp. xci-cxcviii.

————. *On the Nature and Structural Characteristics of Cancer, and of Morbid Growths Which May Be Confounded with It.* Translated by Charles West. London, 1840.

————. *Rede zur Feier des zwei und vierzigsten Stiftungstages des Koeniglichen medicinish-chirurgischen Friedrich-Wilhelms-Institutes am 2sten August, 1836.* Berlin, n.d.

————. "Ueber den feinern Bau der krankhaften Geschwuelste." *Monats. Kgl. Preuss. Akad. Wiss. zu Berlin,* 8 December 1836, pp. 107-113.

————. *Ueber den feinern Bau und die Formen der krankhaften Geschwuelste.* Berlin, 1838.

Naegeli, Carl Wilhelm. *Mechanisch-physiologische Theorie der Abstammungslehre.* Munich and Leipzig, 1884.

Naunyn, Bernard. "Ueber die Entwicklung der Leberkrebse." *Arch. Anat. Phys. wiss. Med.,* 1866, pp. 717-33.

Neuburger, Max. *Die Lehre von der Heilkraft der Natur im Wandel der Zeiten.* Stuttgart, 1926.

Nicholson, G. W. "Sebaceous glands in the cervix uteri." *J. Path. Bact.* 43 (1918): 252-54.

Nicolson, Marjorie H. *Science and Imagination.* New York: Great Seal Books, 1956.

Niebyl, Peter. "The Helmontian Thorn." *Bull. Hist. Med.* 45 (1971): 570-95.

Nordenskiöld, Erik. *The History of Biology.* New York, 1928.

Nussbaum, Moritz. "Zur Differenzierung des Geschlechts im Tierreich." *Arch. mikr. Anat.* 18 (1880): 1-121.

O'Malley, C. D. *Andreas Vesalius of Brussels, 1514-1564.* Berkeley and Los Angeles: University of California Press, 1964.

————. *Michael Servetus: A Translation of His Geographical, Medical, and Astrological Writings, with Introduction and Notes.* Philadelphia: American Philosophical Society, 1953.

Oppenheimer, Jane. *Essays in the History of Embryology and Biology.* Cambridge, Mass.: Harvard University Press, 1967.

————. "The Non-Specificity of the Germ-Layers." *Quart. Rev. Biol.* 15 (1940): 1-27.

Ottley, Drewry. *The Works of John Hunter.* Vol. 1: *The Life of John Hunter.* London, 1835-37.

Pagel, Walter. *J. B. van Helmont: Einfuehrung in die philosophische Medizin des Barock.* Berlin, 1930.

_____. *Paracelsus: An Introduction to Philosophical Medicine in the Era of the Renaissance.* Basel: Karger, 1958.

_____. "The Prime Matter of Paracelsus." *Ambix* 9 (1961): 117-35.

_____. "The Religious and Philosophical Aspects of van Helmont's Science and Medicine." *Suppl. Bull. Hist. Med.* No. 2. 1944.

Paget, James. *Lectures on Surgical Pathology.* 2 vols. London, 1853.

Pander, Christian. *Beitraege zur Entwickelungsgeschichte des Huehnchens im Eye.* Wuerzburg, 1817.

Partington, J. R. *A History of Chemistry.* 4 vols. London, 1961-70.

Pauly, A. *Bibliographie des sciences médicales.* Paris, 1874.

Pearson, John. *Practical Observations on Cancerous Complaints.* London, 1793.

Pechlin, Johannes N. *Observationum physico-medicarum libri tres.* Hamburg, 1691.

Perdulcis, Bartholomaeus. *Universa medicina.* 2d ed. Paris, 1641.

Peyrilhe, Bernard. *A Dissertation on Cancerous Diseases.* London, 1777.

_____. *Dissertatio academica de cancro.* Antwerp, 1775.

Pinel, Philippe. *Nosographie philosophique.* 5th ed. 3 vols. Paris, 1813.

Pott, Percival. *The Chirurgical Works of Percival Pott, F.R.S.: A New Edition.* 3 vols. London, 1779.

Preyer, Wilhelm. "Ueber amoeboide Blutkoerperchen." *Arch. path. Anat. Phys. klin. Med.* 30 (1864): 417-44.

"Queries published by the Society for investigating the Nature and Cure of Cancer." *Edinburgh Med. Surg. J.* 2 (1806): 382-89.

Randall, J. H. *The School of Padua and the Emergence of Modern Science.* Padua: Editrice Antenore, 1961.

Ranvier, Louis, and Cornil, André-Victor. "Contributions à l'étude de développement histologique des tumeurs épithéliales." *J. anat. phys.,* 1866; pp. 271-86.

Rather, L. J. *Addison and the White Corpuscles: An Aspect of Nineteenth-Century Biology.* Berkeley and Los Angeles: University of California Press, 1972.

_____. "Alchemistry, the Kabbala, the Analogy of the 'Creative Word,' and the Origins of Molecular Biology." *Episteme* 6 (1972): 83-103.

_____. "An Early-Nineteenth-Century View of Functional vs. Organic Disease." *A.M.A. Arch. Int. Med.* 108 (1961): 502-06.

_____. *Disease, Life, and Man: Selected Essays by Rudolf Virchow.* Stanford: Stanford University Press, 1958.

_____. "Disturbance of Function (*functio laesa*): The Legendary Fifth Cardinal Sign of Inflammation, Added by Galen to the Four Cardinal Signs of Celsus." *Bull. N.Y. Acad. Med.* 47 (1971): 303-22.

_____. "Georg Ernst Stahl y Friedrich Hoffmann." In *Historia Universal de la Medicina,* vol. 4. Edited by Pedro Laín-Entralgo. 7 vols. Barcelona: Salvat Editores, 1972-75.

_____. "Langenbeck on the Mechanism of Tumor Metastasis and the Transmission of Cancer from Man to Animal." *Clio Medica* 10 (1975): 213-25.

————. "Old and New Views of the Emotions and Bodily Changes: Wright and Harvey versus Descartes, James, and Cannon." *Clio Medica* 1 (1965): 1-25.

————. "Pathology at Mid-Century: A Reassessment of Thomas Willis and Thomas Sydenham." In *Medicine in Seventeenth-Century England,* edited by Allen G. Debus, pp. 71-112. Berkeley and Los Angeles: University of California Press, 1974.

————. "Rudolf Virchow's Views on Pathology, Pathological Anatomy, and Cellular Pathology." *A.M.A. Arch. Path.* 82 (1966): 197-204.

————. "Some Aspects of the Theory and Therapy of Inflammation: From William Harvey to Clemens von Pirquet." In *Proceedings of the Twenty-third Congress of the History of Medicine.* 2 vols. London: Wellcome Institute, 1974.

————. "Some Relations between Eighteenth-Century Fiber Theory and Nineteenth-Century Cell Theory." *Clio Medica* 4 (1969): 191-202.

————. "Systematic Medical Treatises from the Ninth to the Nineteenth Century: The Unchanging Scope and Structure of Academic Medicine in the West." *Clio Medica* 11 (1976): 289-305.

————. "The 'Six Things Non-Natural': Origin and Fate of a Doctrine and a Phrase." *Clio Medica* 3 (1968): 337-47.

————. "Towards a Philosophical Study of the Idea of Disease." In *The Historical Development of Physiological Thought.* Edited by C. M. Brooks and P. F. Cranefield. New York: Hafner, 1959.

————. "Two Questions on Humoral Theory." *Medical History* 15 (1971): 396-98.

————. "Virchow und die Entwicklung des Entzuendungsfrage im neunzehnten Jahrhundert." *Verh. d. 20. Int. Kongr. f. Gesch. d. Med.,* 1966. Hildesheim: 1968.

————. "Virchow und die Entwicklung des Entzuendungsfrage im neunzehnten Jahrhundert." *Verh. d. 20. Int. Kongr. f. Gesch. d. Med.,* 1966. Hildesheim: 1968.

Rather, L. J., and Rohl, Eva. "An English Translation of the Hitherto Untranslated Part of Rokitansky's *Einleitung* to Volume 1 of the *Handbuch der allgemeinen Pathologie* (1846); with a Bibliography of Rokitansky's Published Works." *Clio Medica* 7 (1972): 215-28.

Rather, L. J., and Frerichs, J. B. "The Leibniz-Stahl Controversy. 1. Leibniz' Opening Objections to the *Theoria medica vera." Clio Medica* 3 (1968): 21-40.

Rather, L. J., and Frerichs, J. B. "The Leibniz-Stahl Controversy. 2. Stahl's Survey of the Principal Points of Doubt." *Clio Medica* 5 (1970): 53-67.

Recklinghausen, Friedrich von. "Ueber Eiter- und Bindegewebeskoerperchen." *Arch. f. path. Anat., Phys. klin. Med.* 28 (1863): 157-97.

Reedy, Jeremiah. "Galen on Cancer and Related Diseases." *Clio Medica* 10 (1975): 227-38.

Reichert, Karl B. "Bericht ueber die Fortschritte der mikroskopischen Anatomie in den Jahren 1839 und 1840." *Arch. Anat. Phys. wiss. Med.* (1841), pp. clxii-ccxxvii.

————. "Bericht ueber die Fortschritte der mikroskopischen Anatomie im Jahre 1853." *Arch. Anat. Phys. wiss. Med.,* 1854, pp. 1-80.

Remak, Robert. "Ein Beitrag zur Entwickelungsgeschichte der krebshaften Geschwuelste." *Deutsche Klinik,* 1854, pp. 170-174.

————. *Untersuchungen ueber die Entwickelung der Wirbelthiere.* Berlin, 1855.

Richter, C. S. "Ein Fall von adamantinomartiger Geschwulst des Schienbeins." *Z. Krebsforsch.* 32 (1930): 272-79.

Richter, Paul. "Ueber die Entwicklung des aristotelischen Begriffes der Tumores praeter naturam." *Monat. praktische Derm.* 44 (1907): 65-70.

Riolan, Jean. *Joannis Riolani filii...opera anatomica.* Paris, 1649.

Robin, Charles. *Leçons sur les humeurs normales et morbides du corps de l'homme.* Paris, 1874.

_____. "Mémoire sur les divers modes de la naissance de la substance organisée en général." *J. anat. phys.,* 1864, pp. 152-83.

_____. "Mémoire sur les divers modes de la naissance de la substance organisée en général." *J. anat. phys.,* 1865, pp. 113-52.

_____. Mémoire sur une espèce de tumeur formée aux dépens du tissu des bulbes dentaires." *Compt. rend. soc. de biol.,* ser. 3, 4 (1862): 199-221.

_____. "Sur une variété particulière de tumeur fibreuse provenant du follicule dentaire." *Bull. acad. méd.* 24 (1858-59): 1205-211.

Roemer, Oskar. "Die Pathologie der Zaehne." In *Handbuch der speziellen pathologischen Anatomie und Histologie.* Vol. 4, bk. 2. Edited by Friedrich Henke and Otto Lubarsch. Berlin, 1928.

Rokitansky, Karl von. *Handbuch der pathologischen Anatomie.* 3 vols. Vienna, 1842-46. Translated as *A Manual of Pathological Anatomy* by William Edward Swaine. London, 1849-52.

_____. *Lehrbuch der pathologischen Anatomie.* Vienna, 1855.

_____. *Manual of Pathological Anatomy.* Translated by W. E. Swaine. 4 vols. London, 1849-54.

Rosai, Juan. "Adamantinoma of the Tibia: Electron Microscopic Evidence of Its Epithelial Origin." *Am. J. Clin. Path.* 51 (1969): 786-92.

Rosen, George. "Jacob Henle: On Miasmata and Contagia." *Bull. Hist. Med.* 6 (1938): 907-83.

Roth, Moritz. *Andreas Vesalius bruxellensis.* Berlin, 1892.

Royer-Collard, Hippolyte. "Considérations générales sur les lois d'organisme dans l'état de santé et dans l'état de maladie." *Bull. Soc. Anat. de Paris* 3 (1828): 135-50.

Rudolphi, Karl A. *Grundriss der Physiologie.* Berlin, 1821.

Ruffer, Marc A. *Studies in the Paleopathology of Egypt.* Chicago, 1921.

Russell, E. S. *Form and Function: A Contribution to the History of Animal Morphology.* London, 1916.

Ruszynák, István; Földi, Milhály; Szabó, György. *Lymphatics and the Lymph Circulation.* London: Pergamon Press, 1960.

Schleiden, Matthias. "Beitraege zur Phytogenese." *Arch. Anat. Phys. wiss. Med.,* 1838, pp. 137-76.

Schoener, Erich. "Das Viererschema in der antiken Humoralpathologie." *Sudhoff's Arch. Gesch. Med. Wiss.,* supplement 4. 1964.

Scholem, Gershom. *Sabbatai Sevi: The Mystical Messiah.* Princeton: Princeton University Press, 1973.

Schultze, Max. "Ein heizbarer Objekttisch und seine Verwendung bei Untersuchungen des Blutes." *Arch. mikr. Anat.* 1 (1865): 1-42.

Schwann, Theodor. "Fortsetzung der Untersuchung ueber die Uebereinstimmung in der Structur der Thiere und Pflanzen." *N. Notiz. Gebiete Nat. Heilkunde,* no. 103 (February, 1838), pp. 225-29.

―――――. *Mikroskopische Untersuchungen ueber die Uebereinstimmung in der Struktur und dem Wachstum der Thiere und Pflanzen.* Berlin, 1839. Translated by Henry Smith as *Microscopical Researches into the Accordance in the Structure and Growth of Animals and Plants.* London, 1847.

―――――. "Nachtrag zu den Untersuchung ueber die Uebereinstimmung in der Thiere und Pflanzen." *N. Notiz. Gebiete Nat. Heilkunde,* no. 107 (April, 1838), pp. 21-23.

―――――. "Ueber die Analogie in der Structur und dem Wachstum der Thiere und Pflanzen." *N. Notiz. Gebiete Nat. Heilkunde,* no. 93 (January, 1838), pp. 33-37.

―――――. "Vorlaeufige Mittheilungen, betreffend Versuche ueber die Weingaehrung und Faeulnis." *Ann. Physik Chem.* 41 (1837): 184-94.

Sédillot, Charles. *Recherches sur le cancer.* 2 vols. Strasbourg, 1846. Reprinted in his *Contributions à la chirurgie,* vol. 1. Paris, 1868.

Sennert, Daniel. *Danielis Sennerti...operum in sex tomos divisorum...editio.* Lyons, 1676.

―――――. *Practicae medicae liber quintus.* Wittenberg, 1672.

Shaw, Peter. *Philosophical Principles of Universal Chemistry...Drawn from the Collegium Jenense of Dr. George Ernst Stahl.* London, 1730.

Siegel, Rudolph E. *Galen's System of Physiology and Medicine.* New York and Basel: Karger, 1968.

Simon, Franz J. *Animal Chemistry With Reference to the Physiology and Pathology of Man.* Translated by George E. Day. 2 vols. London, 1846.

―――――. *Physiologische und pathologische Anthropochemie mit Beruecksichtigung der eigentlichen Zoochemie.* Berlin, 1842.

Simpson, James. "Case of Amputation of the Womb Followed by Pregnancy; with Remarks on the Pathology and Radical Treatment of the Cauliflower Excrescence from the Os Uteri." *Edinburgh Med. Surg. J.* 55 (1841): 104-112.

Simson, L.; Lampe, I.; and Abell, M. R. "Suprasellar Germinomas." *Cancer* 22 (1968): 533-44.

Singer, Charles. *A History of Technology.* 5 vols. Oxford: Oxford University Press, 1954-58.

―――――. *A Short History of Science to the Nineteenth Century.* Oxford: Oxford University Press, 1941.

Skinner, Henry Alan. *The Origin of Medical Terms.* Baltimore: Williams and Wilkins, 1949.

Spjut, Harlan J.; Dorfman, Howard D.; Fechner, Robert; and Ackerman, Lauren. "Tumors of Bone and Cartilage." *AFIP Atlas of Tumor Pathology,* ser. 2 fasc. 5, pp. 315-23. Bethesda: Armed Forces Institute of Pathology, 1971.

Stahl, Georg Ernst. *Philosophical Principles of Universal Chemistry...Drawn from the Collegium Jenense of Dr. George Ernst Stahl by Peter Shaw, M.D.* London, 1780.

―――――. *Theoria medica vera.* 3 vols. Edited by J. L. Choulant. Leipzig, 1831-33.

Sudhoff, Karl. "Ueber das primaere multiple Carcinom des Knochensystems." Inaugural dissertation, Erlangen, 1875.

Taylor, A. E. *A Commentary of Plato's Timaeus.* London: Oxford University Press, 1928.

Temkin, Owsei. "The Scientific Approach to Disease: Specific Entity and Individual Sickness." In *Scientific Change, Symposium on the History of Science.* Edited by A. C. Crombie. London: Basic Books, 1961.

_____. "Die Krankheitsauffassung von Hippokrates und Sydenham in ihren Epidemien." *Arch. Gesch. Med.* 20 (1928): 327-52.

Thévenot, Léon. "Des endothéliomes des os." *Rev. Chirur.* 21 (1900): 756-79.

Thiersch, Carl. *Der Epithelkrebs, namentlich der Haut.* Leipzig, 1865.

_____. *Tageblatt der 36. Versammlung deutscher Naturforscher und Aertze im Speyer vom 17. bis 24. September, 1861. Beilage zum Tageblatt. pp. 29, 30.* Speyer, n.d.

Van Helmont, Jean Baptiste. *Ortus medicinae. . .edente authoris filio Francisco Mercurio van Helmont.* Amsterdam, 1652.

Van Swieten, Gérard. *Commentaria in Hermanni Boerhaave aphorismos.* Hildburghausen and Meiningen, 1747.

Vesalius, Andreas. *De humani corporis fabrica.* Basel, 1543; facsimile reprint ed., Brussels: Cultures et Civilisations, 1964.

Virchow, Rudolf. "Cellular-Pathologie." *Arch. path. Anat. Phys. klin. Med.* 8 (1855): 1-39.

_____. *Cellular Pathology As Based upon Physiological and Pathological Histology, by Rudolf Virchow: Translated from the second German edition by Frank Chance, with a new introductory essay by L. J. Rather.* New York: Dover Publications, 1971.

_____. *Die Cellularpathologie in ihrer Begruendung auf physiologische und pathologische Gewebelehre. Zwanzig Vorlesungen gehalten waehrend der Monate Februar, Maerz und April 1858 im pathologischen Institute zu Berlin.* Berlin, 1858; 4th ed., Berlin, 1871.

_____. *Die krankhaften Geschwuelste. Dreissig Vorlesungen gehalten waehrend des Wintersemesters 1862-1863 an der Universitaet zu Berlin.* Berlin, 1863-67. Translated by Paul Aronssohn as *Pathologie des tumeurs.* 4 vols. Paris, 1867-76.

_____. *Die med. Ref.,* no. 51 (June 22, 1849), pp. 271, 272.

_____. "Die neue Auflage von Rokitansky's allgemeiner pathologischen Anatomie." *Wien. med. Woch.,* no. 26 (1855), pp. 401-5.

_____. "Die neue Auflage von Rokitansky's allgemeiner pathologischen Anatomie." *Wien. med. Woch.,* no. 27 (1855), pp. 417-21.

_____. *Gesammelte Abhandlungen zur wissenschaftlichen Medicin.* Frankfurt, 1856; 2d ed., Berlin, 1862.

_____. *Handbuch der speciellen Pathologie und Therapie.* 6 vols. in 9. Erlangen, 1854.

_____. *Hundert Jahre allgemeiner Pathologie.* Berlin, 1895.

_____. "Krankheitswesen und Krankheitsursachen." *Arch. path. Anat. Phys. klin. Med.* 79 (1880): 1-19; 185-228.

_____. "Opinion sur la valeur du microscope." *Gaz. hebdomadaire méd. chirur.* (Paris), February 16, 1855, pp. 124-26.

_____. "Rokitansky, *Handbuch der allgemeinen pathologischen Anatomie."Preuss. Med. Z.,* no. 49 (1846), pp. 237-238.

————. "Rokitansky, *Handbuch der allgemeinen pathologischen Anatomie." Preuss. Med. Z.*, no. 50 (1846), pp. 243-244.

————. "Tuberkulose und ihre Beziehung zu Entzuendung, Skrophulosis, Typhus." *Verh. physikal. med. Gesell. in Wuerzburg* 1 (1850): 81-87.

————. "Ueber die Reform der pathologischen und therapeutischen Anschauungen durch die mikroskopischen Untersuchung." *Arch. path. Anat. Phys. klin. Med.* 1 (1847): 207-55.

————. "Ueber Kankroide und Papillargeschwuelste." *Verh. physikal. med. Gesell. in Wuerzburg* 1 (1850): 106-11.

————. "Ueber Metaplasie." *Arch. path. Anat. Phys. klin. Med.* 97 (1884): 410-30.

————. "Ueber Pachydermia laryngis." *Berlin. klin. Woch.*, August 8, 1887, pp. 585-89.

————. "Ueber Perlgeschwuelste (Cholesteatoma Joh. Mueller's)." *Arch. path. Anat. Phys. klin. Med.* 8 (1855): 371-415.

————. "Zur Entwickelungsgeschichte des Krebses, nebst Bemerkungen ueber Fettbildung im thierischen Koerper und pathologischer Resorption." *Arch. path. Anat. Phys. klin. Med.* 1 (1847): 91-204.

Vogel, Julius. "Gewebe in pathologischer Hinsicht." In *Handwoerterbuch der Physiologie mit Ruecksicht auf physiologische Pathologie*, 4 vols. in 5. Berlin, 1842-53. Vol. 1, pp. 789-859.

————. *Icones histologiae pathologicae.* Leipzig, 1843.

————. *The Pathological Anatomy of the Human Body.* Translated from the German edition of 1845 by George E. Day. Philadelphia, 1847.

Volkmann, Richard. "Die Krankheiten der Bewegungsorgane." In *Handbuch der allgemeinen und speciellen Chirurgie*, vol. 2, pt. 2, 1st half, pp. 234-920. Edited by Franciscus J. Pitha and Theodor Billroth. Stuttgart, 1882.

Voltaire, François Marie Arouet de. "La Pucelle." In *Oeuvres complètes*, vol. 7. Paris, 1887.

Waldeyer, Wilhelm. "Die Entwickelung der Carcinome." *Arch. path. Anat. Phys. klin. Med.* 41 (1867): 470-523.

————. "Die Entwickelung der Carcinome." *Arch. path. Anat. Phys. klin. Med.* 55 (1872): 67-159.

————. "Die neueren Forschungen im Gebiete der Keimblattlehre." *Deutsche med. Woch.* 85 (1885): 305-16.

————. *Eierstock und Ei.* Leipzig, 1870.

————. "Ueber Karyokinese und ihre Beziehung zu den Befruchtungsvorgaengen." *Arch. mikr. Anat.* 32 (1888): 1-22.

————. *Untersuchungen ueber die erste Anlage des Wirbelthierleibes.* Leipzig, 1868.

Walsham, W. J. "On the Osseous Tumors of Bone Formerly Called Osteoid Cancers." *St. Bartholomew's Hospital Reports* 15 (1879): 11-18.

Walshe, Walter H. *The Anatomy, Physiology, Pathology, and Treatment of Cancer.* Boston, 1844.

Wardrop, J. W. *Observations on Fungus Haematodes or Soft Cancer. . . Containing Also a Comparative View of the Structure of Fungus Haematodes and Cancer.* Edinburgh, 1809.

Waterman, Robert. *Theodor Schwann, Leben und Werk.* Duesseldorf: L. Schwann, 1960.

Watson, Thomas. *Lectures on the Principles and Practice of Physic*. London, 1848.

Weber, Carl Otto. *Chirurgische Erfahrungen und Untersuchungen*. Berlin, 1859.

————. "Ueber die Betheiligung der Muskelkoerperchen und der quergestreiften Muskeln an den Neubildungen nebst Bemerkungen ueber die Lehre von der Specificitaet der Gewebselemente." *Arch. path. Anat. Phys. klin. Med.* 39 (1867): 254-69.

————. "Ueber die Entwickelung des Epithelkrebses in inneren Organen, nebst Bemerkungen ueber die Structur der Leber und Lunge." *Arch. path. Anat. Phys. klin. Med.* 29 (1864): 163-89.

————. "Ueber die Neubildung quergestreiften Muskelfasern, insbesondere die regenerative Neubildung derselben nach Verletzungen." *Arch. path. Anat. Phys. klin. Med.* 39 (1867): 216-53.

Weismann, August. *Das Keimplasma: Eine Theorie der Vererbung*. Jena, 1892.

————. *Die Bedeutung der sexuellen Fortpflanzung fuer die Selektionstheorie*. Jena, 1886.

————. *Die Kontinuitaet des Keimplasmas als Grundlage einer Theorie der Vererbung*. Jena, 1885.

————. "Ueber das Wachsen der quergestreiften Muskeln nach Beobachtungen am Frosch." *Z. rat. Med.*, ser. 3, 9 (1861): 263-84.

————. *Ueber die Vererbung*. Jena, 1883.

Willis, Rupert. *Pathology of Tumours*. London: Butterworth, 1948; 4th ed., 1967.

Witschi, Emil. "Migration of the Germ Cells of Human Embryos from the Yolk Sac to the Primitive Gonadal Folds." *Contr. Embryol. Carnegie Inst.* 32 (1948): 67-80.

Wolfe, David E. "Sydenham and Locke on the Limits of Anatomy." *Bull. Hist. Med.* 25 (1961): 193-220.

Wolff, Jacob. *Die Lehre von der Krebskrankheit von den aeltesten Zeiten bis zum Gegenwart*. 2 vols. 2d ed. Jena, 1929.

Wolff, Caspar Friedrich. *De tela quam dicunt cellulosa*. St. Petersburg, n.d.

Wyss, Oskar. "Die heterologen (boesartigen) Neubildungen der Vorsteherdruese." *Arch. path. Anat. Phys. klin. Med.* 35 (1866): 378-412.

Zahn, Friedrich Wilhelm. "Sur le sort des tissus implantés dans l'organisme." Proceedings of the Congrès internationale des sciences médicales, Geneva, 1877; *Compt. rend. mém.*, 1878, pp. 658-64.

Zanobio, Bruno. "Micrographie illusoire et théories sur la structure de la matière vivante." *Clio Medica* 6 (1971): 25-40.

Zenker, Friedrich. *Ueber die Veraenderungen der willkuerlichen Muskeln im Typhus*. Leipzig, 1864.

BIBLIOGRAPHIC SUPPLEMENT

Ackerknecht, Erwin H. *Rudolph Virchow: Doctor, Statesman, Anthropologist*. Madison: University of Wisconsin Press, 1953. The most complete account of Virchow's achievements.

Broca, Paul B. *Traité des tumeurs*. 2 vols. Paris, 1866-69. An informative survey of theories of tumor genesis, from Galen through Virchow, constitutes the first chapter (1: 1-44) of Broca's treatise.

Churchill, Frederic B. "Rudolf Virchow and the Pathologist's Criteria for the Inheritance of Acquired Characteristics." *J. Hist. Med. and Allied Sci.* 31 (1976): 117-48. Among the topics discussed in this extensive paper are Mueller's cultivation of the analogy between embryonic and tumor cell growth, and Virchow's substitution of connective tissues for Schwann's cytoblastema as the source of new cells, both normal and neoplastic.

Florkin, Marcel. *Naissance et déviation de la théorie cellulaire dans l'oeuvre de Théodor Schwann.* Paris: Hermann, 1960. The best account of Schwann's achievements in biology.

Holmes, Frederic L. "The *Milieu Intérieur* and the Cell Theory." *Bull. Hist. Med.* 37 (1963): 315-35. Bernard's synthesis of cell theory with his own theory of the *milieu intérieur.*

Huntington, R. W., and Huntington, R. W. III. "Classification of Neoplasms: A Critical Appraisal." *Perspect. Biol. and Med.,* Winter, 1977, pp. 215-22. A critique of the current system of tumor classification tentatively proposing an alternative scheme based on the assumption that all cells, including those that give rise to neoplasms, not only contain the total genome but may express it over a wider range than is generally admitted.

Maulitz, Russell C. "Rudolf Virchow, Julius Cohnheim, and the Program of Pathology." *Bull. Hist. Med.,* in press. An informed account of the complex relationships actually obtaining between the Virchovian and Cohnheimian research programs, with a critique of the received view. Includes a survey of the development of inflammation theory in mid-nineteenth-century Germany.

Sontag, Susan. "Illness as Metaphor," "Images of Illness," and "Disease as Political Metaphor." *New York Review of Books,* January 26 and February 9 and 24, 1978. An interesting, historical approach to a somewhat neglected topic: the use, abuse, and interchange of certain metaphors in the language of medicine, politics, and general literature, with emphasis on cancer, tuberculosis, and syphilis.

Triolo, Victor A. "Nineteenth-Century Foundations of Cancer Research: Advances in Tumor Pathology, Nomenclature and Theories of Oncogenesis." *Cancer Research* 25 (1965): 75-106. A fully documented study.

ABBREVIATIONS

A.M.A. Arch. Int. Med. American Medical Association Archives of Internal Medicine
A.M.A. Arch. Path. American Medical Association Archives of Pathology
Am. J. Clin. Path. American Journal of Clinical Pathology
Anat. Anzeig. Anatomischer Anzeiger
Anat. Rec. Anatomical Record
Ann. Physik Chem. Annalen der Physik und Chemie
Ann. sci. nat. Annales des sciences naturelles
Ann. Surg. Annals of Surgery
Arch. Anat. Entwickelungsgeschichte Archiv fuer Anatomie und Entwickelungsgeschichte
Arch. Anat. Phys. wiss. Med. Archiv fuer Anatomie, Physiologie und wissenschaftliche Medicin
Arch. gén. méd. Archives générales de médecine
Arch. Gesch. Med. Archiv fuer Geschichte der Medizin und Naturwissenschaften (Sudhoff's *Archiv*)
Arch. klin. Chirur. Archiv fuer klinische Chirurgie
Arch. mikr. Anat. Archiv fuer mikroskopische Anatomie
Arch. path. Anat. Phys. klin. Med. Archiv fuer pathologische Anatomie Physiologie, und fuer klinische Medizin (Virchow's *Archiv*)
Arch. Phys. Archives de physiologie
Arch. phys. Heilkunde Archiv fuer physiologische Heilkunde
Arch. phys. norm. pathol. Archives de physiologie normale et pathologique
Australian and New Zealand J. Surg. Australian and New Zealand Journal of Surgery
Beitr. z. klin. Chirur. Beitraege zur klinischen Chirurgie
Berlin. klin. Woch. Berliner klinischer Wochenschrift
British and Foreign Medico-Chirur. Rev. British and Foreign Medico-Chirurgical Review
Bull. Hist. Med. Bulletin of the History of Medicine
Bull. Acad. méd. Bulletin de l'Académie de Médecine
Bull. Acad. Roy. Méd. de Belgique Bulletin de l'Académie Royale de Médecine de Belgique
Bull. École Méd. de Paris Bulletin de l'École de Médecine de Paris
Bull. N.Y. Acad. Med. Bulletin of the New York Academy of Medicine
Bull. soc. anat. de Paris Bulletin de la Société Anatomique de Paris
Centrb. allg. path. Anat. Centralblatt fuer allgemeine pathologische Anatomie
Clin. Orth. Clinical Orthopedics
Compt. rend. Acad. Sci. Comptes rendus de l'Académie des Sciences
Compt. rend. Soc. Biol. Comptes rendus de la Société de Biologie
Cong. int. sci. méd. Congrès internationale des sciences médicales, 1877
Contr. Embryol. Carnegie Inst. Contributions to Embryology, Carnegie Institution of Washington, D.C.
Deutsche med. Woch. Deutsche medicinische Wochenschrift
Deutsche Z. Chirur. Deutsche Zeitschrift fuer Chirurgie
Die med. Ref. Die medicinische Reform
Edinburgh Med. Surg. J. Edinburgh Medical and Surgical Journal
Edinburgh New Phil. J. Edinburgh New Philosophical Journal
Ergeb. allg. Path. Anat. Ergebnisse der allgemeinen Pathologie und pathologischen Anatomie
Frankfurt. Z. Path. Frankfurter Zeitschrift fuer Pathologie
Gaz. hebdomadaire méd. chirur. Gazette Hebdomadaire de médecine et de chirurgie

249

Gaz. méd. de Strasbourg Gazette médicale de Strasbourg

Jahrb. in-und auslaend. gesam. Med. Jahrbuecher der in-und auslaendischen gesammten Medicin

Jenaische Ann. Phys. Med. Jenaische Annalen fuer Physiologie und Medicin

Jenaische Z. Med. Naturw. Jenaische Zeitschrift fuer Medicin und Naturwissenschaft

J. Hist. Med. Allied Sci. Journal of the History of Medicine and Allied Sciences

J. anat. phys. Journal de l'anatomie et de la physiologie

J. Path. Bact. Journal of Pathology and Bacteriology

London, Edinburgh and Dublin Phil. Mag. J. Sci. London, Edinburgh and Dublin Philosophical Magazine and Journal of Science

L'Union médicale l'Union médicale

Lyon méd. Lyon médicale

Medico-Chirur. Trans. Medico-Chirurgical Transactions

Mém. Acad. Roy. Chirur. Mémoires de l'Académie Royale de Chirurgie

Monat. prakt. Derm. Monatsschrift fuer praktische Dermatologie

Monats. Kgl. Preuss. Akad. Monatsberichte der Koeniglich preussischen Akademie der Wissenschaften zu Berlin

Month. J. Med. Sci. Monthly Journal of Medical Science

Muench. med. Woch. Muenchner medizinische Wochenschrift

N. Notiz. Gebiete Nat. Heilkunde Neue Notizen aus dem Gebiete der Natur-und Heilkunde

Perspect. Biol. and Med. Perspectives in Biology and Medicine

Phil. Trans. Roy. Soc. Philosophical Transactions of the Royal Society

Preuss. med. Z. Preussische medicinal-Zeitung

Proc. Roy. Soc. of London Proceedings of the Royal Society of London

Quart. Rev. Biol. Quarterly Review of Biology

Rev. Chirur. Revue de chirurgie

Rev. méd. Hosp. gen. México Revista médica del hospital general México

St. Barth. Hosp. Rep. St Bartholomew's Hospital Reports

Sudhoff's Arch. Gesch. wiss. Archiv fuer Geschichte der Medicine

Suppl. Bull. Hist. Med. Supplement, Bulletin of the History of Medicine

Trans. Linn. Soc. Transactions of the Linnaean Society

Trans. Medico-Chirur. Soc. of Edinburgh Transactions of the Medico-Chirurgical Society of Edinburgh

Verh. deutsch. path. Gesell. Verhandlungen der deutschen pathologischen Gesellschaft

Verh. physikal. med. Gesell. Verhandlungen der physikalisch-medicinischen Gesellschaft in Wuerzburg

Verh. 20 Int. Kongr. Gesch. Med. Verhandlungen des XX. Internationalen Kongresses fuer Geschichte der Medizin, 1966

Wien. med. Blaett. Wiener medicinische Blaetter

Wien. med. Woch. Wiener medicinische Wochenschrift

Z. Anat. Entwickelungsgeschichte Zeitschrift fuer Anatomie und Entwickelungsgeschichte

Z. Biol. Zeitschrift fuer Biologie

Z. Krebsforsch. Zeitschrift fuer Krebsforschung

Z. rat. Med. Zeitschrift fuer rationelle Medicin

Z. wiss. Zool. Zeitschrift fuer wissenschaftliche Zoologie

INDEX

Abernethy, John, 70-71, 193 *n.*103, 215 *n.*69
Abscesses, 136
Accidental tissue, 61, 62, 64, 67, 75
Actuality, 96
Adamantinoma. *See* Tibial cancroid
Addison, William, white cell emigration and, 224 *n.*169, 225 *n.*170
Aetius of Amida, 16
Albertini, A. von, 161-62
  histogenesis and, 222, *n.*162
Albinus, Bernard, 54
Albumen, 65, 66, 68
Alchemy, Paracelsus and, 26
Alibert, Jean, 107, 112, 209 *n.*145
Amici Giovanni, 82
Anatomy, 29, 35, 186 *n.*79, 189 *n.*1
  classical Greek knowledge of, 47-48
  injection specimens in, lymphatic system and, 32
  macroscopic, 92, 211 *n.*5
  microscope and (Bichat), 55
  microscopic, 51-52, 55, 92
  pathological, 39, 59, 60-61, 64, 74, 75, 211 *n.*24
  in prehistoric times, 46-47
Anaxagoras, 47
Andral, Gabriel, 75, 94, 106, 192 *n.*93, 193 *n.* 112, 194 *n.*128
  on cancer, 69-70
Angiosarcomas, 156, 167. *See also* Sarcoma
Aniline dyes, 111, 139, 155, 168, 213 *n.*46, 229 *n.*213.
Aristotle, 11, 15, 19, 21, 22, 47, 48, 49, 51, 52, 56, 64, 182 *n.*24
Arteries, 14, 19-20, 22, 23, 24, 25, 30, 34
  Bichat and, 56
  Galen on, 49, 50
Aselli, Gasparo, 30
Astruc, Jean, 39-40
Atossa, 9
Aurelianus, Caelius. *See* Caelius Aurelianus
Avicenna, 16, 48, 49

Bacteriology, 35
  in late 1800s, 168-69, 225 *n.*182
Baer, Karl Ernst von, 86, 119
  germ-layer theory and, 78, 79-81
Baillie, Matthew, 59, 61

Bard, Louis, 176-78, 229 *n.*210, 229 *n.*211
Bartholin, Thomas, 31
Bassi, Agostino, 203 *n.*101
Bayle, Gaspard-Laurent, 53, 59, 62-63, 106, 191 *n.*60
Beard, J., 229 *n.*215
Béclard, P. A., 59
Bennett, John Hughes, 67, 111
  on cancroids, 114-15
  laboratory methods of, 207 *n.*132, 209 *n.*134
Bergmann, Ernst von, 215 *n.*66
Berres, Joseph, 198 *n.*30
Bichat, François-Xavier, 10, 39, 45, 48, 70, 72, 92, 118, 199 *n.*41, 215 *n.*69
  disease and, 60
  pathological anatomy and, 61, 212 *n.*24
  tissue concept of, 52-58
  tumor theory and, 58-59
Bile, 184 *n.*56, 184 *n.*58. *See also* Black bile
  humoralism and, 11, 13, 15, 16, 29
  Stahl on, 32
Billroth, Theodor, 148, 162, 163, 174, 177, 217 *n.*89
  epithelial cancer and, 141-42
Biopsy, Kuess and, 110, 206 *n.*126
Black bile (Atra bilis/melancholy humor), 11, 13, 14, 15-16, 29, 34, 45, 182 *n.*19, 184 *n.*58. *See also* Bile
Blastema, 94, 104, 109, 110, 113, 114, 115, 119, 120, 129, 131, 138, 200 *n.*51, 217 *n.*100. *See also* Cytoblastema
  cell generative behavior of, 95
  Foerster and, 125
  Liebig and, 65
  Rokitansky and, 99-100
  Virchow and, 101-4
Blastema theory, 42, 90-92, 115, 118-24, 128, 200 *n.*62, 203 *n.*94
  abandonment of, 95
  in England and France, 144
Bleeding (therapeutic). *See* Bloodletting
Blood, 68, 95, 104, 183 *n.*42, 184 *n.*56, 184 *n.*58, 188 *n.*118
  clotting of, blastema and, 200 *n.*66
  Harvey and, 42
  humoralism and, 11, 12, 15, 16, 27, 65, 66
  lymph and, 31, 32, 45
  microscopy of, 77
  tumors produced by, 39

251

Blood circulation, 32, 75, 184 n.50
    Aristotle on, 48
    Galenical theory of, 19-21
    Harvey and, 21-26, 30, 32
    Plato on, 47
    use of term, 23
Bloodletting, 19, 20, 24, 25, 27
Blumenbach, Johann, 57, 129
Boerhaave, Hermann, 28, 32, 34, 41, 182 n.19,
    204 n.109
Boll, Franz, 174
Bone
    carcinoma of, 156, 157, 220 n.146
    paleopathological, tumors in, 8
    tumors, 15, 158, 159
Bordeu, Théophile, 53, 57
Bouillaud, Jean-Baptiste, 106
Brain tumors, 167
Breast cancer, 9-10, 13, 39, 40, 68, 71, 126
    description of clinical course of untreated
        (Bayle/Cayol), 191 n.60
    Gendron's remarks on, 36, 37-38
    Hodgkin on, 73-74
    Hunter on, 45, 188 n.126
    origin of (Cornil), 144
    Pechlin on, 182 n.19
    surgical removal of, Stahl on, 33-34, 35
    Virchow on, 213 n.55
    Waldeyer on, 150-51
Breuer, Robert, 214 n.59
Brock, A. J., 189 n.4
Broussais, François, 67
Brown, Robert, 67, 84, 85, 196 n.16
Bruch, Carl, 111, 207 n.131
Brunner on Fischer's tumor, 158
Buffon, Georges, 67
Buhl, Ludwig, 148-49
Burns, John, 71, 72
Burton, Robert, 50

Caelius Aurelianus, 11
Caesalpinus, Andreas, 22-23, 24
Cancer. See also Carcinoma; Epithelial theory
    of cancer; Metastasis; Neoplasia; Sar-
    coma; Tumors; names of specific sites
    Andral on, 69-70
    Billroth on, 174
    cell identification, 108-9
    cells in, 90-91, 101, 102-3, 107, 108-12, 114-
        15, 117, 118, 132, 135, 142, 146, 147, 149,
        150, 151, 152-54, 159, 161, 162, 166-67,
        202 n.84, 204 n.113, 206 n.122, 206 n.127,
        207 n.128, 207 n.129, 209 n.148, 219 n.131,
        223 n.164
    cell specificity in, debates over, 104-12
    cellular structure of, 87-88
    chemical basis for, 98-99, 102, 103, 111, 132,

    136, 171
    contagiousness of, 107, 204 n.110, 206 n.121
    deep-lying, epithelial origin of, 113
    as disturbance of nutritive process, 102
    embryology and, 88, 119-24, 139, 145
    emotions and, 11-12, 34, 182 n.19, 187 n.106
    epithelial, 113, 121, 128, 134, 138, 140, 141,
        144, 145-46, 147, 148, 149-54, 216 n.81,
        217 n.89
    Fallopio on, 14-19
    Fernel's description of, 14
    Galen and, 13, 21
    Gendron on, 35-39, 41
    genesis, solidistic account of, 35-39
    Helmont on pathophysiology of, 28
    in Hippocratic writings, 9-10, 183 n.36
    Hunter's coagulating lymph and, 41-45
    infectious theory of, 140, 151-52, 166, 171
    inflammatory process and, 21, 32-34
    lymphatic humoralism and, 39-41
    metaplasia and (Virchow), 174-76
    microscopic structure of (Mueller), 105
    Mueller's classification of, 198 n.34
    occult, 9-10, 33
    pain of advanced, 187 n.92
    Paracelsus on, 27, 184 n.55
    as parasitic growth, 72-73, 76, 78, 194 n.127
    pathogenesis of (Lobstein), 67
    questions concerning (England, early
        1800s), 70, 193 n.97
    recognition of, 62-64
    "seeds," 32-35, 90-92, 185 n.60
    Sennert on, 29
    spread of, 63, 74, 140, 142, 146, 150-51,
        153-54
    Stahl on, 32-35
    transplantation experiments, 107-8, 109,
        132, 140, 173, 226 n.195, 227 n.197, 228
        n.206
    trauma and, 157, 160, 171
    "true," and skin lesions, 112-17
    Virchow on, 103-4, 132-37, 174
    as a "virus" (Peyrilhe), 41
    "viruses," 168
Cancerous degeneration, 38, 90, 109, 140. See
    also transformation entries
    Laennec and, 63-64
Carcinoma, 34, 44, 150, 151. See also Cancer;
    Metastasis
    of bone, 156, 157, 220 n.146
    cell growth and (Foerster), 126, 127-28
    descriptions of, 220 n.146
    epithelial origin of, 157, 162-69, 217 n.89,
        223 n.164
    histogenesis of, 113
    medullary, 109
    origin of (Virchow), 135

spread of, 106, 154
of stomach (Waldeyer), 151
Virchow on, 174
Volkmann on, 156
Waldeyer on, 152-54, 156, 162-69
Carcinoma rests, 163. *See also* Rests
Cancroids, 112-17, 144, 148, 174, 209 *n*.145.
    See also Tibial cancroid
cells of, 122, 147
Virchow's views on, 134, 209 *n*.149, 210
    n.151, 217 *n*.89
Carmichael, Richard, 194 *n*.127
Carswell, Robert, 74-76, 102
Cato the Elder, 10
Cauterization, 9
Cayol, Jean-Bruno, 62-63
on cancer of the breast, 191 *n*.60
Cell globes, 198 *n*.33
Cells. See also Cancer, cells in; Cell theory;
    Pathology, cellular; *names of specific types
    of cells*
"aberrant germ," 174
Bichat and, 56
in cellular tissue, 58
as closed unit (Virchow), 228, *n*.206
cysts and (Bichat), 54
developmental potencies of (Billroth), 142
division of, 81, 119, 121, 123, 125, 133, 153,
    164, 177-78, 200 *n*.62, 214 *n*.59, 229 *n*.213
division between species of (Klebs), 146
as embryo of tumor, 105
emigrated ameboid blood, 162, 164, 224
    n.169, 225 *n*.170
in eye, 86
fibers as, 189 *n*.4
genesis of tumor, 10
genetic substance in (Bard), 177, 179, 227
    n.201
germ, 178, 204 *n*.113, 229 *n*.215
Hooke's "discovery" of, 51
incapability of interconversion of (Bill-
    roth), 142, 148, 174
in chorda dorsalis of larval frog, 93
as morphological units, 87, 102
Mueller's, 88-90, 197 *n*.28
origin of, 85, 87, 91, 94, 101, 103, 115, 118-
    24, 133, 137, 196 *n*.16, 217 *n*.89, 223 *n*.165
reproduction of, 85
somatic, 178-79
as *spatiola*, 189 *n*.20
specificity, limits of, 148-78
tagging of (Cohnheim), 143
transplanted, 109
tumor
    Cohnheim on, 170-71
    Mueller on, 90
tumor tissue and, 82, 83

Virchow on size of, 175
Cell theory. *See also* Cells
    genesis of cells in tumors and, 95-104,
        120-22
    history of, 87
    Mueller and, 88-92
    Schwann and, 10, 84-88, 90, 91, 92-95, 105,
        108, 113, 118, 119, 120, 122, 125, 130,
        197 *n*.22, 200 *n*.62, 210 *n*.1, 211 *n*.5, 211
        n.17
    tumors and, 82-117
    Vogel and, 97
"Cellular membrane"
    as connective tissue, 43
    tumors of, 44
"Cellular tissue." *See also* Tissue
    Andral on, 69-70
    Bichat and, 52-56
    Carswell on, 75
    fibers and, 52
    in lists of tissues (early 1800s), 57
    Schwann on, 197 *n*.22
    structure of, 58
    tumors and, 58-59
    Virchow on, 129-30
Celsus, 10, 11, 181 *n*.12, 183 *n*.36
Cesalpino, Andrea. *See* Caesalpinus, Andreas
Changus, G. W., 159
Chemistry, 39, 65, 186 *n*.79
    Paracelsus and, 28
    Sennert and, 29
    spagyrical (hermetic), 28-30, 33, 45, 64
    terms of, replacing humors, 26-30
Chevalier, Charles, 82
Chimney-sweepers' cancer (sootwart), 112,
    209 *n*.138
Chomel, August, 65
Chromosomes, 230 *n*.219. *See also* Cells, ge-
    netic substance in
Classen, August, 162, 223 *n*.164
Cleavage. *See* Embryo
Coagulating lymph. *See* Lymph, coagulating
Cohnheim, Julius, 164, 168, 169, 174-75, 177
    infectious tumors and, 225 *n*.189
    on tumor function, 225 *n*.187
    on tumors and embryonic "rests," 122,
        169-74
    tagging of cells by, 143
Columbus, Realdus, 22
Condie, Francis, 209 *n*.135
Connective tissue, 150, 151, 164, 176, 200 *n*.62,
    207 *n*.129, 224 *n*.166. *See also* Tissue
    Bichat and, 56
    "cellular membrane" as, 43
    "cellular tissue" as, 54
    embryonic, 88
    Michel's criticism of Virchow and, 137

Remak's concept of, 130-31
Virchow's concept of, 126, 129-30, 132-34, 135, 162, 175
Virchow's theory concerning, decline of, 138-48
Cooper, Astley, 182 n.19
Cornil, André-Victor, 144, 153, 162, 219 n.131
Cruveilhier, Jean, 59, 102
"cancer juice" of, 68
Cullen, William, 194 n.120
Cysts, 44, 125, 194 n.122, 194 n.128, 217 n.84, 229 n.210
Bichat on, 54, 58-59
Hodgkin on, 73, 76, 194 n.115
hydatid, described by Hunter, 188 n.124
of ovaries, 76
Cytoblastema, 93, 94, 95, 100, 103, 109, 124, 200 n.51, 200 n.62, 202 n.86. See also Blastema
Vogel and, 95-99
Cytogenesis, 91, 118
Schwann's solution to, 93
Virchow and, 123-24
Cytological methods. See Pathology laboratory methods

Darius the Great, 9
De Beer, Gavin Rylands, 228 n.209
Degeneration. See Cancerous degeneration
De le Boë, Franz [pseud. Sylvius], 30, 64
Democedes, 9
Dental tumors, 156, 220 n.143. See also Jaw, tumors of
Diet
as cause of flux, 17
as source of humors, 12
as source of scirrhous tumors, 15
Dimas, Altamirano, 159
Disease. See also Humoralism; names of specific diseases
germ theory of, 137, 143, 228 n.206
Hermeticists's classification of, 29-30
inflammation and, 43
Laennec's classification of, 60-61
lymph and, 34
materia peccans and, 105-6
nervous system and, 65
Paracelsus and, 26-27
as parasitic form of life, 72-73, 76, 78, 194 n.127
Pinel's classification of, 52-53
"seeds of contagion" and, 104-5, 106, 186 n.86, 203 n.95
solidistic approach to, 65
zymotic theory of, 132, 137, 142, 185 n.61
Doellinger, Ignaz, 57, 78, 129

Donné, Alfred, 87
Dumortier, Barthélemy, 87
Dupuytren, Guillaume, 53, 57, 59-60, 74, 77, 215 n.69

Ecker, Alexander, 113
Ectopic tumor, 158
Edwards, Milne, 67, 77, 82
Ehrlich, Paul, 168
Embolism, 132, 142, 214 n.56
Embryo, 139
blood and heart in chick, 42
cells and, 178-79, 229 n.215
cells in eye of, 86
cleavage in, 119, 121
generating membranes and, 76
new formations in (Foerster), 125
Schwann's investigation of cells in, 86
tissue implants in, 173
transformation in, 75
Embryology, 77-78, 142, 163, 165, 174-76, 215 n.69
cancer and, 88, 119-24, 139, 145
cellular, 86-87
experimental, Fischer on, 221 n.149
germ-layer theory and, 78-79, 224 n.166, 228 n.209
the microscope and, 80-81
Embryonal cell rests, Cohnheim's theory of, 169-74, 229 n.211
Embryonal cells, 173, 227 n.200, 227 n.201
Embryonal germs, displaced, 157, 158
Emotional disturbances
disease and (Laennec), 61
etiological role of, 182 n.19
Emotion and causes of cancer
Galen's doctrine of temperaments and, 11-12
melancholy (sadness) and, 34, 182 n.19
Peyrilhe and, 187 n.106
Endothelial cells, connective tissue and, 165
Endotheliomas, 156, 157, 158, 159
Endothelium, 145, 174, 218 n.106, 224 n.166
Epidermal cells, 93, 116, 122
Epidermal tumors, 113
Epidermoid cells, Virchow on, 115, 122
Epithelial cells. See also Cancer, epithelial; Epithelial theory of cancer; Tumors, epithelial
in breast acini, 150-51
cancer and, 140, 153, 207 n.128
cancroids and, 113-17
connective tissue cells and, 141, 223 n.164
displaced embryonal, 158
endothelial cells and, 165
Langhans and, 147

metamorphoses of, 152
origin of (Mueller), 198 n.33
primal cells and (Waldeyer), 164
Remak's derivation of, objections to, 130-35
reproducing of, by division (Waldeyer), 164
Schwann's description of, 199 n.44
Spjut and, 160
traumatic irritation and, 149
tumors and, 126, 127, 159
Epithelial theory of cancer, 112-17
  Billroth and, 141-42
  Cornil on, 144
  debate in Germany over, 145-48
  Foerster on, 127-28
  Remak on, 121-22
  Thiersch and, 139-41
  tibial cancroid and, 156-60
  Virchow on, 130-35
  Waldeyer and, 149-56, 162-67, 222 n.164, 229 n.215
Epithelial tissue
  breast cancer and, 151
  cancroids and, 113-17
  carcinoma and, 165
  Schwann's definition of, 93
  tumors and, 126, 127-28
Epithelioma, 112, 118
  Hannover on, 116-17
  Remak on, 122
Epithelioma adamantinoma. See Tibial cancroid
Epithelium. See also Cancer, epithelial; Epithelial theory of cancer; Tumors, epithelial
  connective tissue and (Remak), 156
  Ham's classification of, 199 n.45
  Hicks and, 158-59
  of lymph vessels, carcinoma and (Koester), 165
  Schwann's definition of, 93
  "simple" papilloma and, 127
  Thiersch's derivation of cancer from, 139-41, 142, 145, 151, 156, 223 n.164
  use of term, origin of, 199 n.41
Erasistratus of Alexandria, 20, 22, 23, 47, 51, 189 n.4
Exudates, 103-4, 119-20, 121, 125, 129

Fabricius ab Aquapendente. See Geronimo Fabrizio
Fallopio, Gabriele, 22
  on benign and malignant tumors, 16-19
  on cancers, 14-16
  on parts (organs), 49
Ferments, 45, 204 n.110
  Stahl and, 35, 37

Fernel, Jean, 14, 49
Fever, bloodletting and, 20
Fibers, 14, 37, 47-52, 65-66, 102
  cells and, 88, 90, 91, 189 n.4
  "cellular tissue" and, 52, 54
  of connective tissue, 129-30
  formative molecules and, 68
  of Haller, 92
  muscle, 148-49, 170, 194 n.131
  tissue and, 77, 82, 200 n.66
Fibrin, 42, 65-66, 68, 102, 187 n.110, 188 n.116, 202 n.79
Fibrous tumors, 75
Fischer, Bernhard, 157-58, 221 n.149
Fleming, Donald, 183 n.42
Flemming, Walther, 177, 224 n.168, 229 n.213
Flux, 17, 26, 35, 183 n.42
  defined, 21
  Riolan on, 24, 25
Foerster, August, 134, 138, 139, 142, 213 n.39
  cellular pathology and, 124-26
  epithelial cancer and, 127-28
Food. See Diet
Force plastique. See Plastic force
Foster, Michael, 183 n.42
Foulds, Leslie, 161, 222 n.161, 222 n.162, 228 n.209
Fracastorius, Girolamo, 105
Frerichs, Friedrich Theodor, 210 n.151
Friedrich III, 201 n.76, 215 n.66
Froriep, Robert, 110
Fuchs, Leonhard, 49
Fungoid growths, 197 n.28, 202 n.79
  and tumors, 44, 188 n.125
Fungus haematodes, 71, 72, 74

Galen, 15, 16, 17, 55, 64, 183 n.42, 185 n.70, 189 n.4
  blood circulation theory of, 19-21, 22, 23, 24, 25, 48
  cancer genesis and, 13
  dermatology and, 14
  doctrine of temperaments and, 11-12
  inflammation and, 11, 12-13, 21, 25-26, 181 n.12
  on parts (organs), 47, 49-51
Galenical humoralism. See Humoralism
Galileo, 22
Gallini, Stefano, 57
Gaub, Jerome, 186 n.86
Gendron, Claude-Deshaies
  pain in advanced cancer and, 187 n.92
  solidistic lymphatic theory and, 35-39, 41, 45
Genitals, female
  cysts of, 76
  tumors in, 39, 40, 75, 175

ulcers of, 9
Gerhardt, Karl, 215 n.66
Germ-layer theory, 77-81, 140, 150, 164, 176, 228 n.209
  Remak and, 121, 131, 139, 141
  Virchow on, 175-76
Geronimo Fabrizio [pseud. Fabricius ab Aquapendente], 22, 42
Globes concentriques, 116
Globes épidermiques, 116, 129, 152, 217 n.89
Globules, 83, 84, 108, 109, 185 n.75
Gloor, F., 159
Gluge, Gottlieb, 83, 84, 108, 214 n.59
Goethe, J. W., 78, 80, 195 n.143
Goring, C. R., 196 n.6
Grew, Nehemiah, 51
Growths, tumor theory in classical Greece and, 9, 10
Gueterbock, Ludwig, 199 n.47
Gulliver, George, 200 n.66
Gutiérrez, Díaz, 159

Haeser, Heinrich, 183 n.42
Haller, Albrecht von, 46, 52, 54, 55, 129
  fibers of, 92
Ham, Arthur W., 199 n.41, 199 n.45
Hannover, Adolph, 109, 110, 127, 129, 209 n.145
Hard tumors (*tumor durus*). *See* Scirrhus
Harvey, William, 215 n.69
  blood and, 42
  blood circulation and, 19, 21-26, 30, 32
Hasse, Carl, 174
  tissue formation and, 227 n.205
Heart, 183 n.42
  classical Greek view of, 19, 20, 23, 48
  in embryo, 42
  Vesalius and, 22
Hecker, Karl Friedrich, 205 n.118
Helmont, J. B. van, 35, 64, 184 n.57, 184 n.58
  humoralism and, 27-28
Henle, Jacob, 87, 102, 103, 106, 130, 199 n.44, 199 n.48, 202 n.79, 207 n.131, 211 n.17
  nucleated cells and, 86, 93
  "seeds of contagion" and, 104-5
Hermeticists. *See* Chemistry
Herodotus on breast tumor, 9
Herophilus, 20
Hertwig, Oscar, 195 n.133
Heteroplasia, 174
Hewson, William, 65, 215 n.69
Hey, William, 71, 72
Hicks, J. Douglas, 158-59
Hildebrand, Otto, 156
Hippocrates, 23, 33, 34

Hippocratic writings, 64, 183 n.36, 202 n.92
  blood circulation and, 19-21
  the four humors and, 11-12
  terms used in, 9-10
His, Wilhelm, 141, 142, 145, 163, 185 n.70, 226 n.190
Histogenesis, 91, 118, 155
  Albertini on, 222 n.162
  Bichat on tumor, 58-59
  of carcinoma (Waldeyer), 154
  Carswell on tumor, 75-76
  Hodgkin on tumor, 72, 75
  Lobstein on tumor, 66
  Remak on tumor, 122
  of tumors, 95, 118-79, 215 n.69
  of tumors, "cellular tissue" and, 52
Histological substitution (Virchow), 214 n.63
Histological techniques, 155. *See also* Pathology laboratory methods
Histology, 49, 52
  of Bichat, 53, 54, 55, 56
  Malpighi as founder of, 51
  use of term (1819), 195 n.143
Hodgkin, Thomas, 227 n.197
  fiber theory and, 82
  generative membranes and, 72-74
  on tumor histogenesis, 75-77
Hoffmann, Friedrich, 32, 34
Hohenheim, T. B. von [pseud. Paracelsus, Philippus Aureolus], 35, 64, 184 n.55, n.57
  humoralism and, 26-27
Home, Everard, 83
Hooke, Robert, 51
Horner, William E., 65
Horst, Gregor, 184 n.50
  humoralism and, 25-26, 29
Humoralism, 99
  blood circulation and, 19-26
  changes in theory of, 18-19
  early development of, 11-13
  Galenic theory of, 1-45
  Gendron's cancer theory and, 35-36, 39
  iatrochemical, 26-30, 33
  inflammatory process and, 21
  lymphatic cancer theory and, 39-41
  parts (organs) and, 47-51
  psychosomatic orientation of, 182 n.19
  Stahl and, 32-34
  third version of, 64-67
Hunter, John, 65, 71, 122, 188 n.120, 188 n.124, 209 n.139, 215 n.69
  on cancer of the breast, 188 n.126
  coagulating lymph and, 41-45, 188 n.116
  on fungoid growths and tumors, 44, 188 n.125

Hunter, William, 42
Husson, Henri-Marie, 53
Hydatids. *See* Cysts
Hyperplasia, Virchow and, 134, 135, 175
Hypertrophy, 69, 175

Ibn Ishaq (Joannitius), 48
Idioplasm, 178-79
Infiltration, 63-64
Inflammation, 93, 136, 167-69, 181 *n*.12, 188
     n.120, 188 *n*.121, 192 *n*.93, 217 *n*.100
  bloodletting and, 19, 20
  Cohnheim and, 143
  Galen and, 12-13, 21, 25-26
  Gendron on, 35
  Hunter's ideas on, 41, 43, 45
  of membranes, 53
  neoplasia and, 142-43, 167-69
  Stahl on, 32-35
  tumors and, 11, 18
Inflammatory tumors, 25, 26, 39, 61, 71,
     135-36, 167, 215 *n*.69
Intercellular substance, 94, 200 *n*.51
Irritability, neural pathology and, 65

Jaw, tumors of, 156, 157. *See also* Dental
     tumors
Junker (Juncker), Johannes, 204 *n*.110

Keele, Kenneth D., 188 *n*.117
King, E. S. J., 228 *n*.209
Kircher, Athanasius, 105
Klebs, Edwin, 146, 162, 163, 168, 223 *n*.164
  on cellular pathology, 228 *n*.206
Klencke, P. F., 109, 118
Koch, Richard, 168
Koelliker, Rudolf Albert, 120, 149, 178-79,
     195 *n*.133, 230 *n*.220
Koester, Karl, 162, 165
Kuess, Émile, 110, 113, 115, 206 *n*.126

Laennec, René, 53, 59, 63, 72, 74, 75, 77, 90,
     133, 190 *n*.57
  classification of lesions and diseases by,
     60-64
Lamarck, J. B., 58
Langenbeck, Bernard, 106-8, 109, 132, 134,
     141, 226 *n*.195
Langhans, Theodor, 147-48
Lauche, Arnold, 158, 159
Laughlin, William, 189 *n*.1
Laurentius, 50
Lavoisier, Antoine, 64, 65
"Law of analogous formation" (Vogel), 99,

103, 137
Leaf
  of germinal membrane, 79, 86, 93, 195 *n*.133
  germ-layer theory and, 79, 80
Lebert, Hermann, 109-10, 129, 130, 133, 149,
     152, 207 *n*.129
  cancer cells and, 206 *n*.123
  on cancroids, 114, 115-16, 209 *n*.145
  tumor investigation and, 206 *n*.122,
Lederer, H., 159
Leeuwenhoek, Anthony van, 31
Leibniz, G. W., 186 *n*.79
Lemmens (Lemnius, Lemnie), Levinus, 27,
     32, 184 *n*.56
Leopold, G., 173, 227 *n*.197
Lesions. *See also* Cancer; Tumors
  anatomic, categories of (Dupuytren), 59-
     60
  Andral's opinion on, 69
  bloodletting and, 19
  Burns on, 71
  in cancer of the breast, 34
  cancerous degeneration and, 38
  cancerous, recognition of, 62-64
  Fallopio on, 15
  Fernel on, 14
  heteroplastic, 68
  Laennec's classification of, 60-62
  metastatic, 140
  skin, 44, 112-14, 116, 131
  "tubercle" (Vogel), 98
  tumor theory in classical Greece and, 9,
     12-13, 25-26
Liebig, Justus, 65-66, 132, 185 *n*.61
"Life-force," 96, 109
Light metaphysics, Helmont and, 28
Lipomas, 75, 123, 135
Lister, Joseph J., 77, 227 *n*.197
  fiber theory and, 82
Liver cancer, 145-46
Lobstein, J. F., 94, 97, 102, 215 *n*.69
  formative molecules and, 67-68
  tumor histogenesis and, 66-67
Locke, John, 82
Lubarsch, Otto, 220 *n*.146
Luecke, Georg, 162, 171, 226 *n*.190
Lung cancer, 147
Lymph, 104, 185 *n*.70, 185 *n*.75
  coagulating, 41-45, 66-67, 76, 188 *n*.116,
     194 *n*.128, 194 *n*.129
  plastic, 58, 65, 71, 75, 76, 129
  tumors produced by, 39, 40
Lymphatic circulation, 30-32, 41, 223 *n*.164
Lymphatic theory, solidistic, 35-39, 187 *n*.110

Maas, Hermann, 173, 226 n.195
Macartney, James, 181 n.12
MacCallum, W. G., 161, 222 n.162
Mackenzie, Morell, 215 n.66
Maier, Carola, 156-57, 160
Maier, Rudolf, 162
Malignancy. See also Tumors, malignant
    "grade of" (Rokitansky), 100
    Vogel's concept of, 97
    Waldeyer's concept of, 152
Mallory, F. B., 222 n.162
Malpighi, Marcello, 30, 51
Mandl, Louis, 105
Marchand, Felix, 218 n.106
Mayor, Georges-François, 113, 114
Meckel, Heinrich, 110
    cancer cells and, 206 n.127, 207 n.129
Meckel, Johann Friedrich (1781-1833), 57, 78,
    129
Melancholy. See Emotion and causes of cancer
Melancholy humor (succum melancholicum).
    See Black bile
Melanoma, 194 n.120, 197 n.25
Membranes
    Bichat on, 53-54
    cell, 199 n.47
    "cellular," as connective tissue, 43
    cysts as (Bichat), 59
    Hodgkin's generative, 72-74, 76
    leaf of germinal, 79, 86, 93
Metaphorical terms
    cancer and
        Andral on, 69
        Fallopio on, 16
    cancer's resemblance to crab, 13, 16, 18, 34
    inflammation as, 69, 192 n.93
    leaf, 80
    seed, 104
Metaphorical thorn (spina metaphorica), 203
    n.101
Metaplasia, Virchow on, 174-76, 228 n.208
Metastasis
    Henle and, 203 n.94
    inflammatory disease and, 135-36
    Langenbeck's tumor cell transfer theory
        and, 134
    liver cancer and, 145-46
    mechanism of, 104-12, 173
    transplanted cancers and, 226 n.195
    Virchow and, 210 n.152
    Virchow's connective tissue theory and, 132
    Waldeyer and, 166
    wandering cell and, 142
Metastatic tumors, 67, 140
Metchnikov, Ilya, 168-69
Michel, Eugène, 137
Microscope, 10, 51, 112, 137, 155, 206 n.122,

206 n.125, 209 n.134. See also Microscopic
    examination
    Berres and, 198 n.30
    Bichat and, 55
    cancer diagnosis and, 108, 110-12
    cell study and, 84
    doubts concerning, 101-2
    electron, 159
    Goring and, 196 n.6
    Hodgkin and, 77
    Lister and, 227 n.197
    Mueller's use of, 88, 91, 196 n.9, 196 n.13,
        197 n.28, 207 n.130, 208 n.133, 209 n.135,
        215 n.69
    Pander and, 78
    Recklinghausen and, 224 n.168
    Rokitansky and, 99
    tumor study and, 82-84, 122
    Virchow and, 80-81, 110, 124, 155, 201 n.76,
        209 n.135
Microscopic examination. See also Micro-
    scope; Pathology laboratory methods
    of cancer (Mueller), 105
    of cancerous tissue, 209 n.135
    of carcinoma of bone, 157, 159
    of eggs and embryos, 119
    of fibers, 51
    of germinal membrane, 93
    of kidney tumor, 170
    of lip lesions, 113
    "molecules" and, 67
    of nodules from tumor cells, 107-8
    of tumor cells, 89
    of tumors, 97, 206 n.122
    of Virchow's amorphous substance, 102
    of wandering cells, 224 n.168
Minot, C. S., 228 n.209
Mintz, Beatrice, 229 n.215
Molecular biology, 178-79
"Molecules," formative, 67-68
Montfalcon, Jean-Baptiste, 55
Morgagni, G. B., 61, 65
Morphology, 195 n.143
Mueller, Johannes, 10, 58, 100, 101, 103, 108,
    110, 111, 112, 120, 121, 122, 125, 129, 137,
    197 n.25, 204 n.113
    cancer "seeds" and, 90-92
    on cancroids, 114
    the cell and, 83-84, 88-92, 207 n.131, 230
        n.220
    classification of cancer by, 198 n.34
    microscope and, 88, 91, 196 n.9, 196 n.13,
        197 n.28, 207 n.130, 208 n.133, 209 n.135
    microscopic structure of cancer and, 105-6
    Schwann's papers of 1838 and, 84-88
"Mueller's law," 101, 102
Mueller, Wilhelm, 166

Mulder, Gerard, 66

Naegeli, Carl Wilhelm, 179
Naunyn, Bernard, 145
Needham, John, 67
Neoplasia, 10-11, 12, 41, 45. *See also* Cancer;
    Tumors
    and inflammation, 142-43, 167-69
    Virchow on, 174-76
Nervous system, disease and, 65
Neumann, Ernst, 162, 163
Nicholson, G. W., 228 *n.*209
Noli me tangere, 112, 114
Nuck, Anton, 32
Nuclei, 130, 196 *n.*16
    in cancer cells, 206 *n.*119
    demonstration of, 93-94
    division of, 133
"Nuclein," 179
Nussbaum, Moritz, 178

O'Malley, Charles D., 51
Oppenheimer, Jane, 228 *n.*209
Organs. *See also* Parts
    classification of diseases based on, 61
    instrumental parts and, 49

Padua, University of, 22
Pagel, Julius, 183 *n.*42
Pagel, Walter, 26-27, 35
Paget, James, 140
Paleopathology, 8
Palmer, James, F., 187 *n.*109, 188 *n.*116, *n.*125
Pander, Christian, 78, 79
Papillomas, Foerster on, 126, 127-28
Paracelsus, Philippus Aureolus. *See* Hohen-
    heim, T. B. von
Pardoux, Barthélemy, 49, 50, 51
Parts. *See also* Organs
    instrumental, 49
    similar and dissimilar, 47-52, 92
Pasteur, Louis, 202 *n.*86, 210 *n.*1, 212 *n.*23
Pathology, 39, 55, 59, 65, 75
    cellular
        Foerster on, 124-28
        Klebs on, 228 *n.*206
        Virchow on, 124-37
    humoral, Rokitansky on, 99-100, 124
    neural, irritability and, 65
    Remak on, 121
    Virchow's view of, 103
Pathology laboratory methods. *See also* Mi-
    croscopic examination; Staining
    of Bennett, 111, 207 *n.*132, 209 *n.*134
    current, 160

injection experiments, 32, 204 *n.*109
    late 1800s, 168-69
    of Thiersch, 139
    of Waldeyer, 150
Paul of Aegina, 16
Pearson, John, 204 *n.*110
Pechlin, Johannes, 182 *n.*19
Peck, A. L., 48
Pecquet, Jean, 30
Perithelial cells, 167
Peyrilhe, Bernard, 39, 40-41, 112, 187 *n.*106
Phlegm, humoralism and, 11, 12, 16, 27, 31
Physiology, 121
    the microscope and (Bichat), 55, 56
Pinel, Philippe, 52-53
Plastic force, 66
Plato, 47, 51
Polyps, 38, 44, 58
Porphyry, 46
Potentiality, 96
Pott, Percival, 209 *n.*138
Pouchet, Félix, 212 *n.*23
Praxagoras of Kos, 19
Prochaska, Georg, 57, 129
Prostatic cancer, 145
Protein, 66
Pus, 202 *n.*89
    corpuscles, 93, 143, 149, 199 *n.*47, 216 *n.*73
    formation, 132

Ranvier, Louis, 144
Rather, L. J., 182 *n.*19
Recklinghausen, Friedrich von, 142, 143, 224
    *n.*168
Reichert, Karl, 120, 124, 129, 130, 211 *n.*5
Remak, Robert, 128, 138-39, 149, 153, 156,
    163, 176, 211 *n.*11
    and cell potency, 122
    on genesis of tumors, 121
    germ-layer theory and, 121, 131, 140, 141
    on origin of new cells, 120-24
    on tissue development, 131
Rests
    carcinoma, 163
    embryonal cell (Cohnheim), 169-72
Richerand, Anthelme-Balthasar, 57
Richter, C. S., 158, 159
Richter, Paul, 14, 182 *n.*24
Rindfleisch, Georg, 162, 163
Riolan, Jean, blood circulation and, 24-26
Robin, Charles, 144, 162
    dental tumors and, 220 *n.*143
Roessle, Robert, 219 *n.*139
Rokitansky, Karl von, 94-100, 102, 103
    Virchow's attack on, 100-101, 200 *n.*73
Rosai, Juan, 159, 160

Rosen, George, 203 n.94
Roth, Moritz, 51
Royer-Collard, Hippolyte, 58
Rubin, Charles, 133
Rudbeck, Claus, 31
Rudolphi, Karl, 57, 129
Rusconi, Mauro, 119
Ruysch, Frederik, 218 n.106

Saavedra, Albores, 159, 160
Sarcoma, 38, 72, 147, 149, 154, 157, 170,
    188 n.125, 193 n.103, 213 n.39
  Abernethy on, 71
  Fernel on, 14
  Foerster on, 128
  Hodgkin on, 74
  Waldeyer on, 167
Schleiden, Matthias, 108
  cells and, 84, 85-86, 87, 89, 90, 91, 94, 204
    n. 113
Schoener, Erich, 11
Schwann, Theodore, 81, 102
  cell theory and, 10, 84-88, 90, 91, 92-95,
    105, 108, 113, 118, 119, 120, 122, 125, 130,
    197 n.22, 200 n.62, 210 n.1, 211 n.5, n.17
  embryonic connective tissue and, 88, 89
  spontaneous generation and, 202 n.86,
    210 n.1, 211 n.17
  tissue and, 92-95, 207 n.131
Scirrhus, 150, 191 n.60
  Andral on, 69-70
  Astruc on, 40
  Fallopio on, 15-17, 19
  Galen on, 13
  Galen's melancholy humor and, 29
  Gendron on, 36-37, 38
  Hoffmann on, 34
  Hunter on, 44
  Laennec on, 62
  Lobstein on, 68
  Peyrilhe on, 39
  Stahl on, 33
Sédillot, Charles, 110 113, 207 n.129
Sennert, Daniel, 29
Servetus, Michael, 23
Sigerist, Henry, 184 n.54
Simpson, James, 205 n.118
Sinclair, A. J., 159
Skin cancer, 139-41, 148, 152, 219 n.131. See
    also Cancer, epithelial
Skin tumors, 44, 112-14, 116, 126, 127, 131
Society for Investigating the Nature and
    Cure of Cancer, 70
Sootwart. See Chimney-sweeper's cancer
Soranus of Ephesus, 11
Speed, J. S., 159

Spjut, Harlan, 160
Spontaneous generation, 124, 144, 148, 202
    n.86, 210 n.1, 211, n.17, 212 n.23
  of new cells from blastemas, 137
Stahl, Georg Ernst, 28, 185 n.75, 186 n.79,
    188 n.120
  cancer "seeds" and, 32-35
Staining, 143, 150, 155, 168, 202 n.84, 219 n.138.
    See also Pathology laboratory methods
  Lebert and, 206 n.122
  Thiersch and, 139
Stethoscope, 60
Stewart, F., 159
Strato, 20
Stroma, 146, 150, 151, 154, 207 n.129
Sudhoff, Karl, 156, 220 n.146
Swieten, Gerard van, 182 n.19
Sydenham, Thomas, 30, 82
Sylvius. See De le Boë, Franz

Temperaments. See Emotion and causes of
    cancer
Tendeloo, Nicholas, 181 n.12
Thiersch, Carl, 142, 144, 145, 146, 147, 148,
    151, 156
  epithelial theory of cancer and, 139-41
Thompson, D'Arcy Wentworth, 47-48
Throat cancer, 9
Tibial cancroid, 217 n.89, 221 n.152
  histogenesis of (1850-1971), 154-62
  Remak and, 153
  Virchow and, 115, 122, 128, 138, 140
  Willis's view on, 222 n.162
Tissu cellulaire. See Cellular tissue
Tissues. See also Microscopic examination;
    Staining; names of specific tissues
  Bichat's list of, 55-56
  Bruch on, 207 n.131
  Cohnheim on tumor, 172-73
  cytohistogenesis of (Vogel), 95-99
  development of, 85-87, 91, 93-94, 200 n.62
  embryonic, 89
  formation of
    Buhl on, 148-49
    Hasse on, 227 n.205
    Rokitansky on, 100
  genesis of tumor, 10
  "globules" and, 185 n.75
  Ham's classification of, 199 n.45
  lists of, early 1800s, 56-57
  organization, 66
  Remak on tumor, 122
  Schwann and, 86, 88, 118
  Schwann's cell theory and, 92-95
  structure of, 95
  theory of, 52-58
  transplants of, 226 n.195

tumors and, 58-70, 82, 83
Virchow and, 102-4, 130-31, 174, 175
Tommasini, Giacomo, 57
Transformation of cells, 160, 163
Virchow on, 133, 134
Waldeyer on, 153, 154
Transformation of tissues. *See also* Cancerous
degeneration
Andral on, 69
Carswell on, 75
germ-layer theory and, 80
Laennec on, 63-64
Mueller on, 90
Virchow on, 117, 121, 174
Transplantation experiments, 102-8, 109, 132,
140, 173, 226 n.195, 227 n.197, 228 n.206
Transplantation hypothesis, 142
Thiersch and, 140
Trauma and cancer, 157, 160, 171
Tubercles, 98, 105, 123, 132, 135, 176, 202
n.79
genesis of, 133
Tuberculosis, 98, 104, 133, 137
Tulley, William, 82
Tumors. *See also* Cancer; Malignancy; Metas-
tasis; Neoplasia; *names of specific sites;
names of specific tumors*
Abernethy's classification of, 70-71
Astruc on, 39-40
Bard on, 177, 229 n.210, 229 n.211
benign, 9, 10, 16-19, 38, 75, 84, 88, 96, 108
126, 133, 152, 154, 215 n.69
Bennett's examination of, 207 n.132
Bichat on, 58-59
bloodletting and, 19, 25
Carswell on, 75-76
cell genesis in, 95-104, 120-22
cells in, 88, 90-91, 177, 229 n.211
cell size in (Mueller), 89
cell theory and, 82-117
chemical analysis of, 111
classification of, 70-71, 97-98, 125-27, 147-
48, 161-62, 215 n.69, 222 n.161, 225 n.189,
226 n.190
Cohnheim on, 169-72, 225 n.189
epithelial, 112-17, 118, 121, 122, 126-32,
134-35, 137, 138-42, 144-47, 154, 156-67,
174-75
Fallopio on, 16-19
Fernel on, 14
Foerster's classification of, 125-27
Formation of (Hunter), 43
fungoid growths and, 44, 188 n.125
Gendron on, 35-39
genesis of (Lobstein), 67
growth rate of (Cohnheim), 170-71
histogenesis of, 95, 118-79

Hodgkin on, 75-77, 194 n.118
human nails and, parallels between, 36-37
Hunter on, 43-44
identification of, 161-62, 169
infections (Cohnheim), 225 n.189
inflammatory and neoplastic, demarcation
between, 10-11
Langhan's classification of, 147-48
malignant, 9, 16-19, 34, 69, 74, 84, 88, 96,
97, 108-9, 126, 133, 136, 152, 220 n.79,
205 n.118, 215 n.69
microscope and study of, 82-84, 122
Mueller on, 88, 103, 196 n.9
Peyrilhe on, 49, 40-41
theory of
classical Greece, 9-13, 21
Renaissance Europe, 13-19
tissue theory and, 52-70
Virchow's views on, 100, 132-37, 175-76
Vogel's classification of, 97-98
Wardrop on, 72
Turpin, Pierre, 87

Uhrglas theory (Schleiden), 85
Ulcers
cancerous, distinguished from true cancer,
112
of female genitals, 9
fungated, 44

Van Helmont. *See* Helmont, J. B. van
Van Swieten. *See* Swieten, Gerard van
Veins, 14, 17, 19-20, 22, 23, 24, 25, 30, 34
Bichat and, 56
Galen on, 49, 50
Venesection. *See* Bloodletting
Vesalius, Andreas, 22, 25, 51
Virchow, Rudolf, 112, 143, 153, 164, 169, 170,
171, 173, 177, 181 n.12, 190 n.57, 202 n.86,
203 n.94, 210 n.1, 215 n.66, 217 n.89, 226,
n.195, 228 n.206
blastema and, 101-2, 103
blastema theory and, 123
on breast cancer, 213 n.55
on cancroids, 115, 116-17, 122, 155
cells and, 87, 207 n.128, 207 n.129, 223 n.165,
228 n.206
cellular pathology and, 124-25, 128-37,
204 n.107, 211 n.11
decline of connective tissue theory of,
138-48
epithelial theory of cancer and, 130-35
on histological substitution, 214 n.63
metaplasia and, 174-76
metastasis and, 132, 136

the microscope and, 80-81, 110, 124, 155, 201 *n.*76, 209 *n.*135
pathological anatomy and, 61
Rokitansky and, 100-101, 201 *n.*73
tissue and, 102-4, 126, 130-31
Vogel, Julius, 95-99, 102, 103, 110, 113, 137, 199 *n.*46, 200 *n.*62, 204 *n.*107, 211 *n.*11
Volkmann, Richard, 156
Von Albertini. *See* Albertini, A. von
Von Baer. *See* Baer, Karl Ernst von
Von Haller. *See* Haller, Albrecht von
Von Recklinghausen. *See* Recklinghausen, Friedrich von

Wagner, Ernst, 162
Wagner, Rudolf, 95
Waldeyer, Wilhelm, 155, 156, 160, 223 *n.*165
chromosomes and, 230 *n.*219
epithelial theory of cancer and, 149-56, 162-67, 223 *n.*164, 229 *n.*215
Waller, Augustus, 164
Walshe, Walter, 105, 121, 205 *n.*117
Walther, Philipp von, 57

"Wandering cell," 142, 146, 162, 164, 166-67, 216 *n.*73, 224 *n.*168, 224 *n.*169, 225 *n.*170
Wardrop, James, 72
Warts, 44
Watson, Thomas, 209 *n.*135
Weber, Carl Otto, 145, 149, 216 *n.*81
Weismann, August, 149, 178, 230 *n.*220
White blood cells, 143, 217 *n.*100, 224 *n.*169, 225 *n.*170
Willis, Rupert, 222 *n.*162
Willis, Thomas, 30, 64
Witschi, Emil, 229 *n.*215
Wolff, Caspar Friedrich, 57, 78, 79, 129
Wolff, Jacob, 9, 187 *n.*110
Wotton, Edward, 48
Wyss, Oskar, 145

Zahn, Friedrich Wilhelm, 172-73, 226 *n.*195, 228 *n.*206
Zanobio, Bruno, 82
Zenker, Friedrich Albert von, 148
Zymotic theory of disease, 132, 137, 142, 185 *n.*61

Ceteris typothetarum σφάλμασι quae aciem oculorum fugerunt, lector bene-
volens ignoscat et ipse ea corrigat.